THE
ULTIMATE
WOMEN'S
GUIDE TO
BEATING
DISEASE

AND LIVING A HAPPY, ACTIVE LIFE

2021

FROM THE EDITORS OF BOTTOM LINE

**The Ultimate Women's Guide to Beating Disease
and Living a Happy, Active Life**

Copyright © 2020 by Bottom Line Inc.

10   9   8   7   6   5   4   3   2   1

All rights reserved. No part of this book may be reproduced, scanned, distributed
or transmitted in any form, by any means, electronic or mechanical, without
written permission from the publisher.

ISBN 0-88723-839-4

Bottom Line Books® publishes the advice of expert authorities in many fields. These opinions
may at times conflict as there are often different approaches to solving problems. The use
of a book is not a substitute for legal, accounting, investment, health or any other professional
services. Consult competent professionals for answers to your specific questions.

Offers, prices, rates, addresses, telephone numbers and websites
listed in this book are accurate at the time of publication,
but they are subject to frequent change.

Bottom Line Books® is a registered trademark of Bottom Line Inc.
3 Landmark Square, Suite 201, Stamford, CT 06901

BottomLineInc.com

Bottom Line Books is an imprint of Bottom Line Inc., publisher of print periodicals,
e-letters and books. We are dedicated to bringing you the best information from the most
knowledgeable sources in the world. Our goal is to help you gain greater wealth,
better health, more wisdom, extra time and increased happiness.

Printed in the United States of America

CONTENTS

Contents

Contents

12 • PAIN AND AUTOIMMUNE DISORDERS

13 • PHYSICAL INJURY AND BONE HEALTH

14 • PREGNANCY AND REPRODUCTION ISSUES

Contents

PREFACE

We are proud to bring to you *The Ultimate Women's Guide to Beating Disease and Living a Happy, Active Life 2021.* This essential volume features trustworthy and actionable life-saving information from the best health experts in the world—information that will help women beat the most deadly conditions.* In the following chapters, you'll find the latest discoveries, best treatments and scientifically proven remedies to keep you living a long, happy and active life.

Whether it's heart care, the latest on stroke, breast cancer prevention and treatment, breakthrough treatments for hot flashes or cutting-edge nutritional advice, the editors at Bottom Line Inc. talk to the experts—from top women's health doctors to research scientists to leading alternative care practitioners—who are creating the true innovations in health care.

Over the past four decades, we have built a network of literally thousands of leading physicians in both alternative and conventional medicine. They are affiliated with the premier medical and research institutions throughout the world. We read the important medical journals and follow the latest research that is reported at medical conferences. And we regularly talk to our advisors in major teaching hospitals, private practices and government health agencies for their insider perspective.

*"Leading Causes of Death in Females," Centers for Disease Control and Prevention (*http://www.cdc.gov/women/lcod/2017/index.html*).

In this 2021 edition, we've gone beyond diseases and have included several chapters of life-enhancing health information on pregnancy, pain, depression, fitness, nutrition, quality medical care, sexuality and aging...all of which are essential to living a happy, active life. And it's all backed by breaking studies and top health experts. Also note that respiratory diseases, according to the Centers for Disease Control and Prevention, are now considered one of the top three causes of death in women of all ages (same percentage as stroke).

The Ultimate Women's Guide to Beating Disease and Living a Happy, Active Life 2021 is a result of our ongoing research and connection with these experts, and is a distillation of their latest findings and advice. We trust that you will glean new, helpful and affordable information about the health topics that concern you most...and find vital topics of interest to family and friends as well.

As a reader of a Bottom Line book, be assured that you are receiving well-researched information from a trusted source. But please use prudence in health matters. Always speak to your physician before taking vitamins, supplements or over-the-counter medication...stopping a medication...changing your diet...or beginning an exercise program. If you experience side effects from any regimen, contact your doctor immediately.

Be well,
The Editors, Bottom Line Inc.
Stamford, Connecticut

Chapter 1

AGING WELL

Natural Tricks for More Youthful Skin

I am enthusiastic about the boost in self-esteem that patients gain from cosmetic surgery, but I encourage my patients to try preventive measures first and view surgery as a last resort. A number of natural methods can delay or reduce wrinkling and other signs of aging of the face and body with techniques that not only are simple but also inexpensive.

•**Train your muscles to contract less—without Botox.** Repeated contractions of the facial muscles lead to a creased appearance of the skin. I would never advise someone to smile or laugh less often—those lines are evidence of a life well-lived. But there is no reason to go out of your way to make repetitive movements you don't need. Repeatedly furrowing your brow, for example, etches lines over time.

Instead, do the opposite—train your muscles to contract less. Isolating the small muscles involved in forehead furrows, crow's feet or frown lines is challenging but gets easier with practice. If you ever learned to roll your tongue or flare your nostrils as a child, you already have experience in the type of concentration needed.

While breathing slowly and gently, imagine the muscles of your face softening and widening, even melting. Do this for one to two minutes at least five times a day and whenever you think of it.

Helpful: Frownies (available at Frownies. com or Amazon.com) are lightweight patches that you wear overnight or while relaxing at home to help smooth wrinkles. You stick the patch gently over the lines on your forehead or around your lips, and it acts as a kind of splint, preventing you from contracting those muscles. It also makes you more aware of what happens when you engage the small muscles, so that after a few weeks, you learn to contract them less, even when you are not wearing the patch.

Note: Working out your facial muscles will not stave off sagging and wrinkles. Aging faces droop because they are losing collagen and elastin—two proteins that are the skin's major building blocks—not from lack of exercise. In fact, overexercising your face can cause more wrinkles.

Anthony Youn, MD, FACS, board-certified plastic surgeon. Named a "Top Plastic Surgeon" by *U.S. News & World Report*, Dr. Youn is assistant professor of surgery at Oakland University William Beaumont School of Medicine in Rochester, Michigan. He is author of *The Age Fix: A Leading Plastic Surgeon Reveals How to Really Look 10 Years Younger.* DrYoun.com

•**Sleep on your back.** You may have noticed creases on your face the morning after you slept on your stomach or your side. Skin creases are the result of gravity pulling your facial muscles downward as your skin presses against the pillow. Sleep wrinkles are temporary, but over months or years, repeated pressure from your face against the pillow can make these creases permanent, especially as the elastin in your skin diminishes with age, reducing its ability to "bounce back" to shape.

In contrast, when you sleep on your back, gravity works in your favor. If back-sleeping feels awkward, try using a cervical neck pillow to cradle your neck and keep your head gently in place. A memory foam mattress also may help you feel more comfortable by conforming to your body shape and providing extra support.

Important: Put a pillow under your knees to prevent lower-back strain.

If you cannot fall asleep on your back, invest in a silk pillowcase. They're available on Amazon.com for around $25. Silk doesn't cling to the skin the way cotton or synthetic fabrics do, so you will have less creasing.

An option for side sleepers is the JuveRest pillow, $160 (JuveRest.com). It is designed to reduce skin compression by minimizing contact with the face.

•**Lower the water temperature.** A long, hot shower or bath may feel comforting in the winter, but hot water dries out the skin, whether you are bathing or washing your face. Keep water lukewarm, and don't stay in too long.

•**Lighten sunspots with homemade lemon-juice ointment.** Dark spots from sun exposure on the hands, face and arms will make anyone look older. To lighten those spots, mix equal parts soy milk, lemon juice and honey. The mixture should have a pasty consistency so that it does not drip when applied to your face and body. Apply the mixture to your skin, and leave it on for 20 to 30 minutes. Rinse off with lukewarm water. Use daily until you see improvement.

Why it works: Lemon juice contains citric acid, a natural skin lightener, while proteins in soy milk inhibit the skin's production of the darkening pigment melanin. Honey binds the two ingredients and is a good moisturizer.

Important: Soy milk spoils quickly, so only mix as much of this blend as you will use right away. Start with one teaspoon of each. Note that lemon juice can irritate skin and cause photosensitivity, so wear sunscreen.

•**Wear sunglasses—even on winter days.** You know you should wear sunscreen to protect your skin from premature aging and skin cancer, but your eyes are at risk, too, and the skin around your eyes is too delicate for sunscreen. Protect the area with sunglasses that filter out UVA and UVB rays. By keeping you from squinting, sunglasses—especially those with wraparound frames—also delay and reduce wrinkling.

•**Smooth out crow's feet with a mayonnaise mask.** For a quick eye-lift, use your fingers or a cotton ball to apply a small amount of mayonnaise to your crow's feet. After 30 minutes, wash off gently with lukewarm water. Apply in the morning to look better all day.

Why it works: Mayonnaise contains eggs and oil. The albumin in eggs tightens skin almost immediately, and oil moisturizes it. This treatment won't banish crow's feet forever, but it will make a noticeable difference for a day or so.

•**Mix your own chemical peel at home.** Chemical peels refresh the skin's appearance by removing the top layer of dead or dying skin cells and stimulating the body to produce new cells more quickly. Older skin looks duller than younger skin because this natural process of skin-cell turnover simply slows down with age.

Instead of going to the doctor's office for costly chemical peels, create your own gentle exfoliant by mixing three tablespoons of apple juice, two tablespoons of milk and one egg white. Apply the mixture to your face, and gently rinse off with water after 15 minutes.

Why it works: The malic acid in apple juice and the lactic acid in milk help to remove dead skin. Egg white tightens the skin.

Caution: Exfoliating too often irritates skin and can cause it to age faster, so don't do it every day. If you have normal skin, you can apply this treatment two or three times a week. If your skin is sensitive or if you notice redness after the treatment, don't exfoliate more than once a week.

• **Avoid foods that age you.** One of the worst offenders is sugar, including refined starches such as white bread and white rice, which turn to sugar. Sugar molecules bind to collagen and elastin through a process called glycation, making these skin proteins stiffer and leading to premature wrinkles and sagging. Although avoiding sugar can't reverse damage that has already occurred, it can help slow further aging.

The other major offender is fat—specifically, saturated and trans fats, which increase inflammation. Opt for monosaturated fats, found in olive oil and most nuts, and for omega-3 fatty acids, found in salmon and other cold-water fish, flaxseed and tofu. Over time, these fats calm inflammation and improve the skin's elasticity, and they even may reduce the damage from sun exposure.

Note: You also can add a collagen supplement to your daily regimen.

Beyond Wrinkles...Top Treatments for Thinning Skin

Abigail Waldman, MD, instructor of dermatology at Brigham and Women's Hospital and Harvard Medical School, both in Boston. She is also director of Mohs surgery at VA Boston Healthcare System.

Wrinkles may get most of the attention, but thinning skin is another age-related skin issue you'll want to pay attention to. Thinning skin not only makes you look older but can cause other skin problems as well.

Fortunately, there are some exciting new advances as well as some effective well-established treatments that can help make your skin thicker and restore its smoothness and elasticity.

Why Skin Gets Thin

Skin is composed of a scaffold called the extracellular matrix, which is made up of proteins including collagen and elastin. This matrix is what gives durability and resilience to skin, allowing it to "snap back" and keeping it from being easily damaged.

As we age, some of the components that make up the extracellular matrix break down. Eventually, fibroblast cells within the skin no longer make enough collagen...and the old, "worn out" proteins that make up the extracellular matrix don't get replaced. The result is skin that is thinner and more fragile, which can look saggy, crepey and wrinkled, especially on the face and hands.

Sun Exposure, Gender and More

In addition to age, a main cause of thinning skin is UV radiation from sun exposure. UV radiation causes oxidative damage to DNA, skin proteins and the extracellular matrix. People who have had a lot of sun exposure are at increased risk of having thinner skin at an earlier age.

At greater risk: People with very pale skin have less protection from UV radiation, so they are more susceptible to thinning skin. Smoking—another powerful source of oxidative damage—also increases the risk for thin skin.

At less risk: On average, men's skin is thicker than women's because men have a higher testosterone-to-estrogen ratio, which helps stimulate collagen production and other skin proteins. So while men's skin is susceptible to the same factors as women's skin, it will take longer to be affected.

Risky medication: Prescription-strength topical corticosteroid creams also can thin the skin where they're applied, and long-term use of oral steroids can cause thinning as well—and the thinning can be permanent. Areas of special concern are places where the skin is already thin, such as the face, or areas that absorb medication more easily, such as in the armpits or groin. Always follow a doctor's instructions when using a prescription corticosteroid.

Note: Over-the-counter (OTC) hydrocortisone cream is generally safe and not a risk for thinning skin.

To Improve the Look of Your Skin

While you can't regain the skin of your 20s, there are more options than ever for turning back the clock…

My top advice: Hydrate! The outer layer of skin (the stratum corneum) acts as a kind of brick wall to prevent water from leaving the body. As we get older—and if you have skin damage from the sun or cigarette smoking—that brick wall gets holes in it, which makes it harder for the skin to retain moisture, resulting in a dry, sallow appearance.

Water is the best all-around hydrator, but any liquid you drink counts, even coffee and tea. It's a myth that the diuretic effect of caffeine offsets hydration. Of course, you'll want to avoid soda and other sweet drinks.

To help trap water in skin, I advise an emollient ointment, such as petroleum jelly or Aquaphor (if you prefer not to use a petroleum-based ointment, look for a glycerin-based ointment)…or a product that contains hyaluronic acid, a natural compound that preserves moisture. Many drugstore products containing hyaluronic acid (such as Neutrogena Hydro Boost Water Gel) are as effective as more expensive creams.

• **Use the following topical, cream, serum and/or supplement.** As with any skin-care regimen, the key is consistency and patience. *Your skin didn't thin overnight—it could take weeks or even months before you see a difference when using these therapies…*

Topical retinoids are chemical compounds derived from vitamin A. They have been shown to boost the activity of the extracellular matrix, increasing production of collagen and elastin and making the skin measurably thicker. Topical retinoids are available by prescription or OTC (retinol).

Note: A retinoid can cause irritation, so begin by using it for just two to three nights per week until the skin adjusts.

Glycolic acid creams and **vitamin C serums** increase collagen by combating oxidative stress. Many OTC creams and face washes contain glycolic acid, including Glytone. For vitamin C serums, look for brands that contain vitamins C and E and ferulic acid.

Note: Use these products in the morning if you are also using a retinoid, as the combination can be irritating.

Newest treatment: Nicotinamide, a form of vitamin B-3. Research has shown that nicotinamide can actually reverse sun damage that causes skin cancer. A typical dose to combat skin damage from UV radiation is 500 mg of OTC nicotinamide, taken orally, twice a day. Check with your doctor before taking this (or any) supplement.

• **Try skin treatments.** There are a wide variety of treatments available to help thinning skin. A board-certified dermatologist or plastic surgeon can evaluate your condition and recommend the most appropriate treatment based on your skin and discuss possible risks. Some treatments could be painful, so pain medication or anesthesia may be advised, and you may require more than one treatment to achieve desired results. All treatments should be performed by or under the supervision of a board-certified dermatologist or plastic surgeon.* *Examples…*

• Laser treatments use pulses of light to remove damaged skin, correct imperfections and stimulate production of collagen. Different lasers and frequencies are used for differ-

*Check with your doctor for costs—they will vary depending on your location.

ent problems. For example, some lasers target areas of skin discoloration...others correct surface wrinkling...and others penetrate more deeply to correct heavy wrinkles.

- Microneedling works to stimulate collagen production via tiny needles that poke minuscule holes in the skin.

- Ultrasound uses high-frequency sound waves to boost collagen. The result is tighter skin in areas where the ultrasound is used.

- **Guard against injury.** People who have thin skin do tend to bruise more easily, especially on the tops of the hands. The greatest risk is when the fragile skin tears open, leaving it vulnerable to infection. These tears should not be covered with an adhesive bandage—removing it may cause more injury. Instead, I advise applying an emollient ointment several times a day to keep the tear moist until it heals.

- **Wear sunscreen.** To avoid further sun damage, be sure to use a sunscreen with an SPF of at least 30 every day...and wear a wide-brimmed hat when outdoors. Also, avoid being out in the sun during the warmest part of the day (10 am to 2 pm).

PRP Magic: Look Younger, Feel Younger with Platelet Rich Plasma

Laurie Steelsmith, ND, LAc, licensed naturopathic physician and acupuncturist in private practice in Honolulu. She writes Bottom Line's "Natural Healing Secrets for Women" blog and is coauthor of three books—the best-selling *Natural Choices for Women's Health*, the critically acclaimed *Great Sex, Naturally* and her latest, *Growing Younger Every Day*. DrSteel smith.com

---

Blood may not be the sexiest topic but your own blood may be the secret to health and vitality.

Sound bizarre? Think again. Here in the realm of naturopathic medicine, we live by the tenet that our bodies are built to heal themselves. Proof of this emerges in myriad ways, from scabs that eventually form fresh skin to an (albeit exasperating) itch—a sure sign that blood is moving towards a wound in the name of healing. Overall, the human body is a miraculous creation, designed for curing itself and tremendous resilience.

And we can harness this power even more by using platelet-rich plasma. The therapy, widely known as PRP, utilizes injections of a patient's own blood to jumpstart the healing process and rejuvenate specific areas of concern. First discovered in the 1970s in the field of hematology, PRP began to be used a decade later, initially in maxillofacial surgery before moving into a variety of medical procedures, including cardiac surgery, gynecology, oral surgery and ophthalmology.

But what, exactly, is PRP—and how does it work?

In PRP, a small amount of blood (30-60 milligrams, or two to four tablespoons) is drawn from the patient and placed into a centrifuge. As the blood spins at a very fast rate, red blood cells are separated from plasma (the clear liquid that transports blood throughout the body) and platelets. The removal of red blood cells leaves us with platelet-rich plasma—plasma so rich in platelets, in fact, that it contains 10 times as much as whole blood. In PRP therapy, the platelet-rich plasma is either injected into the region of the patient's body that requires treatment, applied topically or administered through microneedling—a minimally invasive procedure in which ultra-fine needles are inserted into the skin.

So what does this platelet-rich plasma do? Plenty. Platelets play a variety of roles in your body, from encouraging blood to clot to encouraging wounds to heal—or, as the National Institutes of Health frames it, they're on "continual 'call of duty' because inside of them lies one of the most powerful reservoirs of factors responsible for tissue repair." This is thanks to the fact that they're jam-packed with properties that aid in regeneration, including platelet-derived growth factor, transforming-growth factor B, fibroblast activation, insulin-like growth factor, epidermal growth factor and cytokines—cell-signaling proteins that impact immunity and inflammation (among other functions). Ultimately, platelets affect the stem cells in our tissues and stimulate them to produce whatever they're programmed to make—whether it's cartilage, connective tissue, elastin or hair.

As expected, the applications of PRP are broad and exciting, offering the potential of tissue regeneration in everything from sexual wellness to orthopedics. *Here's a closer look at how PRP has helped others—and how it might one day help you...*

Orthopedics

Kari, a 68-year-old woman, arrived at my office suffering from chronic ankle and knee pain, which had been plaguing her since a motor vehicle accident 18 years earlier—a truck hit her as she was standing outside her car while looking in her purse. It dragged her 15 feet and caused multiple ligament tears, broken bones and contusions. I treated her joints with PRP three times, with each session one month apart.

I was confident Kari would benefit enormously from these sessions and I was right. By the end of our time together, she reported an increased range of motion and radically reduced pain. The science is there, too. Therapeutic PRP injections for joints, ligaments and tendons have been studied extensively, and show particular promise in the arena of cartilage repair.

Indeed, PRP can be an absolute windfall for those suffering from osteoarthritis, a form of arthritis that affects 27 million Americans. It can be due to wear and tear of the joint or, as in the case of Kari, from trauma. When cartilage breaks down inside a joint—whether it's from a car accident, heredity, obesity or another cause—it can cause pain, swelling, inflammation and a limited range of motion. PRP has the capacity to aid in this by fueling new cartilage production. It can also help repair chronically inflamed tendons and partially torn ligaments. In some cases—including Kari's—patients can forgo surgery after receiving PRP injections.

Ophthalmology

My esteemed associate, naturopath and acupuncturist Dr. Kristen Coles, has had three patients with severe dry eye disease. Otherwise known as dry eye syndrome, the malady is marked by a chronic lack of sufficient lubrication and moisture, the results of which manifest as constant irritation, inflammation and even scarring.

For Bree—who had severe dry eye disease secondary to Graves' ophthalmopathy—Dr. Coles recommended one PRP drop per eye, once a day, for eight weeks. Bree began to experience relief nearly immediately—as in, within the first two weeks of treatment. At the end of her regimen, her ophthalmologist noted that she had increased moisture in her eyes.

Another patient, a woman named Leila, developed dry eye disease as a result of rheumatoid arthritis. Following 10 days of treatment, which consisted of one drop per eye once a day, Leila was able to wear mascara for the first time in 10 years.

Finally, there was Alexandria, whose symptoms stemmed from an unknown cause. After six weeks of PRP treatment—again, one drop per eye per day—Alexandria's dry eye syndrome was completely resolved.

Why do I mention all of these cases here? To underscore the prodigious benefits PRP has in ophthalmology. Dr. Coles' patients, of course, aren't alone. A 2017 study published in *Ophthalmology Therapy* evaluated the topical use of PRP in 368 patients with dry eye syndrome. The results were startling—and fantastic. After six weeks of treatment, symptoms improved in 322 cases. The authors stated that PRP is an "effective treatment to improve signs and symptoms in patients suffering from moderate-to-severe chronic dry eye syndrome." Another 2017 study, this one published in the *Journal of Ophthalmology*, demonstrated that PRP can mend dry eye syndrome post-LASIK surgery. In short, PRP may be a godsend for anyone suffering from the debilitating side effects of severe dry eye disease.

Sexual Wellness and Gynecology

Menopause often arrives with a series of symptoms that can dramatically affect a woman's sex life. Such was the case with Stella, who, at 57, was suffering not only from vaginal dryness but also incontinence and "reduced" sexual sensation. Following a PRP treatment—affectionately known as an O-Shot® (as developed by Charles Runels, MD)—her libido was revived and her orgasms were "better than ever."

Hers was far from an isolated case. One of PRP's biggest claims to fame is the impact it can have on one's sexual health. During these sessions, PRP is injected into the intimate areas of women and men (in which case, they're called "P" shots). In men, PRP is injected into the shaft of the penis to support girth and enhance sexual sensation, and in women it is injected into the vulva and the area around the urethra to decrease urinary incontinence and to also enrich sexual pleasure.

Sound painful? Don't despair! A patient is prepped with a numbing cream and given a nerve block that prevents pain. Indeed, the most "painful" part is the idea of having any kind of injection "down there." But I can assure you, if it's done right, it doesn't hurt—and the results can be nothing short of rejuvenating.

I have been doing PRP injections for sexual wellness primarily on women and, in fact, "rejuvenated" is the most frequent feedback I receive. Every woman I have treated—from post-menopausal women to a 30-year-old who wanted to boost her sexual enjoyment—has reported positive effects, from increased sensation to greater vaginal lubrication. With data showing that more than 40% of sexually active women experience some degree of sexual dysfunction in their lives, PRP can be a vital adjunct to supporting sexual wellness.

This is thanks, again, to PRP's rich concentration of important growth factors, which can help invigorate the nerves, muscles, connective tissues and blood vessels of the lower pelvic floor (including the clitoris, urethra, vulva and vaginal wall). Because of the structural support that PRP provides, many women also report resolution of their stress and urge incontinence after a PRP treatment. Mary, for example, was experiencing incontinence so frequently she was considering surgery. After a single PRP treatment, her symptoms became a thing of the past.

And it isn't only sexual wellness that may result from PRP therapy. In a 2018 study published in *Case Reports in Women's Health*, PRP was found to restore tissue histologically (that is, on a microscopic level) in a case of Lichen sclerosus (a rare skin condition that typically affects the genitals) in a 38-year-old premenopausal woman. PRP might also help women with uterine prolapse. What's more, given that the treatment is derived from a woman's own body, authors of a 2017 study argued that there is no risk of a reaction to foreign bodies. (To which we women say, hallelujah!)

Aesthetics

Aside from the distinction PRP has earned in the world of sports medicine—Tiger Woods, Kobe Bryant and Reggie Jackson are just a few of its fans—PRP's utmost renown may be in the field of aesthetics. The technique for a PRP facial utilizes either the relatively pain-free (and aforementioned) microneedling or it can be injected. In some cases, the PRP is applied simultaneously with a facial filler, applied directly to the problem with a syringe or smeared on following microdermabrasion or a laser treatment. The end results, meanwhile, can be downright dramatic.

As Mona Gohara, MD, puts it, "PRP theoretically acts as a matrix that promotes collagen production, parlaying into softer wrinkles, firmer skin, more hair and, in some endorsements, lifted breasts." Numerous studies published in the *Journal of Cosmetic Dermatology* confirm this. The data also demonstrates that PRP can significantly reduce the appearance of brown spots, diminish wrinkles, increase skin firmness and, overall, have a "significant, reproducible, positive impact on biological facial rejuvenation." PRP can also be used to offer volume to cheekbones and nasolabial folds.

Following a PRP procedure, your cells will continue to regenerate for three to six months, with the effects lasting up to a year. It's a swell side effect (and deal), considering that my 65-year-old patient Shauna claimed a series of facial PRP treatments took 10 years off of her face—and she was just one of many patients who saw a major transformation.

Once-a-year treatments are recommended to maintain healthy collagen production. If a woman is older, she may choose to do a series of six treatments one month apart. It is about creating and maintaining healthy, vibrant-looking skin, and supporting collagen, which, as we age, tends to break down.

As for that above-mentioned "more hair?" Yes. PRP is making waves—literally—in the domain of hair regrowth. Again, this comes down to the growth factors it boasts, which, when inserted into the scalp, can activate hair follicles and foster hair regrowth. According to Neil Sadick, MD—a dermatologist in New York City and the director of the Sadick Research Group, studying and treating hair loss (an issue that affects one in five Americans, and can take a huge emotional toll on both men and women)—the use of PRP is "a great treatment option for hair loss because it has a number of scientifically based articles showing its efficacy in increasing hair count, hair thickness and the growth phase of the hair cycle."

What About Cost?

You may be wondering about insurance coverage for PRP procedures. My practice does not take insurance, so I never considered the question. I doubt that PRP currently is covered. And PRP procedures can be expensive. For example, treating one joint in my office using a 30mL kit costs $550...a 60mL kit costs around $650. The facial PRP cost is about $650 per treatment. Cost for the O shot is $1,200. But prices vary depending on where you live (most doctors on the mainland charge more than we do).

Yet these costs may not sound so high when you consider the magical results that PRP treatments can yield. Dr. Andrew Weil was right when he said that our own bodies are our best hope for recovery—and we can experience this, profoundly, with PRP therapy.

The Truth About Body-Sculpting Treatments

Anthony Youn, MD, FACS, Youn Plastic Surgery, Troy, Michigan. He specializes in noninvasive, holistic techniques and is author of *The Age Fix*. DrYoun.com

As we age, some pockets of fat on the body are extremely difficult to eliminate—even with a very healthy lifestyle. Noninvasive treatments such as CoolSculpting and SculpSure promise fat loss in specific areas without dieting, exercise or surgery, and in my experience, they generally do provide modest results.

Both are FDA-approved for basically the same areas—the abdomen, including "love handles," inner and outer thighs, back and double chin—and in studies have been shown to reduce fat by about 25%. With CoolSculpting, an applicator freezes fat cells underneath the skin...and with SculpSure, a laser (heat) disrupts fat cells. In both treatments, the fat cells are naturally eliminated from the body.

These procedures can be mildly uncomfortable but are not typically painful. Swelling and/or bruising is common afterward, but goes away quickly. To date, few serious side effects have been reported. It costs about $1,500 to $3,000 for either treatment, depending on where you live in the US, and it takes about a half hour.

Note: SculpSure can treat up to four small areas at the same time.

It can take two to three months to see the final result, but the result should be permanent provided the patient maintains a healthy lifestyle.

Consult a board-certified plastic surgeon to see if you're a good candidate. Treatments should be performed by a trained technician who could be a doctor, nurse or aesthetician.

Help for Undereye Circles

The herb arnica can do more than just ease sore muscles and reduce bruises. Apply a thin swipe of arnica (gel or cream) under the eyes to combat puffiness and dark circles.

Caution: Avoid getting it in your eyes.

Andrew Rubman, ND, founder and medical director, Southbury Clinic for Traditional Medicines, Southbury, Connecticut. SouthburyClinic.com

Can You Treat Cataracts with an Eyedrop?

Marc Grossman, OD, LAc, doctor of optometry and licensed acupuncturist in New Paltz and Somers, New York. He is coauthor of *Natural Eye Care: Your Guide to Healthy Vision.* A holistic eye doctor, his multidisciplinary approach uses nutrition, lifestyle changes and Traditional Chinese Medicine to tackle eye problems. NaturalEyeCare.com

Cataract surgery is now so streamlined and commonplace, it can almost seem like an inevitable part of aging. However, the procedure isn't risk free—and some people can't have the surgery. Wouldn't it be wonderful if cataracts could be treated with something as simple as an eyedrop? That may be more than wishful thinking!

About 20% of people over age 60 and 80% over age 75 have cataracts. It's the leading cause of blindness worldwide, largely because cataract surgery, the only approved treatment, requires highly trained surgeons and high-tech surgical equipment that are not available in many parts of the world. In the US, however, cataract surgery is a simple, painless, outpatient procedure that is usually covered by insurance. (*Note*: Certain kinds of corrective implantable lenses may not be covered.) However, the procedure can have complications, especially for patients with other eye conditions, such as macular degeneration or glaucoma. Even without other eye conditions, while most of the time one procedure is sufficient, it's not uncommon to need additional surgeries to adjust vision.

Cataracts 101

Cataracts form when oxidative stress—such as from sun exposure, diabetes, high blood pressure, smoking or simply aging—damages protein molecules in the lens of the eye, causing them to clump together. Normally, the protein molecules are arranged in a way that lets light pass through. When the molecules clump, they cloud areas of the lens…and as the clumps grow, larger areas of the lens cloud, making it harder and harder to see.

Antioxidants can reduce or prevent cell damage caused by oxidative stress. One antioxidant in particular, N-acetylcarnosine (NAC), is a strong antioxidant that occurs naturally in the heart, muscles and brain. Human studies have demonstrated that NAC eyedrops can improve cataracts.

What the Research Shows

Most of the research on NAC eyedrops for cataracts has been done in Russia, and the most impressive study comes from Hemholtz Research Institute of Eye Disorders in Moscow and was published in *Journal of Anti-Aging Medicine*. For the study, 49 patients (average age 65) with cataracts received either NAC eyedrops or placebo eyedrops twice daily. After 24 months, 90% of the NAC group had significant improvement in their cataracts… compared with significant progression of their cataracts in nearly 90% of the placebo group. The researchers found that adding an acetyl molecule to NAC allowed it to be absorbed through the front (anterior chamber) of the eye, where it could counteract oxidative stress in the eye lens.

The FDA will need more research, such as large studies, before approving NAC eyedrops for treating cataracts. However, eyedrops approved as moisturizing drops that contain 1% NAC, the same strength used in the study, are available now without prescription. People with cataracts—and some eye doctors—have been treating cataracts with the drops and reporting good results. Brands include Can-C, which contains the same formula that was used in the Russian trials, and OcluMed, which contains additional nutrients that are beneficial for treating cataracts.

Should You Try NAC Eyedrops?

It's important to note that NAC drops are most effective for nuclear cataracts—age-related cataracts that form in the center of the lens—that are still at an early stage. The drops will not improve cataracts present at birth...subcapsular cataracts (cataracts that form at the back of the lens, often from diabetes or taking high doses of steroid medications)...or cortical cataracts (cataracts that form at the edges of the lens). While NAC drops may slightly improve advanced cataracts, they are unlikely to improve vision enough to avoid the need for surgery.

The usual treatment is one drop twice a day and can be continued as long as there is vision improvement. The only side effect experienced by some people is a few seconds of slight stinging when applying the drops, especially if eyes are dry. People who wear contact lenses should wait 15 minutes after applying the drops before putting on contacts.

Check with your eye doctor before using this or any other kind of eyedrops. As there are no known risks, medical condition warnings or other contraindications, NAC drops may be worth trying, particularly if your cataracts are at an early stage. If the drops are going to help, you should see an improvement within the first three months. Even if your cataracts aren't completely reversed, NAC drops may at least keep them

from progressing...or slow their progression so that you can hold off longer on surgery. Taking oral supplements of glutathione, n-acetyl cysteine, alpha-lipoic acid and vitamin C also can help slow down the progression of cataracts.

Besides NAC eyedrops, remember that healthy vison also depends on a healthy lifestyle...

- **Don't smoke.**
- **Wear sunglasses.**
- **Eat plenty of fruits and vegetables to get more antioxidants.**
- **Work with your doctor to control diabetes and/or high blood pressure.**
- **Limit alcohol.**

Car Exhaust Linked to Eye Damage

People exposed to high levels of the pollutants carbon monoxide or nitrogen dioxide, major components of automobile exhaust, were 84% and 91%, respectively, more likely to develop the potentially blinding condition age-related macular degeneration (AMD) than those exposed to the lowest levels, according to a study of nearly 40,000 women and men ages 50 and older.

If you live in a heavily trafficked area: Avoid the outdoors during peak traffic time.

Suh-Hang Hank Juo, PhD, researcher, Graduate Institute of Biomedical Sciences, China Medical University, Taichung, Taiwan.

Statins May Reduce Glaucoma Risk

Glaucoma-free people age 40 and older who took statins for five years or longer were 21% less likely to develop the most common form of glaucoma than were people who never used statins. This might be due to statins' ability to affect enzymes that play a role in blood flow to the eye.

Louis Pasquale, MD, site chair of the department of ophthalmology and professor of ophthalmology at Icahn School of Medicine at Mount Sinai Hospital, New York City, and coauthor of the study published in *JAMA Ophthalmology*. MountSinai.org

Protecting Your Eyes in a Screen-Focused World

Marc Grossman, OD, LAc, doctor of optometry and licensed acupuncturist in New Paltz and Somers, New York. He is coauthor of *Natural Eye Care: Your Guide to Healthy Vision & Healing*. A holistic eye doctor, his multidisciplinary approach uses nutrition, lifestyle changes and Traditional Chinese Medicine to tackle eye problems. NaturalEyeCare.com

Before the age of technology, nearsightedness was found primarily among professions that required a lot of reading, such as accountants, lawyers and college professors, and hardly ever found among, for instance, farmers. Now nearsightedness is reaching epidemic proportions. For example, in China and Japan up to 90% of students (teenagers and older) are nearsighted…while in parts of Africa and among other cultures that don't spend extended periods of time doing close work far fewer people are nearsighted.

Why Eyeglasses Aren't the Answer

Nearsightedness is associated with other ocular problems, such as higher risk for glaucoma, cataracts and macular degeneration…and increased likelihood of developing those conditions at an earlier age. There is evidence, in fact, that our near-focus habit is damaging our eye tissue and aging our eyes faster. Studies have linked computer overuse to glaucoma risk…while other research links exposure to blue light (the kind of light emitted by our electronic devices) to macular degeneration and cataracts.

Eyeglasses, contact lenses and surgery, including Lasik and PRK, can bring distant objects into focus, but these don't address the other ocular problems. *Technology is not going away, nor would we want it to…but following these 10 steps can keep your eyes healthier in a near-focused world…*

1. Use smartphones the smart way. Smartphones strain eyes more than do computer screens or tablets. Smartphones are typically held closer to eyes and the font is smaller, both of which concentrate focus, making eye muscles have to work harder.

Solution: Hold your phone as far away as you can to comfortably read the screen.

2. Get outdoors. Being outdoors changes what you're looking at (that is, not a screen and something farther away), and also gives you a chance to exercise your peripheral vision.

Tip: As you walk around, keep your eyes forward but maintain awareness of your whole visual field rather than focusing on a particular object. Do this effortlessly—don't strain!

3. Take breaks. Rest your eyes periodically by letting them wander and rest on the horizon.

Rule of thumb: For every 20 minutes of close work, rest two minutes…for every 30 minutes of close work, rest five minutes… and for every hour of close work, rest 10 minutes.

4. Blink, breathe…and smile! People unconsciously blink less and breathe more shallowly when looking at a screen. Your eyes need to blink to maintain a healthy tear film and protect against dry eye. Taking deep breaths keeps blood flowing so that sufficient oxygen gets to your eyes.

Try this: Blink rapidly six times…then close your eyes and take two slow, deep breaths. Repeat four times.

Easy way to prevent eyestrain: Make a small smile. When you smile you can't put strain on your eye muscles.

5. Try rose water. Rose water is especially good for your eyes, as it has a relaxing effect and helps tired eyes feel more hydrated. Spray rose water around your head and eyes (close your eyes first).

6. Watch TV from a safe distance. Ideally, the distance between your eyes and the screen should be at least seven times the width of the screen. For a 40-inch screen, that would be about 23 feet away. If the ideal distance isn't practical, even half that distance is still better than sitting two feet away from the screen.

7. Keep neck muscles loose. Tense muscles in the neck and shoulders can affect nerves at the back of the neck that lead to eye pain. Neck strain also can cause ocular headaches.

What helps: Do neck rolls, put warm compresses on your neck...and avoid hunched postures!

8. Avoid extremes of light/dark contrast. In darkness, your pupils dilate to let more light into your eyes so you can see better...and in bright light, the pupils contract to keep light out. When you look at a bright screen against a dark background it gives the eyes a mixed message. Try to keep screen brightness at 50% for smartphones, tablets, laptops and monitors. Avoid looking at brightly lit screens against total darkness—such as watching TV with all the lights turned off.

9. Lounge "consciously." Avoid slouching in bed or on the couch to watch TV, read or work on a laptop. Instead, sit up and have what you're focusing on at a comfortable level for your eyes—ideally 20 degrees below eye level. Use a lap desk to elevate a laptop, book or tablet.

10. Look up! Looking up from near work and into the distance relaxes your eyes' extraocular muscles (the muscles that move your eyes to the left, right, up and down) and ciliary muscles (which help the eyes to focus) and helps those muscles stay flexible.

Too Much Screen Time Can Age You

Blue light from screens may accelerate aging. Fruit flies exposed to 12 hours of blue light and 12 hours of darkness lived significantly shorter lives than those kept in total darkness or exposed to light with blue wavelengths filtered out. Blue-light–exposed flies had damaged retinal cells and brain neurons and developed difficulty climbing the walls of their enclosures. Human blue-light exposure is increasing quickly through widespread use of LED lighting and electronic devices.

Study by researchers at Oregon State University, Corvallis, published in Aging and Mechanisms of Disease.

What You Don't Know About Night Sweats

Adam Perlman, MD, MPH, director of Integrative Health and Wellbeing at Mayo Clinic in Jacksonville, Florida. He is board-certified in internal medicine.

You wake up drenched...pajamas sopping wet, sheets clammy beneath you...and it's not the first time. But the bedroom is relatively cool, and you aren't dressed too warmly—in other words, all that heat is coming from you.

Contrary to popular opinion, menopause isn't the only cause of night sweats. But if you're a woman (or a man) not affected by menopause, you may be scratching your head at the same time you're mopping your brow. Why are you getting these nightly soakings?

Little-Known Culprits

Menopause is the main cause of chronic night sweats, but other health conditions and factors can be to blame for excessive sweating that occurs at night (and sometimes during the day). *These include...*

●**Medications.** Various drugs, used long term or even for just a few days, are a lesser recognized cause of night sweats. These include antidepressants…pain relievers including aspirin, *acetaminophen* (Tylenol) or opioids…niacin/vitamin B-3, often taken to help lower cholesterol…*tamoxifen* (Nolvadex) to reduce breast cancer risk…steroids…*hydralazine* (Apresoline) to lower blood pressure…nitroglycerin for angina pain…and erectile dysfunction drugs such as *sildenafil* (Viagra).

●**Thyroid problems.** An overactive thyroid, in which the gland produces too much thyroid hormone (hyperthyroidism), can rev up metabolism, triggering night sweating. But paradoxically, night sweats also can stem from an underactive thyroid (hypothyroidism) or cancer of the thyroid gland.

●**Low testosterone.** This one is a men's issue. Drops in testosterone, dubbed "manopause," prompt hot flashes and night sweats that are similar to those that plague menopausal women. Hormone treatment for prostate cancer also can be to blame.

●**Other hormone problems.** In addition to thyroid and sex hormone fluctuations, various hormone disorders might be at play. These include carcinoid syndrome, which results in the overproduction of chemicals, including serotonin, in the presence of a rare, slow-growing cancer that may occur in the lung or digestive tract…or a type of adrenal gland tumor that ramps up hormones called catecholamines.

●**Infections.** If you've had the flu, you may have felt the wrath of night sweats on top of classic symptoms such as fever, cough and achiness. But many infections can soak your sheets, including urinary tract infections (UTIs)…abscesses in the skin, tonsils, gut or appendix…and less commonly, tuberculosis, HIV, and heart valve inflammation known as endocarditis.

●**Low blood sugar.** Among people with diabetes, those taking insulin or pills to help control blood sugar sometimes experience drops in blood sugar during sleep that trigger sweating.

●**GERD.** Gastroesophageal reflux disease (GERD), a common cause of heartburn, can trigger night sweats.

●**Neurologic disorders.** While an unusual trigger for night sweats, brain conditions such as Parkinson's disease, stroke or autonomic neuropathy (a condition that damages nerves controlling involuntary body functions such as digestion) may be the culprit.

●**Cancer.** Night sweats are an early symptom of certain cancers—particularly lymphoma and leukemia. But in this less common scenario, other symptoms are usually also present, including fever and unexplained weight loss. Chemotherapy to treat certain cancers can cause night sweats as well.

●**Food.** Certain foods may provoke sweating at night. Spicy foods, caffeine and alcohol are among the most common triggers. However, these foods are more likely to cause hot flashes right after eating them than night sweats.

●**Stress or anxiety.** These largely overlooked triggers can greatly contribute to night sweats by promoting the release of additional epinephrine, the body's "fight-or-flight" hormone.

●**Excess body weight.** People who are overweight or obese are more likely to suffer night sweats than those of normal weight—due, in part, to body fat acting as insulation that traps heat and raises the body's core temperature.

Pinpointing the Cause

Unless it's a clear case of menopause, night sweats should never be dismissed. That's because they're a symptom of something else, so it's crucial to see a doctor to get to the bottom of it.

Important: If you're a menopausal woman suffering from night sweats, work with your primary care doctor and gynecologist to ensure that the symptom is due to menopause and not one of the conditions described earlier.

To find the cause, your doctor should…

•**Take a thorough medical history,** including a travel history, to determine if you visited a region where tuberculosis is prevalent.

Other questions may include: What medications, vitamins or supplements are you taking? Were you ill recently? Are any other unexplained symptoms occurring? This step is key because it tells the doctor how aggressively to pursue additional testing.

•**Perform a complete physical exam,** checking weight and for signs of disease such as nodules on the thyroid or loss of muscle mass in a male, which might indicate low testosterone.

•**Order blood tests to check hormone levels or rule out various infections or certain types of cancer.**

•**Perform other tests,** such as a Mantoux tuberculin skin test for tuberculosis and, when appropriate, evaluate for certain cancers, such as leukemia, through blood work.

•**Order imaging tests,** such as X-rays or a CT or MRI scan, to rule out malignancies such as thyroid cancer.

•**Review your medications.** Because certain drugs, including those described earlier, can trigger night sweats, it's important for your doctor to review all medications and supplements you're taking. In some cases, a different drug can be prescribed.

Caveat: After exhausting every possible avenue to figure out why the waterworks turn on while you sleep, it's possible that your doctor may find…nothing. In this case, night sweats are deemed a case of idiopathic hyperhidrosis, which means your body sweats too much at night for no identifiable medical reason.

Important: If a cause is not determined and night sweats continue, be sure to report any new symptoms, such as weight loss and/or fever.

How to Get Relief

If there's an underlying medical cause, treating that condition should eliminate night sweats. But if that's not the case, you'll want to take the obvious steps to get some relief, such as using fans, dressing in easy-to-peel-off layers and lowering the temperature in your bedroom. *Beyond that, try these additional strategies…*

•**Invest in newer high-tech bedding or nightwear.** These products include quick-drying or moisture-wicking sheets or pajamas and are available online.

Note: A device called BedJet includes a fan that is installed beneath the bed to blow cool (or warm) air into the bedding.

•**Freeze an icy gel pack during the day… and place it under your pillow at bedtime.** You can flip the pillow periodically during the night to sleep on the chilled side.

•**Try stress-busting techniques,** such as acupuncture, meditation, deep breathing and/or yoga.

Smart idea: Do these close to bedtime, when it's helpful to quiet down the nervous system prior to going to bed.

•**Consider taking vitamins and other supplements believed to combat night sweats.** These include B-complex vitamins, vitamin E, black cohosh, red clover and evening primrose oil.

Important: Get your doctor's advice on which supplement(s) would be most appropriate for you—some may interfere with medications you're taking.

•**Decrease sugar in your diet.** This advice is ideal for overall health, of course, but is believed to also reduce inflammation in the body, which may contribute to hot flashes and night sweats.

•**Ask your doctor about medications to battle night sweats if all else fails.** This may include off-label use of a low-dose antidepressant, such as *paroxetine* (Paxil)…or the blood pressure drug *clonidine* (Catapres).

Licorice Root for Hot Flashes

Laurie Steelsmith, ND, LAc, medical director of Steelsmith Natural Health Center in Honolulu. She is author of *Natural Choices for Women's Health, Great Sex, Naturally* and *Growing Younger Every Day* and writes the "Natural Healing Secrets for Women" blog at BottomLineInc.com. DrSteelsmith.com

Probably the most well-known use of licorice root is as a sweetener in candies (it's also often used as a sweetener in herbal tea formulas). But you might not know that this herb has been used for medicinal purposes for centuries—including for the relief of hot flashes.

As women go through the transition of menopause, estrogen levels fall, which is thought to trigger hot flashes. Up to 80% of women experience hot flashes during menopause, and a study found that the uncomfortable symptoms can last for up to 14 years. Licorice root can help reduce both the frequency and severity of hot flashes because it's a phytoestrogen, which means that it contains very weak estrogens.

Recent finding: In one small study, women who took a 330-milligram licorice root capsule three times a day reported a decrease in the frequency and severity of hot flashes over eight weeks. And no significant side effects were reported.

If you would like to try licorice root for hot flashes, be sure to consult a naturopathic doctor to get the dosage that's right for you.

Caution: Licorice root can cause high blood pressure, irregular heartbeat and low potassium levels in some people. A chemical called glycyrrhizic acid is responsible for these effects, so choose a deglycyrrhizinated licorice supplement, which has this chemical removed.

Drinking a daily cup of licorice root tea is another way to help mitigate hot flashes, but this also can increase blood pressure in some people, due to the glycyrrhizic acid. If you're prone to high blood pressure, choose other teas rich in phytoestrogens such as red clover or evening primrose.

Additional alerts on licorice: Besides the blood pressure caution above, if you have a hormone-sensitive condition, such as breast, uterine or ovarian cancer, endometriosis or uterine fibroids, you should avoid phytoestrogens such as licorice. And a recent study found that several compounds in licorice supplements can potentially interfere with the way the liver processes both prescription and over-the-counter drugs, so if you take medication, check first with your doctor before taking a licorice supplement or drinking licorice root tea.

Adjusting to Hearing Aids

Tina Childress, AuD, CCC-A, audiologist, Association of Late-Deafened Adults, Champaign, Illinois. ALDA.org

Adjusting to new hearing aids is a process. Patience and keeping communication options open are key.

Hearing aids make many sounds more audible, including environmental sounds such as traffic noise or a ringing phone. But speech is much more difficult to hear because it's a more complex sound. Sometimes hearing aids aren't enough—you may need to use assistive devices to communicate in groups, talk on the phone and watch TV.

For better communication with someone who just began wearing hearing aids: When you want to say something to him, give him a tap or slight wave to get his attention and make eye contact before talking to him. It's also helpful to have good lighting and speak face-to-face so that he can interpret gestures and use lip-reading clues.

Be sure to pause between sentences and speak at a normal pace (not too fast or too slow). And don't cover your mouth. Speak in your normal tone of voice, since shouting can distort speech. Moving to a quieter place helps with ease of communication as well. If he or she keeps misunderstanding something, try different words, which he may be able to hear better.

Writing notes can be another effective way to communicate unfamiliar words that may be difficult for your loved one to lip-read.

Important: Talk with your audiologist if you have further questions.

"Tickle Therapy" Fights Aging

Using a small, painless electrical current to "tickle" the ear improves sleep and mental health. In test subjects, the tingling, self-administered current increased activity in the "resting" part of the nervous system by stimulating part of the vagus nerve, which can be reached via the outer ear.

Implication: The therapy's positive effect on sleep and mental health may slow down aging.

Aging.

Losing Your Sense of Smell?

Richard L. Doty, PhD, FAAN, director of the Smell and Taste Center and professor of psychology in oto-rhinolaryngology: head and neck surgery at the Perelman School of Medicine, University of Pennsylvania, Philadelphia. He is author or editor of 11 books, including *The Great Pheromone Myth* and *Smell and Taste Disorders.*

If you've noticed that your sense of smell (aka olfaction) isn't what it used to be, you're not alone. For some 20 million Americans, the ability to detect everyday smells, from baking bread to burning wood, is slipping away...or even gone.

Why this matters: Even though primary care physicians rarely ask patients about loss of smell, it can be an early red flag for certain chronic medical conditions. It is also an early symptom for the new coronavirus.

A Multitasking Sense

Few people appreciate the multitude of daily functions tied to their sense of smell. *This all-too-often neglected sense serves as...*

• **A key to appetite.** Smell is responsible for most of our sense of taste. People with a diminished sense of smell often have a poor appetite, remarking that food is tasteless or just doesn't taste the same. While taste buds can distinguish basic levels of sweet, sour, bitter, salty and umami (a savory, earthy taste), smell also plays an important but often underappreciated role in our ability to taste foods.

• **A harbinger of serious disorders.** A diminished sense of smell is often an early symptom of Parkinson's disease and Alzheimer's disease. In fact, smell dysfunction is the most common early symptom reported by Parkinson's patients even before they suffer motor-related symptoms, such as tremors or walking difficulties.

A Hard-to-Spot Deficiency

Because few primary care physicians test for smell problems, you need to be alert for any suspected loss of this sense.

This can be challenging because the loss of smell that tends to occur with aging happens gradually, and most people with health problems don't recognize that they have lost their sense of smell. For example, loss of smell is present in about 90% of people with Parkinson's disease, but most don't recognize that they have a problem.

Self-defense: Even if you only suspect a change, you should report this to your doctor. If there is no obvious reason for the loss of smell, such as a cold, allergies or nasal congestion, then smell testing is recommended.

Smell Testing

A number of tests are available to assess one's ability to smell. These range from simple three-item scratch-and-sniff screening tests...the 16-item Sniffin' Sticks odor identification test that uses felt-tip pens to dispense odors...to longer tests, such as the 40-item University of Pennsylvania Smell Identification Test (UPSIT).* With the 15-minute UPSIT, you are asked to smell a series of odors (such as rose, pizza, cinnamon and mint) and identify each odor from a list of choices.

The UPSIT, which can be ordered by physicians online for a nominal cost, helps doctors to determine both the absolute and relative (to one's age and sex) degrees of smell loss.

Treatment Options

The first step in treatment is to identify the cause of the smell loss. Olfactory problems related to Parkinson's disease or brain damage are generally believed to be irreversible, but early detection is helpful in planning medical treatment.

There is strong evidence in a 2013 paper published in *JAMA Otolaryngology–Head & Neck Surgery* that regular exercise can help to maintain the ability to smell in later life, much like it can help to avert or delay the onset of dementia. However, it is not known whether exercise can reverse such impairment once it is present.

If the loss is due to simple inflammation, including that caused by chronic sinusitis, then treatment with powerful anti-inflammatories (such as corticosteroids) may bring back some sense of smell. Oral steroids typically restore smell function within about a week. Continued topical therapy with steroid sprays or washes can, in some cases, maintain the restored function. If nasal polyps are to blame, surgical removal can be helpful.

Promising therapy: Some evidence shows that the antioxidant alpha-lipoic acid may help one regain the sense of smell in certain cases, such as long-lasting dysfunction due to

*Dr. Doty is president of Sensonics International, the manufacturer and distributor of the UPSIT.

upper respiratory infections. The suggested dosage is 400 mg to 600 mg daily.

Important: Before trying alpha-lipoic acid, talk to your doctor. This supplement has been shown to lower blood sugar, so people with diabetes need to use caution. It could also interact with some medications, including antibiotics, anti-inflammatories, tranquilizers, heart medications and chemotherapy drugs.

Another option: Small amounts of smell-restoring alpha-lipoic acid can be found in foods.

Good sources: Organ meats (such as kidneys and liver)...spinach...and broccoli.

Are You at Risk?

There are dozens of possible causes for smell loss. *Among the most common...*

•**Aging.** With age, the nerves that are involved in smell weaken, and odor-detecting membranes lining the nose become thin and dry.

•**Smoking.** Because it irritates nasal passages, smoking impairs one's sense of smell. The good news is that normal smelling function can return in less than a year after quitting in light smokers and over the course of several years in heavy smokers—providing another reason to quit.

•**Air pollution.** Research published in 2016 in *Environmental Health Perspectives* noted that the tiny particulates in polluted air enter the nose, cross through the olfactory bulb and actually enter the brain. There the stray microparticles, commonly found in diesel exhaust and air pollutants, can induce an inflammatory response that can lead to brain tissue damage, the development of Alzheimer's-like pathology and a loss of smell.

•**Certain medications.** More than 70 medications can affect one's sense of smell. The list includes heart drugs, such as the cholesterol-lowering medication *atorvastatin* (Lipitor) and blood pressure drugs such as *amlodipine* (Norvasc) and *enalapril* (Vasotec), and some decongestant nasal sprays.

17

Unfortunately, there is not much data indicating whether stopping such drugs will reverse smell loss.

•**Head injury.** Even a relatively minor head injury, as might occur when one hits the back of the head on the pavement after slipping on ice, can permanently damage the delicate nerve connections to the brain that control your sense of smell.

Smell Training Could Improve Your Sniffer...

If you're concerned that your sniffer isn't performing quite up to snuff, be sure to mention this to your doctor. Loss of smell (anosmia) can have a variety of causes, ranging from a common cold or the use of certain medications to a serious underlying medical condition, such as Parkinson's disease or Alzheimer's disease.

Your doctor should get a complete medical history to help determine what's causing your loss of smell and administer a smell test to assess the function of your olfactory system.

If no underlying medical condition is detected, consider trying "olfactory training" (aka smell training). Some research suggests that practice may improve one's sense of smell—something that's closely tied to one's sense of taste and overall life satisfaction. After all, who doesn't enjoy smelling a fresh pot of brewed coffee or a lovely bouquet of gardenias?

Research finding: When 40 study participants with anosmia due to a severe upper-respiratory tract infection, head trauma or unknown cause, were asked to smell four odors (rose, eucalyptus, lemon and clove) for 10 seconds each in the morning and evening for 12 weeks, olfactory function for 30% of them improved while those who did not train reported no change, according to research published in *The Laryngoscope*.

Smell training doesn't guarantee that your sense of smell will improve. It is most likely to help accelerate the recovery of your olfactory function following a viral infection, such as a cold or the flu—both of which can temporarily damage olfactory receptor cells in the nasal cavity.

A simple way to try smell training: Place four bottles of spices (such as clove, mint or cinnamon) and/or extracts (such as vanilla, lemon or maple) next to your bed. Sniff each one first thing in the morning and before going to bed three or four times. Before changing scents, take a few "cleansing" sniffs. Every few days, write down whether you can accurately identify each scent and the potency of the aroma (based on a scale of 1 to 5). If your sense of smell is going to improve with practice, it will typically occur within a few months.

Another practice to follow: Because such illnesses frequently cause loss of smell, take steps to prevent illness in the first place by practicing good hand hygiene—wash your hands for at least 20 seconds with soap and water (or an alcohol-based hand sanitizer if water is not available) before, during and after preparing foods...before eating...after using the toilet...after blowing your nose, coughing or sneezing...after caring for someone who is sick...and after touching an animal.

This is one of the simplest ways to protect your sniffer!

Hydrogen Fights Disease and Delays Aging

Sergej M. Ostojic, MD, PhD, professor of biomedical sciences at University of Novi Sad, and adjunct professor at University of Belgrade School of Medicine, both in Serbia. Dr. Ostojic has published numerous scientific papers on molecular hydrogen in many medical journals, including *Sports Medicine, Annals of Medicine* and *Pharmacological Research*.

Hydrogen (H_2) is the most abundant element in the universe. In fact, we literally bathe in it (H_2O). While tiny, scientists are discovering that the H_2 molecule may have the powerful ability to help counter many of the effects of aging and related diseases with its purported antioxidant and anti-inflammatory effects. Although further research is needed to confirm the health benefits, ready-to-drink hydrogen-infused water and bath tablets are already widely available online.

Why We Age

Research on the science of aging continues to evolve…

• **Free radical theory.** Free radicals are naturally occurring oxygen atoms missing an electron in their outer ring, making them unstable. Seeking stability, free radicals try to bind with other atoms and molecules. Too many free radicals can create what scientists call oxidative stress, a kind of cellular rust that ages us. Proponents of the theory claim that cellular rust is behind many of the conditions and diseases of aging, from arterial disease and arthritis to vision loss and wrinkles.

• **Telomere theory.** Telomeres are tips at the end of chromosomes that protect the genetic information within each chromosome. Throughout your life, every time a cell divides, telomeres become a little shorter. In telomere theory, the shorter the telomere, the more your body shows signs of aging. Scientific evidence links many of the ailments of aging—high blood pressure, diabetes, cancer, dementia—to shorter telomeres.

• **Mitochondrial energy theory.** Mitochondria are the energy factories in every cell. In this theory, broken-down mitochondria cause the body to work less efficiently, leading to accelerated aging and age-related diseases.

The Hope for Hydrogen

Although hydrogen is essential to the formation of all matter, including life-giving water, it was thought to be biologically "inert," with no function in health or healing. But in 2007, Japanese scientists revolutionized the understanding of hydrogen gas. They showed in cellular and animal experiments that H_2 could neutralize free radicals.

Some scientists also believe that H_2 is a key signaling molecule, improving communication between brain cells and blood flow in arteries. It also activates health-protecting genes that promote the burning of fat and sugar. Plus, hydrogen may cool chronic inflammation, which fuels many diseases of aging.

In the last decade or so, there have been more than 400 cellular, animal and human studies on using H_2 for health and healing, showing that hydrogen may help do many things, including…

• **Prevent muscle pain after exercise**

• **Protect skin from sun damage**

• **Protect the brain from stroke damage**

• **Improve memory and cognition in Alzheimer's disease patients**

• **Strengthen the heart in cardiovascular disease patients**

• **Lower "bad" LDL cholesterol and boost "good" HDL**

• **Balance glucose and insulin,** preventing or slowing diabetes

• **Shield the retina from damage,** helping to prevent and control age-related macular degeneration and glaucoma

• **Slow or stop the degeneration of cartilage,** which can lead to osteoarthritis.

Some of the latest studies that demonstrate just how powerful molecular hydrogen can be include…

• **Heart health.** In a study of middle-aged, overweight women, published in the *Iranian Journal of Medical Sciences*, Serbian researchers found that swallowing hydrogen-producing caplets significantly reduced body fat, insulin and triglycerides—risk factors for heart disease and diabetes—during the four-week study. They theorize that H_2 makes cells more sensitive to insulin, thereby improving the burning of blood fats, leading to less body fat and cardiac stress.

In a study in *Circulation Journal*, patients who inhaled hydrogen gas when they arrived at the ER after a heart attack had less long-term heart damage.

In a study in *Vascular Health and Risk Management*, a team of Japanese researchers found that people who drank hydrogen-rich water had improved arterial health within 30 minutes—with 12% greater blood flow.

•**Stroke.** In a study published in *Journal of Stroke & Cerebrovascular Disease*, Japanese scientists studied people who had a stroke, dividing them into two groups. In the 24 hours after the stroke, one group inhaled hydrogen gas for one hour twice a day and one group received a placebo treatment. Those getting the H_2 had less brain injury (as shown by an MRI), less severe stroke symptoms (such as facial palsy, the inability to use limbs and problems with speech) and more and faster benefits from physical therapy, as measured by function in daily living.

•**Arthritis.** In a study published in *International Immunopharmacology* on people with painful rheumatoid arthritis, researchers found that a month of hydrogen-rich saline injections administered intravenously reduced "disease activity" by about 29%—meaning less pain, swelling and tenderness. There was no change in a placebo group.

Hydrogen-ate Your Body

Although most studies to date involve inhaled or injected hydrogen gas (which is not yet approved by the FDA), proponents of hydrogen suggest a much simpler and more accessible method of hydrogen-ating—drink or bathe in it…

•**Hydrogen-infused water.** Ready-to-drink hydrogen water is available. Popular brands include HFactor and Dr. Perricone. To make hydrogen water, manufacturers add odorless and tasteless molecular hydrogen gas to water, then package it in cans or aluminum-lined pouches. (The gas can escape from glass or plastic bottles.) You need to drink the water quickly—within 30 minutes of opening it—or the hydrogen levels will dissipate.

Note: Hydrogen water is different from alkaline water, marketed under brands such as Core and Essentia. Like hydrogen water, alkaline water has been associated with antioxidant properties, but it does not contain hydrogen gas.

You also can buy tablets or powders of electrolyzed hydrogen to dissolve in water (brands include Ultra H_2 and AquaH$_2$). Or you can generate hydrogen water by mixing a powdered magnesium supplement in water and letting the water sit for a few minutes.

Another option: Putting a metallic magnesium stick in your water bottle. The most tested stick is the Dr. Hayashi Hydrogen Rich Water Stick, which uses pure magnesium and is available at Amazon.com.

Optimal dosage of hydrogen-infused water is not yet known. Start with two or three eight-ounce glasses a day.

•**Hydrogen baths.** You can put a hydrogen tablet or powder, available at Amazon.com, into your bath. Bathe in hydrogen-rich water for at least 10 minutes.

Limitations: There are no known side effects of drinking hydrogen-infused water, but more study is needed to determine the possibility of long-term side effects and health benefits. Because there are no dosing guidelines yet, drink in moderation. If using magnesium to make your hydrogen water, limit daily usage to the recommended daily amount of 350 milligrams.

Fast Walkers Live Longer

Researchers found that women who walked at a brisk four-miles-an-hour pace lived about 15 years longer—to age 87—than slow walkers. For men, it was nearly 20 years longer—to age 86. This was regardless of weight or waist circumference, showing that physical fitness may be a better indicator of longevity than body mass index (BMI).

Thomas E. Yates, PhD, professor of physical activity, sedentary behavior and health at University of Leicester, UK, and a lead author of the study using data from 475,000 people, published in *Mayo Clinic Proceedings*.

6 Most Common Problems of Aging Feet

Jonathan D. Rose, DPM, a podiatrist in private practice in Baltimore. He is coauthor of *The Foot Book: A Complete Guide to Healthy Feet.* PodiatryAssociates.org

On average, most people will have walked about 50,000 miles by the time they reach age 50. Active people will have walked or run even more. So it's not surprising that up to 25% of older adults complain of assorted types of chronic foot pain. *Here are six common problems and the simple things you can do to keep your feet healthy…*

PROBLEM: Thinning of the fat pads in the ball of the foot. The fatty padding under your feet naturally wears away over time, which can lead to pain and inflammation in the soles of the feet, a condition known as metatarsalgia. By age 50, many people have lost half of their natural padding. Fat pad atrophy (FPA) affects men and women equally.

What to do: To prevent the fat pads from thinning, wear comfortable walking shoes. Frequent use of high-heeled shoes can cause FPA as well as conditions such as rheumatoid arthritis. If you must wear heels for an event, limit the distance you walk in them. Excess weight also can have an impact on FPA. Staying within a normal body mass index (BMI) range can help maintain your foot padding. Once thinning has begun, you can add gel pads or inserts into shoes to substitute for the loss of your natural padding. If that doesn't do the trick, remove the shoe's existing insert and replace it with a cushioned orthotic insert.

Alternate solution: If the pain persists or gets worse, ask your podiatrist about injections of steroids or, in more extreme cases, a nerve block to relieve the pain.

Not recommended: Injections of fat or synthetic products to repad the sole. These treatments offer only temporary relief and are unproven.

PROBLEM: Corns and calluses. Corns are areas of thickened skin that develop on the tops or sides of the toes, usually due to friction or pressure from wearing shoes that are too tight. Calluses are broader areas of thickening that develop on the bottom of the feet. They're also usually due to friction or pressure, or they can occur in areas where there isn't a lot of fat padding.

What to do: You've probably already tried the corn and callus cushion pads at your local drugstore—possibly with limited success—but the best thing you can do is simply buy new shoes. Corns and calluses often go away on their own if you stop the offending friction and pressure caused by wearing a shoe that squeezes your toes or a shoe that's too small. You may not realize this, but there's a chance you need a larger size shoe at age 60 than you did at 30, as the ligaments and tendons in your feet lose their elasticity, making your feet expand. Choose shoes with soft uppers and wide toe boxes, so your feet don't rub against the shoe.

Tip: Go shoe-shopping late in the day when your feet will be at their widest. Bring the socks with you that you intend to wear with those shoes to make sure they don't rub.

Alternate solution: Rub a pumice stone over the hardened area after taking a shower. Moisturize afterward. And be patient—these types of skin issues can take several months to heal.

Note: Avoid over-the-counter products that contain salicylic acid to eat away corns and calluses—they often take healthy tissue with them. Likewise, don't shave corns and calluses yourself. See a podiatrist if you think the area needs to be exfoliated.

Important: Don't manage corns and calluses or other foot problems yourself if you have diabetes, rheumatoid arthritis or cancer. That can lead to infection.

PROBLEM: Bunions and hammertoes. You usually inherit bunions and hammertoes. Poor shoe choice, however, can increase the speed that the deformity develops. Rheumatological conditions or injury also can contribute to bunion or hammertoe deformities. Despite its appearance, a bunion is not a growth on the joint. It reflects movement of the big toe toward—or over or under, in severe cases—the second toe.

What to do: Ditch the high heels and pointy-toed shoes. You can buy gel and silicone toe separators, splints, wraps or guards for both bunions and hammertoes. Splints are better for bunions at night. Guards, toe separators or pads are helpful for bunions when people are wearing shoes. Pads cushion the deformities, while splints attempt to delay the progression. Avoid overwearing flip-flops and clogs, which increase the risk for hammertoes because they encourage curling of the toe to grip the shoe.

Alternate solution: Use paper tape to gently push down your hammertoe. Apply the tape around the toe to pull it down, and tape it to the bottom of the foot so that it doesn't rub against your shoe. You may be able to get some relief with products such as YogaToes Gems that spread toes apart to stretch weak ligaments. Surgery is a last-resort option, done to correct a deformity that causes you severe pain and functional limitations and that cannot be relieved by other treatments.

PROBLEM: **Toenail thickening.** Toenails tend to become thicker with age, which can make them difficult to cut. It doesn't help that, for many elderly people, bending down to reach the nails becomes increasingly difficult.

What to do: It seems obvious, but many people don't do this—go to a podiatrist or have regular professional pedicures if you are too stiff or inflexible to easily cut your toenails yourself. Using nail softeners also may help make it easier to cut your nails. Cut nails straight across or take small snips in them to prevent painful ingrown toenails. Smooth the ends with an emery board. Clean under the toenails regularly with a nail file.

PROBLEM: **Nail fungus.** Age can make toenails more prone to nail fungus, an unsightly nail infection that is caused by dampness and spread in gyms, pools and public showers. Three-quarters of people over age 60 have had nail fungus at some point in their lives. It is very difficult to treat successfully once you have a fungus—the available drugs and lasers take a long time to work and aren't effective for everybody.

What to do: The best defense is a good offense—wear rubber sandals in public showers, pools and gyms to prevent picking up fungus. If you have machine-washable shoes, wash them with bleach and water to disinfect them. Change to fresh socks every day (or multiple times a day if your feet sweat). Wear acrylic socks that wick away moisture instead of cotton socks. A home remedy to treat nail fungus that you can try is to apply Vicks VapoRub to the affected nail daily for six to 12 months.

PROBLEM: **Dry skin.** The skin on the feet gets drier as you age. When severe, skin fissures can occur.

What to do: Keep things simple. Just wash feet daily, and pat dry. Showering is best. Soaks in the tub are too drying. Regular twice-a-day moisturizing is essential. Apply a moisturizer that contains urea, which helps slough off the dead skin and keeps skin hydrated. Apply at night, and then sleep with socks on. If severe, you can also wrap the foot in plastic wrap at night to increase penetration of the lotion.

Important: Don't apply moisturizer between toes where fungus or bacteria might grow.

Easy Exercises for Foot Health

The right exercises can help keep your toes and feet limber and strong.

Exercise #1: **Pick up marbles.** This will strengthen muscles in the bottom of your feet and may help prevent plantar fasciitis. Place marbles on the floor. Pick up one marble at a time with your toes, and drop it into a nearby bowl or cup. Repeat with your other foot.

Exercise #2: **Grasp a towel with your toes.** This exercise encourages you to do toe curls that will strengthen the tops of your feet. Sit in a straight-back chair with a small towel at your feet. Use the toes of one foot to scrunch the towel and pull it toward you. Repeat with the other foot.

Exercise #3: **Trace the alphabet.** This exercise helps ankle mobility. Sit down and extend your leg. Trace the alphabet in the air with your big toe. Repeat with the other foot.

Supplements Can Be Dangerous

Not a Magic Pill...

Dietary supplements may not extend life. A recent study found that adequate intake of vitamins A and K, magnesium, zinc and copper were associated with a lower risk for death. However, the link was found only when the substances come from food not from supplements. And high doses of some supplements were found to be harmful.

Example: Calcium at a level of 1,000 milligrams or more a day was associated with higher risk for death from cancer, but no association was shown when calcium intake was from food sources.

Fang Fang Zhang, PhD, MD, associate professor of epidemiology, Friedman School of Nutrition Science and Policy at Tufts University, Boston, and senior author of a study of 30,899 people, published in *Annals of Internal Medicine.*

Choking Alert...

Nearly 4,000 people (most over age 65) reported problems swallowing dietary supplement pills during a 10-year period, according to a report from the FDA. Three deaths also were reported.

Self-defense: Swallow supplements with plenty of water...or ask your pharmacist or doctor for a liquid, powder or chewable form.

Cecile Punzalan, MD, MPH, medical officer, Center for Food Safety and Applied Nutrition, FDA, College Park, Maryland.

Exercise #4: **Do toe raises.** This exercise helps to strengthen the Achilles tendon and the arch of the foot. Stand with your hands resting on the back of a sturdy chair, and slowly rise up on your toes and come back down. Toe raises can be done in three sets of 10. Repeat two to three times a week.

Note: Toe raises are not recommended for people suffering with plantar fasciitis. Instead, you want to stretch the calf by bringing the toes and feet upward toward the shin.

Keto Diets Are Risky for Older People

Keto diets can deprive the body of the protein it needs to build and maintain muscle mass. The diets often limit protein to 15% of calories consumed, with the rest of the diet consisting of about 75% fat and 10% carbs. But older people tend to need more protein than these diets allow to avoid frailty, falls and fractures. Keto diets also have effects on people of all ages that may be more serious for older adults, including increasing risk for kidney stones, renal damage and elevated LDL cholesterol. The diets can be difficult to maintain—even with professional assistance.

Roundup of experts on diet, reported at AARP.org.

Reinvent Yourself at Any Age

Marc Agronin, MD, geriatric psychiatrist and chief medical officer of MIND Institute at Miami Jewish Health. He is author of *The End of Old Age: Living a Longer, More Purposeful Life.* MarcAgronin.com

Sadly, many people have a very narrow view of old age and brain health—none more so, perhaps, than those who are aging themselves. While there are many jokes about senior moments, I believe that older brains have enormous potential because of the aging and learning process. How so? Seniors make better decisions and have more informed perspectives on life. Pulling from a broad store of memories and experiences also allows older people to problem-solve more creatively.

Taken all together, aging can be a jumping-off point for a renewed sense of purpose and growth if you are willing to explore some new directions…

• **Try a more creative approach.** Part of problem-solving comes from being able to think divergently, along different pathways. As the brain matures, we get better at doing this and our solutions become more creative. In real terms, this means that if you find yourself facing a challenge, such as being unable to stand for long periods of time, you usually can find a work-around—maybe one that is even better than the original way you had of doing things.

Example: The famous French painter Matisse almost died from an intestinal ailment in the early 1940s. Miraculously, he survived, but not in the same physical condition. He could no longer stand and paint big canvases. So he had a choice to make. He either had to give up his career or find a new way of doing it. In the end, he revolutionized the art world. From his wheelchair, he cut shapes from vividly colored sheets of paper and instructed his assistant on how to paste them up on the wall. Much of what Matisse is best known for comes from the last 10 years of his life.

• **Think of yourself as liberated.** We tend to think that liberation and experimentation are the domain of the young, but that's not true. With age comes fewer inhibitions. In my experience, older people often feel less encumbered by previous approaches, ideologies and ways of thinking than they did when they were younger. It's time to shake up the stereotypes we have about aging and realize that we can take a leadership role in

Make a "Chuck It" List

Don't just have a bucket list. Also create a "chuck it" list of things you want to stop doing. Free yourself of stuff you've always thought you must do, and focus on what's important to you.

Nancy Collamer, career coach, speaker and founder of MyLifestyleCareer.com, Old Greenwich, Connecticut, and author of *Second-Act Careers*.

terms of doing things differently. You even have the freedom to reinvent the type of relationships you have with people in your family—especially the younger generation.

• **Take stock of all your personal assets.** Think of your life as you would a financial portfolio. What are your assets? It could be sewing…it could be your ability to set up and maintain a budget…it could be that you still are a very good driver. Talking to people about your list of unique skills and assets will help to redefine how you see yourself and how you can define your future. This is what I call "re-aging," because then you can start pursuing some of these new activities.

• **Be open to new directions.** Are you happy with the roads you have pursued so far? Look back, and ask yourself, What were some of the most challenging experiences in my life?…How did I get through them?… What pushed me forward? The answers to these questions give individuals a sense of their purpose, and this may drive ideas for what you can do going forward. Just because you have always been an accountant doesn't mean that you now can't pursue your passion for gardening. It's not too late. Make a list of the things you want to do now. This is not a traditional bucket list of travel destinations. It's about how you want to live the coming years…and the legacy you want to leave behind.

Chapter 2

BRAIN HEALTH

Surprising Headache Link to Alzheimer's

We know a lot more than we used to about dementia, which currently affects about 5.8 million Americans. But we still do not have a way to accurately predict who will get it. Now, a new study has found that having a certain type of headache may be a clue to increased risk—especially for Alzheimer's disease. Here's what you need to know...and what you should do if you get these headaches.

Dementia is the most common neurological condition in older adults...while headaches are the most common neurological condition in people of all ages. Considering how common both conditions are, researchers from University of Waterloo in Ontario, Canada, wanted to see if there was a link.

Study: The researchers looked at a severe form of headache, migraines, and dementia among 679 men and women (62% of them were women) age 65 and older who had participated in a long-term study on healthy aging. The data included history of migraine, as well as other factors associated with dementia risk. The participants had no memory problems at the start of the study. The researchers then followed the participants for five years, checking for various forms of dementia, including vascular dementia (dementia that occurs as vessels that supply blood to the brain become blocked, such as following a stroke) and Alzheimer's disease.

Results: 51 participants were diagnosed with dementia over the study period. Those who had reported a history of migraines were three times more likely to be diagnosed with any type of dementia...and four times more likely to have Alzheimer's disease, after considering the effects of age, education, gender, depression, diabetes and cardiovascular conditions such as high blood pressure, stroke and heart attack. However, the association was found only among women, because no men in the study had both migraines and dementia. Migraines and dementia are more common in women. The study authors say larger studies are thus

Suzanne Tyas, PhD, associate professor, School of Public Health and Health Systems, University of Waterloo, Ontario, Canada. She is coauthor of the study titled "Migraine and the risk of all-cause dementia, Alzheimer's disease, and vascular dementia: A prospective cohort study in community-dwelling older adults," published in *International Journal of Geriatric Psychiatry*.

needed to further examine the migraine/dementia association among men.

The researchers also had expected to find a strong association between vascular dementia and migraines, which is considered a vascular condition—blood vessel swelling in the brain is thought to drive the pain. However, no association was found, suggesting that another pathway may be involved in the development of dementia.

What This Means

If further research confirms that migraine history is a risk factor for Alzheimer's disease, it may pave the way toward earlier diagnosis and enhanced prevention efforts, the researchers hope. For instance, doctors may want to screen earlier for signs of cognitive decline in people with a history of migraines in order to treat other risk factors for Alzheimer's disease more aggressively.

Meanwhile, if you have a history of migraines, it might be worth mentioning this research to your doctor. And whether or not you have migraines, it doesn't hurt to keep up healthy, brain-protecting activities, such as staying physically and mentally active and socially engaged…eating a healthy diet…and managing health conditions such as high blood pressure and diabetes that put your brain at risk. If it's good for your heart, it's also good for your brain!

Hot Flashes and Brain Health

Cognitive decline is linked to menopausal hot flashes. Women experiencing menopause often complain of memory loss, and recent studies have found that this tends to be greatest among women who experience frequent hot flashes and/or night sweats. The cognitive issues are believed to be related to hormonal changes occurring in the brain. Speak with your doctor about hormonal and nonhormonal therapies that could help.

Pauline Maki, PhD, professor of psychiatry, psychology and obstetrics and gynecology at University of Illinois at Chicago.

The One-Week Plan to a Better Brain

Dean Sherzai, MD, PhD, and Ayesha Sherzai, MD, neurologists and codirectors of the Brain Health and Alzheimer's Prevention Program at Loma Linda University in California. They are authors of the brain-health book from Bottom Line Inc., The Alzheimer's Solution (BottomLineStore.com), and creators of a free brain-health app at BrainXQ.com. TeamSherzai.com

With researchers clamoring to unlock the mystery of what causes memory loss and related cognitive difficulties, it's easy to assume that some elusive discovery will banish these brain problems forever.

The truth is, the key to a better brain—sharper mental focus, improved memory, clearer thinking, balanced emotions and a lower risk for dementia and stroke—is largely within our control now.

Based on the body of research we have analyzed, nine out of 10 cases of Alzheimer's disease could be prevented by changes in lifestyle—what you do day by day…day after day—to improve the health of brain cells (neurons) and build more connections between them.

After 15 years of treating thousands of patients with Alzheimer's disease and its frequent precursor known as mild cognitive impairment (MCI), we've devised a simple one-week plan that will help you form habits to protect and enhance your brain in the weeks, months and years to come. *Better-brain lifestyle strategies to adopt…*

DAY #1: **Don't rely on supplements to protect your brain.** There are only two supplements we think are worth taking for brain health—an omega-3 supplement with at least 250 mg daily of docosahexaenoic acid (DHA), the most important omega-3 fatty acid for brain health...and 500 micrograms (mcg) daily of vitamin B-12, which is linked to reduced risk for Alzheimer's.*

Our recommendation: Opt for an algae-derived omega-3 supplement over fish oil —it is highly absorbable and toxin- and pollutant-free.

***DAY #2:* Add a "superstar" food to your diet.** A whole-food, plant-based diet reduces brain-damaging inflammation and oxidation...protects the small arteries of the brain that are damaged by saturated fats and cholesterol...supplies the brain with the nutrients and phytochemicals it needs for optimal functioning...and minimizes or eliminates refined carbohydrates and other processed foods—all of which weaken neurons and their connections.

Among plant foods, mushrooms are a surprising superstar. In fact, a study published in *Phytotherapy Research* found that older people with MCI had improved cognitive function after 16 weeks of taking dried mushroom powder. Plus, mushrooms deliver umami—the pleasant, savory taste found mainly in cooked meat, making them a great meat substitute.

Our recommendation: Include mushrooms in your meals at least two to three times a week—button mushrooms, portobello, cremini, porcini, maitake, shiitake, you name it.

If you aren't able to follow a strictly plant-based diet, a Mediterranean diet or MIND diet, which focuses on leafy greens, nuts, berries, beans, whole grains, and fish and poultry, is advised.

***DAY #3:* Choose the right fats.** More than 60% of the brain is comprised of fat, and the brain constantly uses those fats in the process of rebuilding neurons and their support structures. But for optimal brain health, you need to consume the right kind of fats—not saturated fat, for example, but plant-based fats,

*Before taking any supplement, check with your doctor if you have a medical condition or take medication.

such as the mono- and polyunsaturated fats found in nuts, seeds, avocados and olives.

Omega-3 fatty acids—found in nuts, seeds, marine algae and fish—are especially critical for brain health.

Note: We don't recommend fish because it often has high levels of mercury and other toxic chemicals that are bad for the brain. If you must eat fish, stick with small, low-mercury fish such as sardines and anchovies.

Our recommendation: As part of a plant-based diet, get plenty of good fats and limit bad fats. *To do this...*

•Minimize or eliminate sweets...processed junk food...sugary cereals...baked packaged goods...chips and other salty snacks...processed white bread products... meats, processed meats and poultry...and canned soups.

•Maximize fresh and frozen vegetables and fruits...beans and lentils...100% whole grains...seeds and nuts...brain-healthy oils, such as olive and avocado...low-calorie, plant-based sweeteners, such as date sugar and stevia...nondairy plant milks...and spices (turmeric is particularly brain protective at a dose of one teaspoon daily—consult your doctor before adding turmeric to your daily diet if you have a chronic condition, such as a gallbladder problem...or take medication, such as a diabetes drug).

***DAY #4:* Protect sleep.** During sleep, we "consolidate" memory—turning daily experience into long-term memories. Sleep also detoxifies the brain when "janitor" brain cells (microglia) are activated to remove toxins that accumulate during the day.

Our recommendation: Aim for seven to eight hours of sleep a night.

Avoid foods that are particularly disruptive to sleep, such as sugary foods, high-fat foods, and chocolate and other caffeine-containing foods. Stop eating at least three hours before going to sleep at night...and stop drinking fluids at least two hours before.

***DAY #5:* Increase your "klotho" with exercise.** Klotho is a little-known but important antiaging hormone linked in animal studies to protection against cognitive decline. Studies show that klotho levels increase after only 20 minutes of intense aerobic exercise. "Intense" means that you'll have difficulty finishing a sentence.

Our recommendation: Aim for 25 to 30 minutes of intense aerobic exercise, four to five days a week, such as brisk walking, biking or working out on a treadmill, an elliptical, a stair-climber or other type of cardio machine.**

***DAY #6:* Get rid of clutter—and clean out your brain.** Stress exhausts the brain. And a surprising source of stress is a cluttered environment—when our homes or offices become disorderly, we experience more stress and anxiety. A clean, orderly space encourages sustained quiet and self-reflection, both of which positively impact cognition.

Our recommendation: As part of a stress-reducing plan, keep your home and office clean and uncluttered.

***DAY #7:* Put on your dancing shoes.** Brain-protective cognitive reserve develops from any challenging mental activity, such as learning to play a musical instrument or mastering a new language. But one of the best and most enjoyable ways to build cognitive reserve is dancing. When you dance, it activates various parts of the brain such as your motor cortex…your parietal lobe…your frontal lobe…and your occipital lobe. Plus, dancing is a social activity—and research shows social interaction also builds cognitive reserve.

Our recommendation: Find a dance studio and take dance classes—and then go out dancing. Or buy a DVD and learn to dance at home. Ballroom, jazz, folk—the possibilities are endless!

**Speak to your primary care physician before starting this (or any new) exercise program.

Top 20 Brain-Nourishing Foods

Excerpted from *The Alzheimer's Solution* by Dean Sherzai, MD, PhD, and Ayesha Sherzai, MD, published by Bottom Line Books (BottomLineStore.com).

Here are the most brain-nourishing foods (listed in alphabetical order) you can consume, based on a variety of scientific studies.

Avocados: This fruit is packed with mono-unsaturated fats that support brain structure and blood flow.

Beans: Beans are high in antioxidants, phytonutrients, plant protein, iron and other minerals…and have been shown to increase longevity and reduce the risk for stroke (one of the most common neurodegenerative diseases that shares risk factors with dementia).

Blueberries: In a Harvard longitudinal study conducted on 16,000 nurses, the consumption of berries—especially blueberries and strawberries—was associated with a lower risk for cognitive decline. Specifically, the study suggested that regular consumption of berries delayed cognitive decline by two-and-a-half years.

Broccoli: This veggie is rich in lutein and zeaxanthin, carotenoid antioxidants that can cross the blood-brain barrier and reverse damage caused by free radicals and normal aging. A large study at Harvard Medical School of more than 13,000 women found that participants who ate more cruciferous vegetables such as broccoli had less age-related memory decline.

Coffee: The caffeine in coffee is an adenosine receptor antagonist, which stimulates the production of *acetylcholine*, a known neuroprotective agent in the brain. Coffee also contains potent antioxidants in the form of polyphenols (plant-derived antioxidants that fight free radicals) and chlorogenic acid.

Dark Chocolate: Dark, unprocessed cocoa or cacao nibs, the purest forms of chocolate, are incredible sources of flavanol phytonutrients that have been shown to relax arteries and help supply oxygen and nutrients to the brain. In fact, people who eat dark chocolate have a lower risk for stroke.

Extra-Virgin Olive Oil: In small amounts as a replacement for saturated fats, extra-virgin olive oil is an excellent source of monounsaturated fatty acids and polyphenols.

Flaxseed: It contains the highest amount of plant-based omega-3 fatty acids that have been shown to decrease inflammation and reduce LDL ("bad") cholesterol levels. Flax also contains lignans, chemical compounds that protect blood vessels from inflammatory damage.

Herbal Tea: Mint, lemon balm and hibiscus teas are the three most anti-inflammatory beverages available. Iced herbal tea (with added stevia or erythritol for sweetness) can easily replace sugary drinks in the summer.

Herbs: Fresh or dried herbs such as cilantro, dill, rosemary, thyme, oregano, basil, mint and parsley contain 10 times the antioxidants of nuts and berries. Even a small amount boosts your daily antioxidant consumption.

Leafy Greens: Leafy greens are a rich source of polyphenols, folic acid, lutein, vitamin E and beta-carotene—all nutrients that are associated with brain health.

Mushrooms: Whether they're fresh, dried or powdered, mushrooms improve overall immunity and reduce inflammation in the blood vessels of the brain. Cremini mushrooms are an excellent plant source of vitamin B-12, which is linked to a lowered risk for Alzheimer's disease.

Nuts: Nuts provide the highest source of healthy unsaturated fats, which have been shown to reduce the risk for Alzheimer's in multiple studies.

Omega-3 Fatty Acids (derived from algae): High-powered, plant-based omega-3s reduce inflammation and boost the immune system.

Quinoa: One of the most nutrient-rich foods, quinoa is the only grain that's a complete protein source (most grains lack the amino acids leucine and isoleucine). It also contains ample fiber, vitamin E and minerals such as zinc, phosphorus and selenium—all essential building blocks for brain cells and their supporting structures.

Seeds (Chia, Sunflower): Seeds are high in vitamin E and other brain-boosting minerals.

Spices: Spices contain the highest amounts of antioxidants per ounce compared with any other food and are excellent at supporting the brain's innate detox systems. Both spices and herbs such as cinnamon, cloves, marjoram, allspice, saffron, nutmeg, tarragon and others should be a regular part of our diet…not just a once-in-a-while addition. Curcumin, an extract of turmeric, is an antioxidant, anti-inflammatory and antiamyloid powerhouse. In studies of both animals and humans, curcumin has been shown to have a direct effect in reducing beta-amyloid.

Sweet Potatoes: Packed with phytonutrients, fiber, vitamins A and C, and minerals, this tuber actually has the ability to regulate blood sugar. Its anti-inflammatory effects have also been documented in numerous studies.

Tea: Green tea contains green tea catechin, another polyphenol that activates toxin-clearing enzymes.

Whole Grains: Whole grains are packed with cholesterol-lowering fiber, complex carbohydrates, protein and B vitamins. The starch in whole grains such as oats, buckwheat, millet, teff, sorghum and amaranth is the most beneficial type of complex carbohydrate—it both feeds good bacteria in the gut and provides an excellent source of sustained energy for the brain.

Just Thinking About Coffee Can Boost the Brain

People who regularly drink coffee get some of the same effects of being alert, awake and attentive when they simply think about drinking it.

Sam Maglio, PhD, associate professor of management, University of Toronto, Canada, and coauthor of a study published in *Consciousness and Cognition.*

Omega-3 for the Brain

Take an omega-3 supplement to boost B-vitamins' brain benefits.

Background: People with high blood levels of the amino acid homocysteine are at increased risk for Alzheimer's disease.

An underreported finding: In the VITA-COG study, people who took homocysteine-lowering B vitamins (B-12, folate and B-6) for two years had less brain atrophy and slower cognitive decline—but only if they had adequate blood levels of omega-3.

If you're concerned about cognitive decline and have elevated homocysteine: Ask your doctor about taking an omega-3 supplement along with a B-complex.

Richard Podell, MD, MPH, clinical professor, Rutgers Robert Wood Johnson Medical School, New Brunswick, New Jersey.

How Personality Affects Dementia Risk

People who were calm and mature as teens have lower dementia risk later in life. A study of personality tests taken by high schoolers in 1960 and their Medicare records from 50 years later revealed that teens who described themselves as calm or mature as opposed to reckless were less likely to have dementia.

What may help: Develop traits like conscientiousness starting today, especially by managing stress.

Benjamin Chapman, PhD, MPH, associate professor in the departments of psychiatry and public health sciences at University of Rochester Medical Center and lead author of the study published in *JAMA Psychiatry.*

A New Early Symptom of Alzheimer's Disease?

Daniel Z. Press, MD, associate professor of neurology at Harvard Medical School, and a specialist in cognitive neurology at Beth Israel Deaconess Medical Center, both in Boston. His research has been published in *Neurology, Journal of Alzheimer's Disease* and other leading medical journals.

Even though a seizure can be caused by conditions ranging from drug or alcohol withdrawal to stroke, most people associate this surge of electrical activity in the brain with epilepsy.

Now: An increasing body of scientific evidence links seizure activity to Alzheimer's disease. This area of research is so important that it was a major focus of the 2019 Alzheimer's Association International Conference (AAIC) in Los Angeles.

With estimates showing that up to 16 million Americans will be diagnosed with Alzheimer's disease by 2050—and still no cure or effective therapy to slow it down—researchers hope that early treatment of seizure activity may offer a new way to stop the progression of this relentless disease.

What you need to know…

A Different Type of Seizure

Seizures occur in about 10% to 22% of people with Alzheimer's, according to research published in *JAMA Neurology*. These seizures are often less dramatic than commonly known seizures that involve erratic movements and loss of consciousness (see next page).

In Alzheimer's patients who have seizures, their symptoms, including the classic loss of memory and other mental abilities, known as cognitive impairment, are typically more severe.

Cognitive impairment also may occur about five to seven years earlier in these people than in those with Alzheimer's and no seizures. In individuals with early-onset Alzheimer's, for example, which can begin in one's 50s, the likelihood of having seizures is more than 25%.

At the AAIC, research was presented showing that seizures can occur even before other cognitive impairment symptoms are noticeable. For example, a study of close to 300,000 US veterans found that vets over age 55 who had a first seizure had twice the risk of developing Alzheimer's disease within nine years. This research had not been published at the time that it was presented at the AAIC.

Other studies presented at the conference found that…

• **Alzheimer's patients are over six times more likely to have seizures than older adults without Alzheimer's.**

• **Alzheimer's seizures are more likely to be recurrent.** Two-thirds of patients have a second seizure within eight months.

• **The longer a person has Alzheimer's disease, the higher the risk for seizures.**

A Trigger or a Symptom?

Even though the most recent research suggests that seizures can occur before Alzheimer's disease symptoms become apparent, it's not clear whether the seizure is a trigger, a symptom or a risk factor for a more accelerated form of Alzheimer's. It is known, however, that the accumulation of abnormal proteins called amyloid plaques and tau tangles in the brains of people with Alzheimer's destroy brain cells—and loss of brain cells can lead to abnormal brain activity and seizures.

Interestingly, even before seizures develop, 42% of people with Alzheimer's disease (some of whom did not have apparent memory problems) had abnormal brain waves detectable on an electroencephalogram (EEG), known as subclinical epileptic activity, versus 10% of study participants without Alzheimer's, according to research published in *Annals of Neurology*.

As scientists try to sort out the role that seizures play in people with Alzheimer's, the best explanation for now is that the abnormal brain waves of preclinical epilepsy are an early result of Alzheimer's disease. These changes can lead to seizures that cause more damage and speed up the progression of Alzheimer's. As Alzheimer's worsens, it can lead to more seizures…and more damage—in short, a vicious cycle.

What Should You Do?

If you or a loved one has early-stage Alzheimer's—or a diagnosis of mild cognitive impairment (which may become Alzheimer's)—be on the lookout for any seizure activity. These seizures, especially the early ones, may not be the classic grand mal type of epileptic seizure, usually marked by a fall, loss of consciousness and uncontrollable muscle jerking.

Instead, it may be a type of seizure called a partial seizure, which is easy to miss. This type of seizure may be just a brief period (a few minutes) of staring off into space…being confused or unresponsive…fumbling…stumbling…or losing the ability to speak.

Any such behavior should be reported to your primary care physician. An EEG may show abnormal brain waves that indicate seizure activity. If this is the case, a neurologist can be consulted, and antiseizure medication may be prescribed.

Important: Because there are many causes of seizures, any type of seizure activity in an older adult (with or without Alzheimer's) needs to be evaluated. Don't assume that a seizure in an older person means a future diagnosis of Alzheimer's disease.

Currently, there is no evidence that treating a new seizure in a person without Alzheimer's will stop the disease from developing. However, researchers say that any patient with Alzheimer's who has a seizure should be treated, since seizures may make the disease worse.

Promising treatment: A study led by researchers at Beth Israel Deaconess Medical Center (BIDMC) in Boston and published in *Journal of Alzheimer's Disease* found that brain wave activity returned to a more normal pattern in early-stage Alzheimer's patients with subclinical epileptic activity who received a single dose of the antiseizure drug *levetiracetam* (Keppra). Their cognitive function did not improve, but this was not expected after a single treatment.

The BIDMC researchers have received funding from the National Institutes of Health to conduct a larger and longer study in which they hope to find that treating preclinical epilepsy will not only restore normal brain waves but improve or delay cognitive decline. In past studies, levetiracetam and another antiseizure drug, *lamotrigine* (Lamictal), were found to be more effective at controlling Alzheimer's seizures than *phenytoin* (Dilantin) and other older antiepileptic drugs.

Bottom line: Any seizure in a person with Alzheimer's disease should be recognized and treated. Future studies should tell us if treating seizure activity can alter the course of Alzheimer's—something that would be a big breakthrough for this baffling disease. Levetiracetam is currently the best established therapy for seizures in people with Alzheimer's disease.

Alzheimer's Alert: Difficulty Detecting Scams

Susceptibility to scams may be an early sign of Alzheimer's disease and cognitive impairment. Scam awareness taps into a number of complex behaviors such as the ability to detect fraud, evaluate an offer and manage emotions under pressure. Seniors who have difficulty detecting scams should consider a clinical assessment for Alzheimer's and cognitive impairment, particularly if other changes, such as difficulty managing finances, are present.

Patricia A. Boyle, PhD, neuropsychologist, associate professor of behavioral sciences at the Rush Alzheimer's Disease Center, Rush University Medical Center, Chicago, and lead author of a study published in *Annals of Internal Medicine.*

Tests Rule Out Alzheimer's

When 749 women and men, ages 70 to 83, with mild cognitive impairment (MCI) took a test that measures cognition and a test that assesses the ability to identify odors, nearly all (96.5%) who performed well on both tests did not develop dementia over the next four years.

Implication: These assessments, typically used to predict dementia risk, could help older adults with MCI avoid further invasive and expensive diagnostic tests.

D.P. Devanand, MD, professor of psychiatry and neurology, Columbia University Vagelos College of Physicians and Surgeons, New York City.

Beware of Popular Drugs Linked to Dementia

Malaz Boustani, MD, MPH, Richard M. Fairbanks Professor of Aging Research at Indiana University School of Medicine in Indianapolis and research scientist at the Regenstrief Institute, Regenstrief.org, an Indianapolis-based research organization that focuses on informatics and health-care research. Dr. Boustani created and validated the Anticholinergic Cognitive Burden (ACB) Scale.

If there were more than 50 prescription and over-the-counter (OTC) medications that had been linked to an increased risk for Alzheimer's disease and other related dementias, you'd think that everyone would avoid those drugs—especially when safer alternatives are often available. But that's not happening.

Sobering new finding: When medications known as anticholinergics are taken for three or more years, previous research has linked them to about a 50% higher risk for dementia, but a new finding shows that these medications are still being widely used to treat conditions ranging from the common cold, allergies and incontinence to Parkinson's disease, motion sickness and muscle pain. *To protect yourself and your loved ones…*

What Are Anticholinergics?

More than 10 million Americans, age 65 and older, use anticholinergic drugs. The medications block the action of acetylcholine, a neurotransmitter (brain chemical) that activates many key body functions involving muscles, the heart, digestive system, lungs, urinary tract and blood vessels. These drugs, which include medications from various drug classes, also have effects on the brain and are used to treat dizziness, nausea, epilepsy and depression.

Well-documented side effects from these drugs include dry mouth and constipation. Because these medications also affect the brain, they can cause confusion and memory loss. Older adults are at highest risk for dementia from these drugs because they tend to take more of them than younger adults. Older adults also are at increased risk for dementia due to their age—in part, because acetylcholine production declines as people grow older.

New Study Sounds the Alarm

In the study mentioned earlier, which was published in *JAMA Internal Medicine*, the medical records of about 225,000 patients (ages 55 to 100) who had not been diagnosed with dementia were compared with those of about 60,000 dementia patients to see how many in each group had taken a prescription-strength anticholinergic drug during an 11-year period.

The researchers found that 57% of the dementia patients and 51% of the non-dementia patients had been prescribed at least one of the 56 anticholinergic drugs included in the study. The most commonly used drugs were prescribed to treat depression, dizziness, nausea, vomiting and bladder spasms. *Other key findings…*

•**Greater exposure, bigger risk.** Patients who took an anticholinergic on a daily basis for three years had a 49% higher risk of being diagnosed with dementia than patients with no exposure. Those who took one of the drugs for less than three months had a 6% increased risk.

•**Some drugs are riskier than others.** The highest-risk anticholinergics included antipsychotics, such as *olanzapine* (Zyprexa) or *quetiapine* (Seroquel)…overactive bladder medications, including *tolterodine* (Detrol) and *oxybutynin* (Ditropan)…antiparkinsonian drugs, such as *benztropine* (Cogentin)…antiepileptics, including *carbamazepine* (Tegretol) and *oxcarbazepine* (Trileptal)…and antidepressants, such as *amitriptyline* (Elavil) and *paroxetine* (Paxil).

Even though these findings are observational (that is, they do not prove cause and effect), they are consistent with earlier research. For this reason, the researchers recommend that doctors carefully weigh the risks and benefits of prescribing these drugs for patients who are middle-aged and older and strongly urge the use of other effective drugs, that are not anticholinergics, whenever possible.

What Should You Do?

To avoid the potential harms of anticholinergics, you should know which medications have been linked to the greatest dementia risk.

To get a clearer picture of the risk associated with the most widely used anticholinergic drugs on the market, consult the Anticholinergic Cognitive Burden (ACB) Scale (go to BottomLineInc.com/health/dementia/beware-of-popular-drugs-linked-to-dementia), which ranks both prescription and OTC anticholinergic drugs, according to their degree of risk.

If you are taking a prescription drug that appears on the list, talk to your doctor. Ask if you can stop taking the drug…or if there is a suitable substitute that is safer for you. For example, if you are taking an antidepressant on the ACB Scale, *sertraline* (Zoloft) or *citalopram* (Celexa) may be a safer choice, since each has minimal anticholinergic effects.

Caution: Never stop taking a medication that your doctor has prescribed without consulting him/her.

It's also worth noting that many OTC anticholinergics are considered high risk. Among the most widely used are the antihistamines *diphenhydramine* (Benadryl) and *chlorpheniramine* (Chlor-Trimeton)... the cold and allergy medicine *brompheniramine-PPA* (Dimetapp)...and the motion-sickness drug *dimenhydrinate* (Dramamine).

If you take an OTC anticholinergic frequently (one pill for 60 days in a 12-month period), ask your doctor or pharmacist if you really need it. You can also ask if there is a substitute drug that is not an anticholinergic.

Important: Dementia risk linked to these drugs is added to any other risk factors you may have, such as older age...high blood pressure...diabetes...inactivity...a family history of dementia...and smoking. For this reason, your entire risk profile should be considered when discussing the use of these drugs with your doctor.

Extra Weight Could Contribute to Your Brain Aging

Having a higher body mass index (BMI) and wider girth was associated with thinning of the cerebral cortex—a region shown to be associated with cognition—and increased problems with memory and thinking in older adults. The chronic inflammation of obesity could be the connection.

Michelle R. Caunca, PhD, a medical student at the Medical Scientist Training Program at University of Miami Miller School of Medicine and lead author of a study of 1,289 people in their 60s, published in *Neurology.*

Don't Ignore This Overlooked Symptom of Dementia

Nearly half of people with dementia suffer from apathy (a lack of feeling, interest or enthusiasm), according to research involving 4,320 people with Alzheimer's disease. Apathy is often overlooked because it causes less drama than other symptoms, such as wandering or aggression, but should be addressed because it is linked to accelerated cognitive decline and a higher mortality rate. Social interaction and exercise have been shown to help.

Clive Ballard, MD, executive dean of medicine, University of Exeter, UK.

Dementia May Be Linked to Marital Status

Married people are less likely to develop dementia as they age—and divorced people are twice as likely as others to develop the condition. Divorced men are at even greater risk than divorced women.

Hui Liu, PhD, professor of sociology, Michigan State University, East Lansing, and leader of an analysis of more than 15,000 people, published in *Journals of Gerontology: Series B.*

Dementia Affects Vision, Too

Teepa Snow, OTR/L, FAOTA, an occupational therapist and dementia-care educator who works with caregivers and professionals worldwide through her company, Positive Approach to Care, based in Efland, North Carolina.

When a loved one has Alzheimer's disease or another form of dementia, you expect changes in memory and thinking.

But did you know that the brain changes that accompany dementia, combined with aging, can literally change how people see the world?

Four vision changes seen in people with Alzheimer's and other forms of dementia—and how to help them...

•**Poor depth perception.** People with dementia can lose the ability to perceive dimension and see the world in all its 3-D glory. That can affect their ability to judge distances. They might not perceive, for example, that a fan spinning six feet above their heads is too far away to turn off by hand.

Or a picture of an apple may be mistaken for a real one. That can lead to behaviors that caregivers mistake for signs of hallucinations—such as reaching for that fan or trying to take a bite of that apple. It also can lead to accidents, especially with stairs or curbs.

How you can help: You don't have to correct every misperception. In fact, you can build trust by going along with the harmless ones. Let your loved one enjoy the puppies on that YouTube video he/she keeps watching, even if he thinks they are in his yard. But eliminate or lessen hazards, like that ceramic apple he might bite or the bottom step he might miss.

Helpful: Mark the edge of the top and bottom steps with bright tape. Avoid a dark throw rug on a light background—it can look like a hole or step down.

•**A shrinking field of vision.** As we age, everyone loses some ability to see things off to the side, over and under our point of focus. For many people with dementia, this loss of peripheral vision is accelerated and can be severe. In fact, someone with dementia can have a field of vision that is only 12 to 18 inches across, as it takes all the person's ability to take in that amount of visual data and try to figure it out.

How you can help: When approaching a person with dementia, do so from the front—and, if possible, catch his gaze. Put important things, such as food and drinks, right in front of your loved one. Offer guidance in situations where a person with dementia might not see what's obvious to you, such as a handrail on the stairs.

•**Poor color and contrast perception.** A loss of ability to distinguish color and contrast can happen in the earlier stages of dementia, leaving someone unable to tell colored pills apart or respond quickly to traffic signals, especially at sunrise or sunset, when it is dimmer. People with dementia also can have trouble making out objects with inadequate color contrast—an all-white bathroom, for example, can be a nightmare to navigate.

How you can help: Put a colored seat on the white toilet. Make sure food items stand out from the plate—for example, mashed potatoes on a white plate will get lost. One study found that presenting food on a red plate resulted in greater intake for people living with dementia.

•**Need for brighter light.** To see well, people in their 60s need light three times brighter than what's needed by those in their 20s. Someone dealing with vision challenges linked to dementia can have even greater trouble than a similarly aged healthy person in a dim environment.

How you can help: Provide bright light (over 100 watts, in general), but be careful to choose bulbs and fixtures that keep the lighting diffuse—no exposed bulbs or lights that will shine directly into eyes. Use "full-spectrum" bulbs that mimic sunlight. That will help people stay alert and on task.

Important: Vision changes are a primary and early symptom of some types of dementia. In one rare type, called posterior cortical atrophy, people may have little memory loss but serious difficulties with vision, including trouble identifying common objects such as the handle versus the blade of a knife. Vision changes and visual hallucinations also are common early-stage symptoms of a condition known as Lewy body dementia. For these reasons, you should always report changes in vision to your health-care providers.

Brain Games: Have Fun While Keeping Your Memory Sharp

Cynthia R. Green, PhD, a psychologist and assistant clinical professor in the department of psychiatry at Icahn School of Medicine at Mount Sinai in New York City. Dr. Green is president and founder of Total Brain Health and CEO of TBH Brands LLC, which offers Total Brain Health programs to groups and individuals. She also is author or coauthor of five books on memory and brain health, including *Your Best Brain Ever*. TotalBrainHealth.com

Solitary pursuits such as crossword puzzles, Sudoku or even online and app-based games can help you stay mentally sharp, but there's something special about joining friends or family for a fun board, card or tile game.

These real-time, in-person gatherings ratchet up the brain-boosting effects. And regularly engaging in such games and other intellectually stimulating pursuits has been linked to lower rates of dementia. Chess, checkers, bridge and Scrabble are all good contenders—there's no strong research showing that one nonsolitary game is better than another. *But to try something different, consider…*

Mahjong

The game that originated centuries ago in China and caught on in the US in the 1920s is enjoying a new wave of popularity here. This four-person game is played with domino-style tiles. Rules can vary, but the most common American version is played much like the card game rummy.

What you do: Players are dealt a set of tiles—including "suits" decorated with dots, bamboo and Chinese characters—and have chances to discard and pick up tiles, with the aim of collecting sets and pairs. The first player to collect a winning hand calls out "Mahjong" and wins the game. A game typically consists of four rounds of about 45 minutes each. A mahjong set can cost less than $50 to more than $100. *When you play mahjong, the mental muscles you exercise include…*

- **Attention skills.** You need to keep track of your own tiles (typically, 13 to 14) and what the other players are doing.
- **Short-term memory.** As you play, you must keep in mind not only the tiles you have in front of you but also the ones you need.
- **Planning and strategizing.** Each time you hold or discard a tile, you weigh its future value in creating sets and pairs.
- **Mental flexibility.** You need to adjust your strategy as the game progresses.
- **Long-term memory.** If you are a veteran player, you draw on strategies that worked for you in the past.

SET

The card game SET, which was designed by a research scientist, isn't widely known, but it will give your brain a good workout. You can buy this game online for less than $10.

SET consists of a deck of 81 cards, each of which displays four features—a color, number, pattern and shape. Each feature comes in three variations. So, a card can be red, green or purple…with one, two or three objects… with shaded, unshaded or striped patterns… and with diamond, oval or squiggle shapes.

What you do: You lay out 12 cards at a time and race other players to find groups of three cards that make a "set." A set consists of three cards, each having one feature (color, number, pattern or shape) that's either all the same or all different. At the end, the player with the most sets wins.

The concept can be tricky to grasp, but you will get better with practice—a sign that your brain is carving out new neural pathways. *SET works your…*

- **Attention skills.** To identify "sets," you must be attentive to the distinguishing features and variations on each card.
- **Flexible thinking.** Because there are multiple features (color, number, pattern and shape) and variations on each card, your thinking must be nimble enough to move back and forth from one feature and variation to the next.

• **Visual perception skills.** These skills help you identify the features and variations on each card.

• **Processing speed.** The time pressure involved in this game helps build faster mental-processing capacities.

Bonus: SET is a great game to play with kids and groups of varying sizes. You can play solo, too, but the biggest brain boost occurs when you play against others!

Inflammation and the Brain

Inflammation makes the brain less alert. This is the sluggishness or brain fog that many people report when they are ill or dealing with a chronic condition. Inflammation—the body's response to illness—affects the part of the brain responsible for reaching and maintaining a state of alertness. Inflammation also may have an impact on other brain areas, such as those responsible for memory. More study could show that it is possible for anti-inflammatory drugs to improve or preserve cognitive function in some people with chronic conditions such as obesity, kidney disease and Alzheimer's.

Ali Mazaheri, PhD, principal investigator, Centre for Human Brain Health, University of Birmingham, UK, and senior coauthor of a study published in *NeuroImage*.

To Improve Your Memory, Declutter Your Brain

Maureen K. O'Connor, PsyD, assistant professor of neurology at Boston University and director of neuropsychology at Bedford Veterans Affairs Medical Center. She is coauthor, with Andrew E. Budson, MD, of *Seven Steps to Managing Your Memory: What's Normal, What's Not, and What to Do About It.*

If you have always prided yourself on having an excellent memory, chances are you don't make a shopping list or put that weekend dinner with a friend on a calendar. You simply point to your forehead and say, "It's all in here."

Even though this might feel like a good way to continually test your memory, you're likely missing out on more than just an occasional forgotten quart of milk.

People who don't use simple memory aids—everything from handwritten lists to new-fangled phone apps—forgo a key strategy that's embraced by most highly accomplished people. You also are "cluttering" that wonderful brain of yours with a lot of stuff that could be kept elsewhere.

Some people are reluctant to use lists, schedules, alarms and other aids because they think it will make their brains lazy. But that's not true! Using memory aids can, in fact, help reduce the stress and annoyance that inevitably come from age-related memory errors.

Memory aids also can help you establish lifelong habits that will make a big difference when you experience those normal age-related memory lapses, such as losing things from time to time or sometimes forgetting which word to use.

These changes happen to everyone—including people who never develop Alzheimer's disease or other serious memory disorders. What's interesting, though, is that people who use memory aids handle those little memory glitches more easily.

6 Top Memory Aids

Memory aids to choose from…

• **Keep a notebook.** Get a small notebook that you can slip into a pocket or carry in a handbag to jot down grocery lists…questions for your doctor or accountant…and information you get at an appointment or meeting.

Smart strategy: Use a note-taking app on your smartphone.

• **Rely on technology.** In addition to apps, smartphones have built-in features that are easy to use and do wonders to support your memory.

Smart strategy: If you're out running errands and remember something you need to do the minute you get home, call your landline from your cell phone and leave yourself a message. If you use the calendar on your smartphone, ask for alerts a day, an hour or a few minutes before an appointment or phone call.

You can use your phone's alarm feature or timer to remind you to check the cookies in the oven or the wet laundry in the washer. You can even label the alarms you set as "meeting" or customize them for specific tasks (such as "take out neighbor's garbage can").

Also helpful: Your phone's camera is a memory aid, too—use it to take a picture of the street sign near your parking space before walking away from your car.

● **Create a memory table (or bowl or basket).** This is where you toss your keys when you walk in the door—and find them when you go out again. It's also a good spot for the bills you want to mail in the morning and the book you want to return to your neighbor.

Smart strategy: Put a memory table, bowl or basket near the door you use to leave and enter the house. Some people like to pair it with a hook for their keys and a wastebasket for incoming promotional mail.

Important: It will defeat the purpose if you allow this area to become cluttered—it should be a temporary landing spot for a few small essential items.

Also helpful: If you have room, the space above your memory table or basket is ideal for a whiteboard or chalkboard, where you can leave messages for other household members—or for yourself. ("Take out the trash today!")

● **Use a "workhorse calendar."** Some people love an old-fashioned wall calendar with big squares for writing details. Others never use anything but the calendar on their phones. Still others like to blend paper and portability with a planner they tote everywhere. Any of these choices is fine, though a digital calendar has some advantages, including the ability to share your schedule with others and get pop-up reminders before events.

Smart strategy: Use a calendar of your choice—but make sure it's kept in a place you can easily access every day. Wherever your calendar is, make it a workhorse. When you add an appointment, be sure to include When, Who and Where (including, if needed, an address), along with What—what is the appointment for and what do you need to bring? And add a phone number—you will thank yourself if you end up running late or have to cancel at the last minute. Check your calendar every morning and evening.

● **Get a pillbox.** People have all sorts of systems for keeping track of medications, but nothing beats a pillbox. The basic version has a compartment for each day's medications (and/or supplements) and holds enough for one to four weeks. You also can get compartments for morning and evening meds or meds taken three times a day. These are all available online or at your local drugstore, often for less than $10.

Fancier versions have built-in alarms to remind you that it's time to take pills and sensors that link to apps you can set to communicate with others—if, for instance, you want a family member to know you are on track with your pills. You can even get box-

---

Two Simple Practices May Reduce Memory Loss

Memory and cognitive performance improved in 60 men and women with subjective cognitive decline (a strong predictor of Alzheimer's disease) after they practiced a beginner chanting meditation or listened to classical music for 12 minutes a day for 12 weeks, and then as often as they wanted for an additional three months. The gains remained or even increased at six months.

Theory: These practices promote memory and cognition by reducing stress and improving sleep.

Kim Innes, PhD, professor of epidemiology, West Virginia University School of Public Health, Morgantown.

es with vibrating alarms or braille lettering for people with hearing problems or vision challenges.

Smart strategy: Once you have a pillbox, pick a regular refilling day and time (add it to your calendar!)…and put your box where you will see it at medication time.

• **Use sticky notes.** The beauty of these little slips of paper is that you can put them anywhere and move them as needed.

Smart strategy: Whenever you have an errand to run or a task that needs to be done on a certain day, place a sticky note in a visible spot as a reminder. If the sticky note doesn't attach to the surface you're using, tape it to the door (or the handle of your bag) so that you'll see it when you're leaving your house.

The Golden Rules

To get the greatest benefit from memory aids, follow these rules…

RULE #1: **Don't delay.** When you make an appointment, write or type it into your calendar immediately. When the alarm goes off, go get the laundry, take your pill or make your call.

RULE #2: **Keep it simple.** Have one calendar, not four.

RULE #3: **Make it routine**. When you use your memory aids all the time, they become automatic and easier to use—even when you get tired, distracted or rushed.

Can You Still Do Basic Math in Your Head?

Dharma Singh Khalsa, MD, founder, Alzheimer's Research & Prevention Foundation, Tucson, Arizona, and author of *Brain Longevity*.

As we age, the brain naturally takes a bit longer to make decisions or complete basic calculations. However, oth-er factors can contribute to mental slowdown as well.

For example, some chronic health conditions, such as high blood pressure and diabetes, slow blood flow to the brain. Anticholinergic drugs, commonly used to treat allergies and many other conditions, slow brain activity as well—as can proton pump inhibitors (PPIs), used to treat heartburn. If you take one of these drugs, your doctor may be able to change your treatment.

Note: Never stop taking a prescribed drug without consulting with your doctor.

In some people, slowed thinking can signal the very early stages of memory loss that may lead to mild cognitive impairment (MCI) and then possibly dementia. But living a brain-healthy lifestyle may reduce risk for progression.

My advice: Visit your doctor, and start to incorporate the Four Pillars of Alzheimer's Prevention into your life…

#1. Healthy Diet. Cut down on saturated fats, such as those in red meat, and instead eat foods high in omega-3s, like salmon and nuts. Also, eat lots of vegetables and fruit.

#2. Exercise. A brisk 30-minute walk on most days of the week increases blood flow to the brain. Strength training has also been shown to enhance cognition.

#3. Yoga and Meditation. Research shows that a daily, 12-minute yoga/meditation technique called Kirtan Kriya (KK) offers significant brain-boosting benefits. Learn how to do KK at AlzheimersPrevention.org/research/kirtan-kriya-yoga-exercise.

#4. Spiritual Fitness. Staying connected to your spiritual side is also important for brain health. Volunteering, being close to loved ones and/or prayer all help develop spiritual fitness.

Eat This Way to Power Up Your Brain

All recipes excerpted from *The Whole Brain: The Microbiome Solution to Heal Depression, Anxiety, and Mental Fog without Prescription Drugs* by Raphael Kellman, MD. Copyright © 2017.

The same old superfoods aren't enough to keep your brain firing on all cylinders.

To really stay sharp, you need to consume a diet that also feeds other key support systems of your brain—your gut and microbiome, the community of bacteria that populate your digestive tract.

For a day's worth of brain-boosting meals, try the recipes below—excerpted from *The Whole Brain* by Raphael Kellman, MD...

Sample Breakfast:

Quinoa with Pear, Blueberries and Almonds

This energizing hot breakfast contains plenty of fiber to nourish your microbiome, as well as healthy fats to heal your gut wall and feed your brain. Cinnamon balances your blood sugar and reduces inflammation. Makes one serving.

Ingredients:
1 teaspoon clarified pasture-raised butter or ghee
½ cup quinoa, rinsed and drained
1 cup water
1 Tablespoon coconut oil
½ cinnamon stick
⅛ teaspoon freshly grated nutmeg
½ teaspoon peeled and grated fresh ginger
¼ cup coconut milk
½ cup ripe pear, cored and diced into large pieces
Salt
1 teaspoon chopped raw almonds
½ cup blueberries
Pinch of ground cinnamon

Directions:
1. Place the butter, quinoa, water, coconut oil, cinnamon stick, nutmeg and ginger in a small saucepan and stir. Bring to a boil.
2. Lower the heat, and simmer for 10 minutes.
3. Stir in the coconut milk and pear, and simmer for five minutes.
4. Add salt to taste, and sprinkle with the almonds, blueberries and ground cinnamon.

Sample Snack:

Caribbean-spiced Garbanzos

A zesty, addictive snack! Leftover spices can be used for other snacks or as a rub for fish, meat and poultry. The garbanzos are a terrific high-fiber source of protein that your microbiome will love, and turmeric and cinnamon help reduce inflammation, which your brain loves, too. Makes three servings.

Ingredients:
1 teaspoon curry powder
1 teaspoon ground cumin
¼ teaspoon ground turmeric
1 teaspoon ground allspice
¼ teaspoon freshly grated nutmeg

Multitasking Undermines Memory

People who multitask regularly have more difficulty with tasks requiring working memory and sustained attention than people who multitask only minimally. Multitasking apparently leads to attention lapses that, over time, make it more difficult for any single task to sustain a person's attention.

Self-defense: Block out your daily calendar with times in which you will give full attention to a single task. During those times, close all windows on your computer except any needed for that one task...put your phone on silent or airplane mode...remove any other distractions.

Anthony Wagner, PhD, chair, department of psychology, Stanford University, Stanford, California, and coauthor of a study published in *Proceedings of the National Academy of Sciences.*

⅛ teaspoon ground cloves

½ teaspoon ground cinnamon

1 teaspoon ground coriander

½ teaspoon chili powder

¼ teaspoon cayenne pepper

2 (16-ounce) cans organic garbanzos, drained and rinsed

1½ Tablespoons olive oil

2 teaspoons coarse salt

Salt and freshly ground black pepper

Directions:

1. Preheat the oven to 375°F.

2. Combine all the spices in a small bowl.

3. Combine the garbanzos with the oil in a medium-sized bowl. Add two teaspoons of the spice mixture and the coarse salt. The leftover spices will keep well for another batch or as a rub for fish, meat or poultry.

4. Spread the garbanzos on an ungreased baking sheet or shallow roasting pan. Bake until golden and crisp, about 30 to 40 minutes. Remove from the oven and let cool to room temperature. Season with salt and pepper to taste. Store in an airtight container. If the garbanzos get soggy, rebake until crisp.

Sample Lunch:

Frittata of Swiss Chard, Mushrooms, Asparagus and Onion

This Italian egg dish makes a delicious hot lunch or an invigorating breakfast. Although most frittatas include some form of dairy, coconut milk is substituted here for cow's milk, as well as a little sheep's-milk cheese (Pecorino Romano), which is easier for most people to digest than cow's-milk products. Your brain will love the healthy fat! Makes two servings. Serve with a leafy green salad.

Ingredients:

6 large organic eggs, at room temperature

2 Tablespoons coconut milk

1 teaspoon chopped fresh tarragon

½ teaspoon fresh thyme leaves

¼ cup grated Pecorino Romano

½ teaspoon salt, plus more to taste

½ teaspoon freshly ground black pepper, plus more to taste

2 Tablespoons olive oil

1 cup roughly chopped onion

1 cup sliced mushrooms

8 thin asparagus stalks, cut into one-inch pieces

½ pound Swiss chard, washed and torn into one-inch-wide pieces

Directions:

1. Preheat the oven to 475°F.

2. Beat the eggs with the coconut milk in a bowl, and add the herbs, two tablespoons of the cheese and the salt and pepper.

3. Heat the oil in an eight-inch heavy-bottomed, ovenproof skillet over medium heat, and sauté the onion until just translucent, about five minutes. Add the mushrooms and asparagus, and sauté until tender. Add the Swiss chard, and cook until wilted.

4. Spread the vegetables evenly in the skillet, and season with additional salt and pepper to taste. Increase the heat, and when the skillet is very hot, pour in the eggs and cook until they begin to set.

5. Sprinkle with the remaining cheese, and place the skillet in the oven.

6. Bake for five minutes, or until the frittata is firm but not browned.

Sample Dinner:

Seared Fish Fillet with Parsley Caper Sauce

For this dish, use a low-mercury fish, such as haddock, cod, tilapia or salmon. Although the recipe calls for seven ounces, you can increase the fish to 12 ounces and use the extra in a salad for another meal. The sauce is delicious with any seared or grilled fish and vegetables. The fish has thyroid-friendly iodine, brain-friendly fats and a delicious tangy taste from the parsley caper sauce. Serve with Swiss chard and green beans. Makes one serving.

Ingredients for the parsley caper sauce:

2 teaspoons white vinegar

½ teaspoon Dijon mustard

¾ cup fresh parsley leaves

1 heaping Tablespoon fresh basil leaves

2 Tablespoons small capers

¼ cup garlic-infused olive oil

¼ cup olive oil

2 canned anchovy fillets (optional)

Ingredients for the seared fish:

7 ounces fresh fish fillet, about one-inch thick

¼ teaspoon salt

¼ teaspoon freshly ground black pepper

1 teaspoon olive oil

1 teaspoon unsalted butter

Wilted Swiss chard (optional side dish)

Sautéed green beans (optional side dish)

Directions:

1. To prepare the parsley caper sauce, combine the vinegar and mustard in a food processor.

2. Add the herbs and capers, and process until they are roughly chopped.

3. Slowly add the garlic-infused olive oil, olive oil and anchovy fillets, if using. Process until the sauce is very smooth.

4. To prepare the fish, sprinkle the salt and pepper on both sides of the fish.

5. Heat the olive oil in an eight-inch nonstick or cast-iron pan over high heat.

6. If the fillet has skin, place it, skin-side down, in the skillet, and press down for about 30 seconds as it begins to cook, to prevent it from curling. Sear the fish over high heat, flip the fillet, add the butter, and cook until the fish has cooked through, one to three minutes, depending on the thickness of the fish.

7. Serve with the parsley caper sauce and, if desired, wilted Swiss chard and sautéed green beans.

8. Refrigerate leftover sauce for future use.

Noninvasive Treatment for Parkinson's Disease Now Available

Guided focused ultrasound (MRgFUS) uses ultrasound-wave technology in combination with magnetic resonance equipment to destroy targeted brain tissue and stop or reduce tremors. Now available at more than a dozen medical centers, it can be used at an early stage, when medication isn't effective and as an alternative to brain-stimulation surgery.

Gordon H. Baltuch, MD, PhD, professor of neurosurgery at University of Pennsylvania Perelman School of Medicine and a neurosurgeon at Pennsylvania Hospital, both in Philadelphia.

Stuttering Begins in the Brain

A genetic mutation linked to stuttering may decrease the number of astrocytes, cells that supply the brain with oxygen and nutrients, according to a mouse study that tracked pauses in the animals' vocalizations. The discovery could lead to new stuttering treatments.

Proceedings of the National Academy of Sciences.

Make the Ringing Stop!

The phantom sounds of tinnitus—ringing, clicking, roaring, etc.—can be severe enough to disrupt daily life.

Recent research: A small study found that deep-brain stimulation, which involves the use of electrical stimulation to specific areas of the brain, improved symptoms in a majority of patients. More study is under way.

Journal of Neurosurgery

Chapter 3

CANCER BREAKTHROUGHS FOR WOMEN

Heads-Up, Women: Hair Dye and Chemical Straighteners Linked to Breast Cancer

Most women know what increases their odds of developing breast cancer. Some risk factors, such as age or having a family history of breast cancer, can't be changed, while women do have some control over other risks, such as being overweight or not getting enough physical activity.

Now: Recent research is providing more clarity on a possible risk factor that's perplexed scientists for years due to mixed study findings. The new study, published in *International Journal of Cancer,* found that hair dye is associated with higher breast cancer risk—and it goes a step further by uncovering another potentially harmful type of hair product.

Study details: As part of the Sister Study, researchers analyzed data from nearly 47,000 women who filled out questionnaires that included information regarding their use of hair products during the prior 12 months. Study participants were ages 35 to 74 and did not have breast cancer themselves but did have a sister with the disease. By studying sisters who share genes, environments and experiences with a sister who developed breast cancer, the researchers hope to gain a better understanding of the risk factors associated with breast cancer.

Key findings: Overall, study participants who used permanent hair dye during the year before they enrolled in the study were 9% more likely to develop breast cancer during an eight-year follow-up period than those who didn't dye their hair.

When researchers did more analysis, they discovered some intriguing additional associations. For example, the breast cancer link was much stronger among black women who used hair dye—they were 45% more likely to develop breast cancer than non-users of hair dye, while increased risk was 7% for white women who dyed their hair.

The study also found that chemical hair straighteners, when used at least every five to eight weeks, increased breast cancer risk by about 30% in all women studied, although these products are more commonly used by black women. Researchers theorize that the

The study "Hair Dye and Chemical Straightener Use and Breast Cancer Risk in a Large US Population of Black and White Women" was published in the online version of the *International Journal of Cancer.*

chemicals found in hair products may play a role in the development of breast cancer, and the products used by black women may have more carcinogens than those used by white women. The results could also be due to differences in application methods or hair texture.

Even though the researchers stated that the hair products included in the study were associated with increased breast cancer risk, they pointed out that the use of a permanent hair dye or a hair-straightening product doesn't mean that a woman will necessarily develop breast cancer.

Said study coauthor Dale Sandler, PhD, chief of the National Institute of Environmental Health Sciences Epidemiology Branch, "While it is too early to make a firm recommendation, avoiding these chemicals might be one more thing women can do to reduce their risk of breast cancer."

More studies will be done to see if the new findings can be replicated. The research team also noted that little to no increase in breast cancer risk was found in women using semipermanent or temporary dye.

6 Signs That DCIS Is Likely to Become Invasive Breast Cancer

Study titled "Predictors of an Invasive Breast Cancer Recurrence after DCIS: A Systematic Review and Meta-Analyses" by researchers at the Netherlands Cancer Institute, Amsterdam, published in *Cancer Epidemiology, Biomarkers & Prevention.*

Most ductal carcinoma in situ (DCIS) breast cancer will never become life-threatening, even if left untreated. However, there hasn't been a good way to tell when DCIS should be treated and when treatment can be safely skipped—until now. A new study has identified six factors that determine when DCIS is most likely to become invasive breast cancer.

DCIS is cancer that starts in a milk duct and has not spread outside the duct. Often called "stage 0," it's such an early stage of cancer that some experts believe it's actually a precancerous condition rather than actual cancer. DCIS has become increasingly common—possibly because women are living longer, more women are getting screening mammograms and mammograms have become better at finding these small breast cancers. About 20% of all breast cancers are DCIS.

Most women with DCIS have a lumpectomy, and some also have radiation. The risk for DCIS recurrence after lumpectomy alone is about 25% to 30%...adding radiation therapy drops the risk to about 15%. Only half of recurrences are invasive cancer—the rest are DCIS again.

However, as there hasn't been a way to reliably predict which women with DCIS will develop invasive breast cancer, guidelines call for all women with the condition to be treated with either surgery alone or surgery and radiation...and frequently hormonal therapy as well. Doctors are coming to believe that this is overtreatment for the majority of women.

Now: Researchers from the Netherlands Cancer Institute in Amsterdam reviewed 17 studies and identified 26 unfavorable prognostic factors associated with invasive breast cancer developing after DCIS. Six factors in particular emerged as the most significant indicators, with risk for invasive breast cancer after DCIS diagnosis ranging from 36% to 84%. *They were...*

•**Feeling a lump (84% risk).** DCIS does not cause symptoms and 80% of the time is found only by mammography. However, when DCIS causes a palpable lump (one that can be felt), it is likely to be aggressive.

•**Involved margins (63% risk).** When the tumor is removed, if tumor cells are found to extend out to the edge of normal breast tissue, the risk for recurrence increases—because surgery may leave some cells behind.

• **Diagnosed before menopause (59% risk).** Younger women produce more estrogen, which may stimulate tumor growth. They also have more of their lives still ahead, allowing more time for recurrence to occur.

• **High p16 (51% risk).** Overexpression of p16, a protein involved in regulating tumor-cell growth that is detected during biopsy, has been linked to more aggressive tumor growth.

• **Being African-American (43% risk).** For reasons that are not clearly understood, African-American women have higher rates of all types of breast cancer recurrence.

• **High histologic grade (36% risk).** Histologic grade refers to how different from normal cells tumor cells look when studied under a microscope. The more abnormal, or poorly differentiated (meaning that it is hard to tell if the cells are normal or cancer), the higher their grade—and, not surprisingly, the greater their risk for becoming aggressive cancer.

The researchers hope that their findings will be independently validated and help to inform new guidelines...and that future studies will continue to look for other factors that might play a role. In the meantime, if you have been diagnosed with DCIS, it's a good idea to include these six factors in the conversation you have with your doctor to determine the best next steps.

More Women Should Get BRCA Screening

Previously, only women with a family history of a BRCA-related cancer (such as breast, ovarian, fallopian tube or peritoneal, a malignancy of the thin layer of tissue that lines the abdomen) were advised to undergo a risk assessment for the gene mutation that raises risk for these cancers.

Now: Women with a personal history of any breast, ovarian, fallopian tube or peri-

toneal cancer or those whose ancestry puts them at higher risk for BRCA-related breast cancer, such as Ashkenazi Jewish women, should be assessed and may consider BRCA gene testing if indicated after consulting a genetic counselor.

Douglas Owens, MD, chair, US Preventive Services Task Force and professor of medicine, Stanford University, California.

Dense Breasts and Breast Cancer Risk: What You Need to Know

Erin Hofstatter, MD, associate professor of medicine and codirector of the Smilow Cancer Genetics and Prevention Program at Yale School of Medicine in New Haven, Connecticut. She also serves as director of the Breast Cancer Prevention Clinic at Yale New Haven's Smilow Cancer Hospital.

About half of women ages 40 to 74 have dense breasts, which can't be felt when a woman does a self-exam or when a doctor palpates her breasts. This is vital information because dense breasts make it harder to find malignancies on a mammogram.

Even more important, women with dense breasts are four to six times more likely to develop breast cancer than women without dense breast tissue. In fact, high breast density surpasses other known risk factors for developing breast cancer, such as family history or later-in-life childbirth, according to research published in *JAMA Oncology*.

Another important finding: In women with dense breasts, tumors tend to be larger when detected compared with women without dense breasts, according to a study of women ages 50 to 69 published in *Radiology*.

The Detection Challenge

On mammograms, the fibrous and glandular tissue that indicates breast density appears

45

white. To distinguish the degree of breast density, radiologists use four categories—extremely dense (75% or more of the mammogram appears white)…heterogeneously dense (50% to 75% appears white)…scattered areas of density (25% to 50%)…and mostly fatty (0% to 25%). If a woman's mammogram falls within one of the first two categories, her breasts are considered dense.

Even though dense breasts can make mammograms more difficult to read, the test is crucial because many cancers may still be visible. Breast density, along with other risk factors, including personal and family history of breast cancer, should be taken into account when determining mammogram frequency. Women should talk to their doctors to come up with a personalized screening schedule—for both the frequency and types of tests performed.

For women with dense breasts, screening may include one or both of these tests…

• **3-D mammography.** A traditional mammogram is printed on film and is two-dimensional, with two X-ray images taken of each breast—top-to-bottom and side-to-side. With 3-D mammography, also called digital tomosynthesis, the machine takes multiple X-rays, or "slices," and combines them into a 3-D image that the radiologist reads on a computer screen, where breast tissue can be viewed one layer at a time. The resulting images are finer and clearer, showing abnormalities that might otherwise be difficult—or impossible—to see. Both types of mammography require the use of plates that compress the breasts.

3-D mammography delivers only very slightly more ionizing radiation than traditional mammography, but it's still considered safe by the FDA. There are about 40% fewer false positives with 3-D mammography compared with 2-D, preventing unnecessary anxiety in patients and repeated testing to confirm results.

• **Ultrasound.** This technology uses high-frequency sound waves to identify breast cysts or masses. A layer of gel is applied to each breast, and a handheld device called a transducer is placed directly on the skin, transmitting ultrasound waves into the body. A mass will block the sound waves' pathway, signaling a potential cancer. Ultrasound is noninvasive, creates no ionizing radiation and is typically used as a follow-up to any abnormal mammogram.

Important finding: When 3-D mammography and/or ultrasound was given to more than 3,200 women with "dense" or "extremely dense" breasts whose conventional screening mammograms had found no cancer, the additional tests found 24 breast cancers, according to a study published in *Journal of Clinical Oncology*.

One of these cancers was detected by 3-D mammogram alone…11 were detected by ultrasound alone…and 12 were detected by both 3-D mammogram and ultrasound.

Caveats: As part of the same study, there were 53 false-positive results for 3-D mammograms…and 65 false positives for ultrasound. However, researchers considered this disparity to be statistically insignificant.

But do these additional tests actually save lives? That's debatable. Even though the additional screenings have been shown to identify breast cancers that would have otherwise been missed, modern breast cancer treatment is so effective that even if the cancer is detected a bit later, it's still often curable. Even so, the earlier a cancer is detected, the less likely a woman will need chemotherapy. So while an ultrasound may not save lives, it could minimize treatment…or make a treatment regimen less taxing.

The screening decision: This can be a challenging question because professional medical groups have no established screening guidelines based on breast density. These groups do not consider the additional cancers that are detected by ultrasound to be numerous enough to warrant the additional monetary—and potential emotional—cost.

Insurance coverage also has been spotty for both 3-D mammography and ultrasound, so consult your insurer before getting these tests. For those paying out of pocket, a 3-D mammogram costs about $100 more than a

2-D mammogram (about $380 versus $290). An ultrasound can cost several hundred dollars. But if you're one of the women whose cancer is detected with additional testing, it's money well spent.

Note: Women with a strong family history of a BRCA mutation, which increases breast cancer risk, are often advised to also get an MRI, but this scan is typically not recommended for women with dense breasts. For that reason, I usually do not recommend MRI for breast density alone.

Other Breast Cancer Factors

You can't change certain risk factors, such as your family history of breast cancer, but other risk factors are under your control.

Most important steps to take: Strive for a healthy weight, achieved through 150 minutes of moderate-intensity physical activity a week plus a diet rich in plant-based foods and with less than 10% of calories from saturated fat.

There's strong evidence supporting the benefits of these strategies. For instance, nearly a quarter of breast cancers could be avoided by obese and overweight women attaining a body mass index under 25 (for example, a body weight of 140 pounds for a 5'4" woman). That's because fat cells produce estrogen—and an excess of this hormone increases risk for certain types of breast cancer.

Also: Don't smoke…limit alcohol use (to one drink a day or, even better, less)…and be judicious about using hormone replacement therapy, avoiding it if possible or taking it for the shortest course possible if you need it to alleviate menopausal symptoms. Fortunately, most women's breasts become non-dense after menopause.

Poultry Beats Red Meat

According to recent research, women who ate the most red meat, such as beef, were

---

Onion and Garlic Fight Breast Cancer

Women who regularly ate foods that contain onion and garlic more than once a day had a 67% lower risk for breast cancer compared with those who never ate these foods, according to a study of more than 350 women, ages 30 to 79.

Possible explanation: Onions and garlic are rich in flavonoids and sulfur-containing compounds that have anticancer properties.

Lina Mu, MD, PhD, associate professor of epidemiology and environmental health, University at Buffalo, New York.

23% more likely to develop invasive breast cancer than those who ate the least, according to a study of more than 42,000 women who were followed for an average of seven years. Those who substituted poultry for red meat were 28% less likely to develop breast cancer.

Theory: Poultry has lower levels of the saturated fat found in meat, which contributes to the oxidative and DNA damage that can lead to cancer.

Dale Sandler, PhD, chief, Epidemiology Branch, National Institute of Environmental Health Sciences, Research Triangle Park, North Carolina.

Watchful Waiting for Ovarian Cysts

For low-risk ovarian cysts, watchful waiting may be better than surgery. In a two-year study, 2,000 women who had ovarian cysts diagnosed by ultrasound to be at low risk for cancer, rupture or torsion (twisting and cutting off blood supply) had ultrasounds and clinical exams at three and six months. About 20% of cysts disappeared…0.2% had a rupture…0.4% had torsion…16% of the women needed surgery, and of those, less than 1% had ovarian cancer.

Dirk Timmerman, PhD, professor in obstetrics and gynecology, Catholic University of Leuven, Belgium, and lead author of a study published in *The Lancet Oncology.*

Battling Cancer at 65 or Over? This Can Make Chemo More Bearable

Arti Hurria, MD, former director of the Center for Cancer and Aging. Dr. Hurria, who died in 2018, co-authored the report titled "Practical Assessment and Management of Vulnerabilities in Older Patients Receiving Chemotherapy: ASCO Guideline for Geriatric Oncology," published in *Journal of Clinical Oncology.*

The American Society of Clinical Oncology now recommends every cancer patient 65 and older get a geriatric assessment—a questionnaire either done by the patient's own regular doctor and then shared with the oncologist or done by the oncologist him/herself—before beginning chemotherapy.

How it will help improve patients' quality of life during cancer treatment…

Weighing the risks and benefits of therapy involves more than its effect on your cancer. For example, if you have a separate chronic condition, such as high blood pressure, diabetes or even a balance issue, how chemo affects it also needs to be considered. In addition to your medical conditions, a geriatric assessment includes questions about your activity level, diet, social support, depression and anxiety, memory issues and other information about your daily life.

Having the results of your geriatric assessment enables your cancer doctor to know you better, more precisely tailor your treatment plan to you, help predict how severe the side effects of chemotherapy will be, and determine what additional help you might need to get through cancer therapy with the best outcome.

For instance, research has shown that people who suffer from depression can have increased trouble functioning while on chemotherapy. Or, your balance may be worsened by chemo. So, part of your treatment plan may include working with a physical therapist to improve your balance and an occupational therapist to help make your home safer. If you don't have social support, a social worker may be the additional resource you need.

The assessment will help your doctor give you a more accurate prognosis and life expectancy by taking into account not only your cancer, but also your other medical conditions. This, too, may influence your choice of treatment.

Taking the Initiative

You don't have to wait for your doctor to get the process started. You can take the geriatric assessment at the Cancer and Aging Research Group website (MyCARG.org), then print out the results to bring to your oncologist.

Smoked Fish May Raise Cancer Risk

The American Institute for Cancer Research places smoked and cured fish in the same category as processed meats, which are associated with higher cancer risk—and, in some scientists' view, actually can cause cancer when eaten regularly in large amounts.

The New York Times

Faster Lung Cancer Test Available

Compared with a traditional surgical tissue biopsy, a new liquid (blood-based) biopsy called Guardant360 detected biomarkers that can lead to more effective treatments in those with non-small cell lung cancer as accurately and in nearly half the time (nine days versus

15 days). The test identifies patients with gene mutations that can be treated with targeted molecular therapies that result in up to two to three times higher response rates compared with chemotherapy or immunotherapy.

Vassiliki A. Papadimitrakopoulou, MD, professor of medicine, University of Texas MD Anderson Cancer Center, Houston.

Fiber and Yogurt Lower Lung Cancer Risk

According to a recent finding, people who ate the most fiber (about 30 g daily) and yogurt (three to four ounces daily) had a 33% lower risk for lung cancer compared with those who ate the least, according to a study that followed up to 1.4 million men and women for nine years.

Theory: High-fiber foods and probiotic-rich yogurt reduce lung cancer–promoting inflammation.

Xiao-Ou Shu, MD, PhD, MPH, Ingram professor of cancer research, Vanderbilt Ingram Cancer Center, Nashville.

Beware This Hidden Cause of Lung Cancer

Gary G. Schwartz, PhD, chair of the department of population health in the School of Medicine & Health Sciences at University of North Dakota in Grand Forks. Dr. Schwartz is author of more than 100 peer-reviewed papers and coauthor of "Radon and Lung Cancer: What Does the Public Really Know?" recently published in *Journal of Environmental Radioactivity.*

When most people hear lung cancer, they think cigarettes. But that can be a mistake. While cigarette smoking is hands down the number-one risk factor for lung cancer, radon is a very real danger that doesn't get the attention it deserves.

Radon is the leading cause of lung cancer in nonsmokers—and accounts for about 21,000 deaths from the disease each year, according to the Environmental Protection Agency (EPA). Many of these deaths occur in people who never smoked. If you do smoke—and your home has high radon levels—this one-two punch makes your risk for lung cancer especially high. *Facts to know about this silent killer…*

A Widespread Indoor Threat

Radon occurs naturally when uranium, an element found in rocks and soil, decays. As the element breaks down, it releases radon gas. Even though radon can be found outdoors in harmless amounts, it can accumulate in homes and buildings that are constructed on soil with natural uranium deposits, as the air is trapped inside the building.

Radon is an insidious threat because it cannot be seen, tasted or smelled. When radon is inhaled, it causes no symptoms even though invisible particles are attacking the body's cells with cancer-causing radiation.

Thousands of lung cancer deaths would be avoided each year if home and building owners tested and fixed high levels of radon, according to the American Lung Association.

So why are there still so many deaths linked to radon? Over the years, several myths have emerged, undermining efforts to eradicate this pervasive health threat. *For example…*

Don't Be Fooled by These Myths

MYTH #1: **Radon is a concern only in certain parts of the country.**

Fact: It's true that radon exists in higher concentrations near uranium-dense rock deposits, but radon can be found everywhere. In total, nearly one in every 15 homes in the US is estimated to have radon levels that exceed the EPA's recommendation. The EPA has mapped the country into three zones. While the highest levels are generally found in northern states, moderate-risk counties exist in every state except Louisiana. And even in low-risk areas, a single neighborhood might be sitting on a pocket of uranium. For a US map that indicates average radon levels by state and zone, check the EPA Map of Radon Zones (at EPA.gov/radon, search "map of radon zones").

MYTH #2: **I've lived in my home for decades, so there's no point in testing now.**

Fact: Regardless of whether your home was tested for radon when you purchased it, testing should be repeated every five to 10 years. Radon levels can change over the years as your home settles, the ground shifts and new cracks form. And if a test you conduct now indicates that radon levels in your home are high, that doesn't necessarily mean you've had long-term exposure. But because the harmful effects of radon are cumulative, the sooner you address the problem, the lower your risk.

MYTH #3: **I have a brand-new home, so there's nothing to worry about.**

Fact: Some states do require new homes to be radon-resistant, but most don't. Because new homes are built to be more energy-efficient, they're more efficiently sealed. That means new homes can trap whatever radon might emerge from the soil under the house—so they may become even more prone to higher radon levels than older homes.

MYTH #4: **Testing is too expensive and time-consuming.**

Fact: You can buy a basic home test for under $15 at many hardware stores, and some states even provide them for free.

With most tests, you set it up, leave it in place for a minimum of 48 hours and then mail it to a lab for evaluation. Long-term tests may remain in a home for 90 days or more—

This Simple Test Could Save Your Life

Radon testing is simple—and takes only minutes to set up. Stop by your local hardware store or go online to pick up a test kit…place the cannister in the lowest level of your home that you spend time in…give it time (typically 48 hours) to collect an air sample…and mail the cannister to the lab. That's all you have to do! Results are typically mailed and/or e-mailed to you within a week or so.

Here's how to evaluate your test results, based on recommendations from the EPA…

• **Below 2 pCi/L.** Relax, but remember to retest every five or 10 years.

• **Borderline levels (2 pCi/L to 4 pCi/L).** Do a second test. If the second test confirms the first, you have a choice—either begin remediation now or monitor levels by retesting.

• **High levels (4 pCi/L or above).** There are literally no "safe" levels of radon exposure, but the EPA says that you should take action if radon is this high in your home. If DIY sealing doesn't bring down the levels—and a repeat test confirms that they are high—find a radon mitigation contractor. Consult your state's radon office for advice on licenses, registration or certification that may be required for mitigation experts.

Until you can arrange for remediation, keep the windows open. Fresh air will help to dilute the radon concentration indoors. Also, try not to spend significant amounts of time in the basement. Radon levels there are typically two to three times higher than on the first floor.

Important: For the most accurate results, be sure to follow instructions on the test kit carefully. For example, do not move the test device or open doors and windows in the testing area while the air sample is being collected. Weather patterns, such as high winds or storms, can make your results lower or higher than normal.

For more information, read the EPA's "Consumer's Guide to Radon Reduction," which you can find online at EPA.gov. It'll walk you through the process and guide your decision-making.

For renters: Get more information about radon testing and remediation in rental properties from the EPA's report "Radon Guide for Tenants." Both reports can be found at EPA. gov/radon. —Gary G. Schwartz, PhD

these tests are used when home owners want a more stable, average level. However, when researchers at University of Calgary recently compared a five-day radon test against a 90-day test, the longer-term testing was significantly more precise. If you can, use long-term testing.

MYTH #5: **If I test my home and the levels are too high, I won't be able to sell it later on.**

Fact: Radon testing is a routine part of home inspections in many states, so if you have a problem, it could hold things up when you do decide to sell your home. Plus, remediation may be easier than you think. If you have obvious cracks in your basement floor, for example, DIY sealing can be easy and inexpensive—hardware stores sell products made for this purpose. Just retest after performing this type of sealing to ensure that radon levels were adequately reduced.

If the levels are still dangerously high, you may need a remediation system that uses a vent pipe and fan to pull radon to the outside. Such systems cost about $800 to $2,000, depending on your home and location.

Cancer Genetic Testing: Is It Right for You?

Scott M. Weissman, MS, CGC, a board-certified genetic counselor and a clinical faculty member at the Northwestern University Graduate Program in Genetic Counseling in Chicago. He also is the founder of Chicago Genetic Consultants, a personalized genetic-counseling service based in Northbrook, Illinois. His scientific papers have appeared in *JAMA, Genetics in Medicine* and other medical journals.

As cancer treatments become increasingly sophisticated, so too has the testing for this disease. Genetic tests that can determine one's risk for cancer—or help guide treatment in those who've already been diagnosed—are now becoming the standard of care.

For certain patients, Medicare will now cover cancer genetic tests that have been approved by the FDA—tests that detect whether your DNA has a genetic mutation that increases your risk of developing cancer or underlies a diagnosed cancer. Many private health insurers also are picking up the tab.

The testing might show, for example, that you have a mutation (or variant) in the BRCA1 or BRCA2 gene, which increases risk for breast cancer by up to 85% or ovarian cancer by up to 60% (and risk for prostate cancer in men by up to 30% to 40%).

For insights about the new world of cancer genetic testing, we spoke with genetic counselor Scott M. Weissman, MS, CGC, a leading authority on this topic.

What's Available

There are two main types of cancer genetic tests…

•**Germline.** A saliva or blood test is used to detect specific, heredity-based genetic mutations that may predispose you to cancer. If you already have cancer or you're a cancer survivor, the test can detect whether it was tied to a hereditary cause—this will tell you if you're at increased risk for a second occurrence of the same cancer or perhaps another type of cancer…or whether family members should also consider testing. Medicare typically covers this test only if you currently have cancer or are a cancer survivor. Most private insurers also cover people who have not had cancer.

Germline tests can be obtained in three different ways…

•Health-care provider–ordered. Following a risk assessment conducted by a doctor or genetic counselor who documents your personal and family history risk factors, a doctor may order the test. This type of test is 90% to 95% accurate.

•Direct-to-consumer. In this case, you order the test yourself. You receive a kit, provide a saliva sample and send it back to the company. The DNA in the saliva is analyzed, and results are delivered directly to you. For example, 23andMe is the only company offering FDA-cleared direct-to-consumer cancer genetic testing—for BRCA1 and BRCA2 mutations in breast and ovarian cancer...and for MUTYH mutations, which raise the risk for colon cancer. Direct-to-consumer testing is not covered by insurance.

Caution: The 23andMe BRCA test is only for the three genetic variants of the BRCA gene that are prevalent among Ashkenazi Jews—and misses the roughly 90% of people who have other types of BRCA mutations.

•Consumer-initiated, doctor-ordered. With this approach, you order the test from one of several laboratories (see below)—but the lab that conducts the test works with an independent network of genetic counselors and physicians to review the request, with a physician approving the test...or deciding that the test isn't warranted.

This type of testing (typically saliva) can detect dozens of genetic mutations that indicate an increased risk of developing certain cancers (such as breast, ovarian, uterine, colon, pancreatic, prostate, thyroid and brain). Many laboratories across the US now provide this service, but the three most reliable are Color Genomics...Invitae...and Helix/Perkin Elmer.

Helpful: The best laboratories are accredited by the College of American Pathologists, CAP.org, as well as Clinical Laboratory Improvement Amendments, CDC.gov/CLIA. To see if a lab that you are considering using is accredited, check the above websites or the lab websites...or call the lab and ask.

Watch out: Some unscrupulous laboratories are "cold calling" seniors and offering cancer genetic testing—whether the individual needs it or not. Before ordering, talk to your doctor about the benefits of the test.

•**Somatic.** This test uses cancer tissue or blood to see if there is a genetic mutation fueling the cancer. This type of mutation spontaneously develops over the course of a lifetime and cannot be passed on to your children. If a mutation is found, the oncologist can prescribe one of the many "targeted" therapies now available to inhibit the action of the mutated genes.

Examples: The EGFR mutation in lung cancer is targeted by the drug *erlotinib* (Tarceva)...and the BRAF mutation in melanoma is targeted by the drug *vemurafenib* (Zelboraf). Insurance almost always covers a somatic cancer genetic test, which must be ordered by a doctor.

Should You Get Tested?

If you're interested in preventing cancer, it's important to realize that only 5% to 10% of all cancers have a genetic component. When does genetic testing make sense if you have not had cancer? *Some criteria...*

•**When a close relative** (a parent, sibling or child) has been diagnosed with cancer before the age of 50...or a cancer genetic test in a close relative shows a germline cancer mutation...or you have three or more close relatives with the same cancer regardless of age.

•**For a woman,** when there are both breast and ovarian cancers in close relatives...when there is breast cancer in two or more relatives on the same side of the family...when there is a close relative with cancer in both breasts.

•**For colon cancer,** if a colonoscopy detects more than 10 precancerous colorectal polyps regardless of family history.

If you have cancer, you should get a cancer genetic test.

Why this is important: Finding a genetic mutation can determine the best treatment options.

Or if you had cancer years ago, before germline testing was common, and the cancer recurs, that could be a good time to do a risk assessment to see if a germline test is indicated.

Post-Testing Strategy

If your screening test results are positive—meaning that you have a genetic risk for cancer—take action.

Your test results may indicate that you need earlier or more frequent screenings, such as colonoscopies. If you have a genetic risk for breast cancer, for example, along with earlier screening, you might also consider taking an estrogen-blocking drug or getting a preventive mastectomy.

And if you find out that you have a hereditary risk, you should also tell your close relatives (parents, siblings and children), as well as aunts/uncles, cousins and grandparents, that they should consider testing, too.

Important: Even if your test results are negative, if you have a strong family history of cancer, you may need increased monitoring. Ask your doctor for advice.

How Genetic Counseling Helps

It's a complex process to decide whether or not to take a genetic cancer test...choose which test to take and which laboratory to use...understand the results...act on the results...and cope emotionally with positive results. That's why there are genetic counselors—health professionals specially trained in genetics and psychology—to help people in the process of genetic testing.

To find a genetic counselor near you: Go to the website of the National Society of Genetic Counselors, FindAGeneticCounselor. com, and enter your zip code. Some insurers will cover the cost of genetic counseling.

When Cancer Spreads to the Brain

Nduka Amankulor, MD, a neurosurgeon and neuro-oncologist at UPMC Hillman Cancer Center and assistant professor of neurological surgery at University of Pittsburgh School of Medicine.

An astounding 20% to 30% of people with cancer develop metastatic brain cancer (MBC)—cancer that has spread from another organ to the brain.

Cell-Phone Radiation Danger

Cell-phone radiation can cause tumors. Research from the National Toxicology Program has connected radiofrequency radiation with malignant brain and heart tumors in rats exposed to nine hours a day of 2G and 3G radiation.

Best: Don't hold your cell phone against your body...and use headphones. For every millimeter you move the phone away from your body, exposure is reduced by 10% to 15%.

John Bucher, PhD, senior scientist of the National Toxicology Program at National Institute of Environmental Health Sciences, Durham, North Carolina.

Breast cancer, lung cancer, kidney cancer and melanoma are the main types of cancer that invade the brain. But almost any cancer can produce brain metastases, with an estimated 170,000 new cases every year.

Until recently, the prognosis for people with MBC was grim—only 8% of patients were alive two years after diagnosis, and 2% after five years. But those sad statistics are changing.

Now: The treatment of MBC is being revolutionized by targeted drug therapies that attack genetic mutations driving cancer...immunotherapies that stimulate the body's own immune system to fight cancer...and precisely focused radiation.

Immunotherapy more than doubled the average survival time of melanoma patients with MBC—from 5.2 months to 12.4 months, according to a study published in *Cancer Immunology Research*. The effects are even better for melanoma patients with MBC but no other metastases—research found that those who received immunotherapy had an average survival rate of 56 months, compared with 7.7 months for those receiving standard treatment, such as chemotherapy. In other words, MBC patients treated with

53

immunotherapy lived about seven times longer!

What cancer patients and their families need to know…

Many oncologists don't recommend screening for brain metastases, except for certain tumor types that have a significant predilection for spreading to the brain. Of course, if the patient develops neurological symptoms, such as headaches, numbness, blurred vision, balance difficulties, cognitive decline and/or seizures, then brain screening for a brain tumor is recommended, regardless of the type of cancer.

New thinking: Early detection can extend survival time in patients without neurological symptoms who are at high risk of developing MBC.

My advice for who should get screened…

•**Any patient with a new diagnosis of stage II to stage IV lung cancer,** whether it's non-small cell (the most common type) or small cell.

•**A melanoma patient with metastatic disease elsewhere in the body**—because two out of three of these patients will also develop MBC.

•**A breast cancer patient who is positive for HER2** (a gene that plays a role in the development of breast cancer)…or whose tumor lacks hormone receptors (estrogen and progesterone receptors)…or lacks any markers at all (triple-negative breast cancer). The rate of MBC is significantly higher (10% to 15%) in all these breast cancer patients.

The gold standard for early detection is a brain MRI with contrast dye, which can detect brain tumors as small as 2 millimeters in diameter (less than one-tenth of an inch). Especially in patients who are at high risk of developing MBC, insurance may cover the MRI even if there are no neurological symptoms, but be sure to check first. Once MBC is diagnosed, MRIs are obtained roughly every two to four months.

Targeted therapies are drugs (oral or IV) that block or alter specific genes and/or proteins that drive cancer. There have been doz-ens of clinical trials of targeted therapy in patients with brain metastases—with some remarkable results. *For example…*

Researchers from the MD Anderson Cancer Center at University of Texas studied melanoma patients with MBC who had the BRAF mutation, which occurs in about half of patients with this disease. The patients received two drugs—*dabrafenib* (Tafinlar), which targets BRAF…and *trametinib* (Mekinist), which targets MEK, a mutation similar to BRAF. In a group of 76 patients with BRAF who had never been treated for MBC and whose neurological symptoms were under control, 58% had significant shrinking of their brain tumors—and in four patients the tumors vanished, according to the research, which was published in *The Lancet Oncology*. The response lasted, on average, six to seven months.

Immunotherapy drugs are a class of drugs that stimulate a patient's immune system, essentially calling it into action. The most widely used immunotherapies are drugs that block checkpoint proteins, such as PD-1 or PD-L1, which suppress inflammatory responses in the immune system.

Scientific evidence: Impressive results with combined drug therapy—*ipilimumab* (Yervoy) and *nivolumab* (Opdivo)—were cited in a study published in *The New England Journal of Medicine*. In that research, when 94 melanoma patients with MBC took both drugs, 81% were alive after one year and 70% after two years—a dramatic increase over the typical survival rate of four to five months before the introduction of immunotherapy.

In the past, the standard radiation treatment for MBC was whole-brain radiation—multiple treatments of the entire brain with low-dose radiation.

However, whole-brain radiation has significant side effects, such as a marked decrease in memory and other cognitive abilities. Doctors are now using highly focused radiation therapies called stereotactic radiosurgery. Employing a flexible robotic arm to deliver radiation (CyberKnife), or using a helmet with built-in radiation sources (Gamma Knife), this treatment delivers less total radiation…faster…and more accurately. And its cancer-killing efficacy is as good as whole-brain radiation—with less severe side effects.

To take advantage of the breakthrough treatments for MBC, you need a plan of action. *Here are four steps to follow…*

STEP #1: Treat the primary cancer. The key in treating cancer is always minimizing your overall cancer burden using the full range of treatments available—such as chemotherapy, radiation, surgery, targeted therapies and immunotherapy. Controlling the primary malignancy reduces the risk of the cancer spreading to the brain.

STEP #2: Ask your oncologist, "Has my tumor been sufficiently molecularly characterized?" Sophisticated genetic tests will show if you're a candidate for targeted therapy or immunotherapy.

For example, if such testing shows that you have the ALK mutation, treatments for the primary tumor may include targeted therapies such as *alectinib* (Alecensa), *brigatinib* (Alunbrig) or *lorlatinib* (Lorbrena)—all of which also help prevent and/or treat brain metastases.

If a tumor biopsy shows that you have high levels of PD-1 or PD-L1, then you may be a candidate for an immunotherapy drug such as *pembrolizumab* (Keytruda), *nivolumab* (Opdivo) or *atezolizumab* (Tecentriq).

STEP #3: Ask your oncologist, "Are there effective therapies that treat the molecular pathways affecting my cancer—and should we use those therapies to treat my brain cancer?" Once your tumor has been tested for molecular mutations, talk with your oncologist about the targeted and immunological therapies available to treat those problems. You and your doctor should develop a complete list of the targeted therapies and immunotherapies (see examples above) that may be right for you—and then decide which to use.

STEP #4: Demand a multidisciplinary team approach. The best treatment for primary cancer and for MBC is a team approach, typically involving a medical oncologist, a radiation oncologist and a cancer surgeon. The best treatment decisions are made when the entire team talks to one another, face-to-face. This type of multidisciplinary approach is typical of cancer centers that are designated by the National Cancer Institute for offering cutting-edge treatments.

To find such an NCI-designated cancer center near you, go to: Cancer.gov/research/nci-role/cancer-centers/find.

Common Mouth Bacteria Make Colon Cancer More Dangerous

Study titled "Fusobacterium nucleatum promotes colorectal cancer by inducing Wnt/b-catenin modulator Annexin A1" by researchers at Columbia University College of Dental Medicine, New York City, published in *EMBO Reports*.

Colon cancer, a disease that affects one out of 23 adults, has recently been linked to gum disease. But how the one might be driving the other has not been known—until now. A new study has discovered what it is in our mouths that causes colon cancer to become most deadly…and may lead to better tests and new treatments.

Fusobacterium nucleatum is a common bacterium found in the mouth that plays a role in forming dental plaque, which can lead to tooth decay, gingivitis and periodontitis. The bacterium also has been implicated in diseases outside the mouth, including colorectal cancer, atherosclerosis, rheumatoid arthritis and Alzheimer's disease. In fact, research has found that about one-third of colorectal cancer patients test positive for F. nucleatum bacteria—and those patients usually have more aggressive tumors.

Researchers at Columbia University College of Dental Medicine had previously discovered that F. nucleatum produces a molecule called FadA adhesin. They also observed that FadA adhesin interacted with cancerous colon cells but not with healthy colon cells. To learn more, the researchers reviewed cellular data from more than 450 patients with colorectal cancer.

Results: The researchers found that FadA adhesin molecules bind to a protein called Annexin A1 that is produced only in the cancerous cells, not in the noncancerous cells. Annexin A1 stimulates cancer growth and leads to a more aggressive and deadly prognosis. In fact, the patients in the study with the highest levels of Annexin A1 in their cancer cells had the fastest-growing cancers.

Vicious cycle: FadA adhesin molecules bind to the Annexin A1 protein, triggering the cells to produce more Annexin A1. This in turn causes more binding and more cancer growth—a sequence called a "positive feedback loop" in scientific terms.

The researchers hope that the results of their study might lead to development of a test for Annexin A1 levels to identify which cancers are more likely to become aggressive, as well as new treatments for colorectal cancer.

While the researchers were able to show in cell cultures and mouse studies that blocking Annexin A1 prevented F. nucleatum from binding to cancer cells, no research has yet shown that reducing oral F. nucleatum will protect people with colorectal cancer from more aggressive disease. However, it is known that F. nucleatum increases with the severity of gum disease and is also higher in smokers. So, if you have been diagnosed with colorectal cancer it makes sense to be especially persistent about maintaining good oral hygiene. And if you smoke, here's one more good reason to quit.

My Secret for a More Effective and Gentler Colonoscopy Prep

Jamison Starbuck, ND, a naturopathic physician in family practice in Missoula, Montana, and producer of *Dr. Starbuck's Health Tips for Kids*, a weekly program on Montana Public Radio, MTPR.org. She is a past president of the American Association of Naturopathic Physicians and a contributing editor to *The Alternative Advisor: The Complete Guide to Natural Therapies and Alternative Treatments.* DrJamisonStarbuck.com

It's not news that colonoscopy is a wonderful screening and diagnostic tool.

What you may not know: According to the American College of Gastroenterology, bowel preparation is inadequate in up to 20% to 25% of colonoscopies. This means you may get inaccurate results, including missed abnormalities, or you may be asked to reschedule the test involving another round of the dreaded prep!

In the typical colonoscopy prep, patients need to drink a laxative solution anywhere from 12 to 24 hours before the procedure in order to empty the bowels completely. Unfortunately, many patients do not accomplish this goal—sometimes they don't finish the solution due to a strong reaction such as nausea, vomiting and/or painful elimination, they start the prep too late or they don't follow other instructions.

I've developed a plan for my patients that makes typical colonoscopy prep more successful and gentler on the system. The object is to gradually reduce stool volume for a few days before you even begin drinking the prep solution. This helps ensure that the bowels will be well prepared for the test. *What I suggest…*

Four days before your colonoscopy, make your diet simple and clean. Your goal is to have one or two good-sized, complete stools each day during the days prior to drinking the colonoscopy prep solution. *To help achieve this…*

• **Avoid fried and high-fat foods.** Use olive oil and mashed avocado for fats.

• **Become a vegetarian or limit protein to fish or a small amount of turkey.** Eat lots of baked or steamed vegetables. Avoid salads and limit raw vegetables to one or two small servings per day.

• **Avoid corn, nuts, berries and legumes as they can sometimes linger in the bowel.** Whole grains, such as brown rice, are OK.

• **Limit fruit to apples and pears.** Applesauce and baked apples and pears are excellent—delicious and high in fiber.

• **Avoid dairy because it's often not easy to digest.**

Also, cut out any foods with dyes as well as beets, which can discolor your bowel wall. And avoid preservatives and sugar substitutes and alcohols, which can irritate your colon. These ingredients may affect your test results.

Thirty-six hours before your colonoscopy, switch to an all-liquid, low-protein, low-fiber diet.

• **Drink only clear or lightly colored fruit juices,** such as apple or pear…miso…broth…preservative- and color-free, unsweetened electrolyte solutions…and lots of water.

• **Black coffee or tea is OK.** Avoid milk or nondairy milk (soy, almond, etc.).

After using my plan, begin your colonoscopy prep as directed by your doctor. Hydrate with water up until the time your doctor has told you to stop drinking.

After your colonoscopy, load up on probiotics. I advise an acidophilus/bifidus supplement, 20 billion colony-forming units (CFUs), for 14 days.

Caution: If you have a severe illness or a significantly compromised immune system, talk to your doctor before using probiotics—they can increase risk for infection in these individuals. For three days after, rehydrate with lots of water and eat a simple diet of whole foods.

Colonoscopy Alternative

Avoid colonoscopy by using an at-home stool test if you're at average risk, reports Thomas Imperiale, MD. His meta-analysis of 31 studies provides the strongest evidence to date that an annual fecal immunochemical test (FIT), which detects hidden blood in stool, is 75% to 85% effective at detecting cancers. If blood is found, a follow-up colonoscopy is needed. If no blood is found, the test is repeated yearly. Only about 65% of adults ages 50 to 75 comply with screening recommendations. The FIT could boost that.

Thomas Imperiale, MD, research scientist at the Regenstrief Institute, Indianapolis, and lead author of a study published in *Annals of Internal Medicine*.

Aspirin for Colon Cancer

The US Preventive Services Task Force has recommended that aspirin be considered to reduce risk for colorectal cancer in people with advanced colon polyps, after an analysis found that it reduces the risk by 40%.

However: In a study of 84 patients ages 40 to 91, only 42.9% of patients with advanced colon polyps, determined by biopsy, were taking aspirin.

Note: Even if you have been diagnosed with colon polyps, daily aspirin increases bleeding risk. Ask your doctor for advice.

Charles H. Hennekens, MD, DrPH, senior academic advisor, Schmidt College of Medicine, Florida Atlantic University, Boca Raton.

Psoriasis and Cancer Risk

Psoriasis increases risk for many types of cancer by an average of 18%. Esophageal, liver, pancreatic and squamous cell skin cancers were among the highest risks. The exact link is unclear but could be related to inflammation, a hallmark of both psoriasis and cancer. Keeping up with recommended cancer screenings can help with early detection and diagnosis.

Alex M. Trafford, MSc, PhD candidate in the department of biology, medicine and health at University of Manchester in the UK and lead author of a study published in *JAMA Dermatology*.

Don't Make These Sunscreen Mistakes!

Barney Kenet, MD, a board-certified dermatologist and dermatologic surgeon at NewYork-Presbyterian/Weill Cornell Medical Center and in private practice, both in New York City. He is author of *Saving Your Skin* and *How to Wash Your Face*. KenetMD.com

Sobering facts: Fewer than 30% of women (and 15% men) even bother to use sunscreen regularly on their faces and other exposed skin when they are outside for more than an hour, yet the effect can be devastating. In 2020, melanoma, the deadliest type of skin cancer, is expected to be diagnosed in 100,350 Americans. Meanwhile, more than three million Americans are diagnosed each year with other types of skin cancer. *To help protect your precious skin, avoid these mistakes…*

MISTAKE #1: You neglect this vulnerable spot. Your eyelids occupy a relatively small part of your body, but thanks to their combination of extremely thin, delicate skin and near-constant ultraviolet (UV) exposure, about 10% of all skin cancers occur there. Scientists may now have an explanation.

In research published in *PLOS ONE*, study participants failed to cover 10% of their faces, on average. And the most frequently neglected area was—you guessed it—the eyelids… and the area located between the inner corners of the eyes and the bridge of the nose.

Not surprisingly, several study participants said that they left those hot spots unprotected out of concern that sunscreen would sting their eyes.

Solution: Choose a gentle sunscreen lotion or cream.

What to try: SkinCeuticals Physical Eye UV Defense, SPF 50 (SkinCeuticals.com)…or "tear-free" Neutrogena Pure & Free Baby Sunscreen, SPF 50 (Neutrogena.com).

Note: Even though these products can be used on the eyelids, keep them out of your eyes.

Don't forget: Sunglasses also help protect the eyelids—and your eyesight. At least 10% of cataract cases can be directly attributed to UV exposure. Look for sunglasses that block 99% or 100% of UV rays.

MISTAKE #2: **You don't wear sun-protective clothing.** Ask a dermatologist for his/her favorite UV-protection tip, and you might be surprised to hear "cover up with clothing" just as often as you hear "wear sunscreen."

Even though you get some protection from regular shirts and pants—think dark-colored synthetic or tightly woven fabrics—"sun-protective clothing" does a far better job. This clothing is rated with a UPF, which stands for Ultraviolet Protection Factor and represents the amount of UVA and UVB rays that can penetrate a particular fabric. A UPF of 50 allows only one-fiftieth of UV radiation to reach the skin.

What to try: Solumbra by Sun Precautions (SunPrecautions.com) has clothing options for men and women.

Don't forget a hat: Golf and baseball caps don't protect the ears from sun exposure. Both men and women should choose a hat with a minimum two- to three-inch-wide brim. Coolibar (Coolibar.com) offers stylish hats with a UPF of 50+ for men and women.

MISTAKE #3: **You skip your "lips and tips."** Lips are prone to developing precancerous lesions called actinic cheilitis—scaly patches that, when untreated, can turn into squamous cell carcinoma, the second most common form of skin cancer.

What to try: Neutrogena Revitalizing Lip Balm, SPF 20 (Neutrogena.com) is a tinted lip balm with moisturizer. Vanicream Lip Protectant, SPF 30 (Vanicream.com) is gluten-free and free of dyes, parabens and other preservatives.

Don't forget your "tips": Tips of the ears, the scalp and tops of hands also are vulnerable to developing skin cancers due to their cumulative sun exposure.

What to try: A stick that allows precise application, such as Kiss My Face Sport Hot Spots Sunscreen, SPF 30 (KissMyFace.com).

MISTAKE #4: **You ignore the label.** Sunscreen ingredients do matter. The FDA has proposed that zinc oxide and titanium dioxide be considered GRASE (generally recognized as safe and effective). On the other hand, para-aminobenzoic acid (PABA) and trolamine salicylate are not GRASE for use in sunscreens due to possible safety concerns. (Trolamine salicylate, for instance, can interfere with healthy blood clotting.)

An additional 12 ingredients, such as the chemical sunscreen ingredients oxybenzone, avobenzone and octinoxate, fall somewhere in between—some experts are concerned about the potential for endocrine disruption, for instance—and more research is needed to determine safety.

Recent finding: After four thorough applications, the popular chemical sunscreen ingredients avobenzone, oxybenzone, octocrylene and ecamsule were detected in volunteers' blood in concentrations that exceeded the FDA's testing threshold, according to a study published in *JAMA*. For oxybenzone, the threshold level was detected just two hours after the first application and it accumulated at higher rates than the other ingredients. More safety testing will be done.

What to try: Badger's Clear Zinc Sunscreen, SPF 30 (Badgerbalm.com) blends with your skin tone and has 98% certified organic ingredients. Or try Aveeno Baby Continuous Protection Sensitive Skin Zinc Oxide Sunscreen, SPF 50 (Aveeno.com).

Also, pay close attention to terms on the label. *Be sure to choose…*

• **"Broad spectrum."** This means that it protects against UVA rays (which contribute to premature skin aging) and UVB rays (sunburn). Both can lead to skin cancer.

• **"Water-resistant" or "very water-resistant."** This means that it protects wet or sweaty skin for 40 or 80 minutes, respectively.

Also: Throw out sunscreen that is expired…or showing signs of expiration, such as changes in consistency, smell or color. If a product doesn't show an expiration date, use a permanent marker to write the date of purchase on the bottle and use that as a guide. (Sunscreen formulas should last up to three years, according to FDA guidelines.)

MISTAKE #5: **You use a combination sunscreen-insect repellent.** Insect repellent ingredients (DEET, in particular) can slash SPF by more than 30%.

What to do: Use a separate sunscreen and insect repellent, and follow the manufacturer's recommendations for each. Apply insect repellent first and wait at least a minute before applying sunscreen. One ounce (two tablespoons) of sunscreen needs to be reapplied every two hours, but insect repellent does not, so be sure you don't apply too much.

Tumors Hate Happy Vibes

Study by researchers at Technion-Israel Institute of Technology, Haifa, published in *Nature Communications*.

Feeling good may slow tumor growth. When the brains of mice were stimulated

Often-Overlooked Areas in Skin Checks

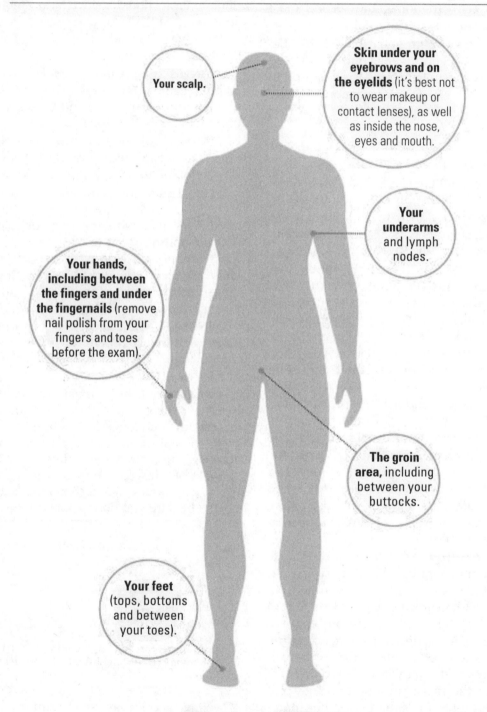

Your scalp.

Skin under your eyebrows and on the eyelids (it's best not to wear makeup or contact lenses), as well as inside the nose, eyes and mouth.

Your underarms and lymph nodes.

Your hands, including between the fingers and under the fingernails (remove nail polish from your fingers and toes before the exam).

The groin area, including between your buttocks.

Your feet (tops, bottoms and between your toes).

© 2019 Bottom Line Inc. BottomLineInc.com

after the animals had cancer cells implant-ed, they released dopamine, which disabled some cells that promote tumor growth—and the mice's immune systems responded more effectively against the tumors.

The Ultimate Guide to Skin Checks

National Institutes of Health, medlineplus.gov/lab-tests/skin-cancer-screening/.

Frequent head-to-toe self-exams are one of the best ways to detect skin cancer early, when it is most treatable. Be sure to check the areas that are often over-looked, which are indicated in the graphic on page 60. A skin-cancer screening per-formed by a doctor (see below) should also include these areas.

To perform a self-check: You'll need to fully undress and do the exam in a well-lit room in front of a full-length mirror (and have a hand mirror available).

To ensure that you are checking your skin correctly, follow these steps…

1. Stand in front of the mirror and look at your face, neck and stomach. (Women should look under their breasts.)

2. Raise your arms and look at your left and right sides.

3. Look at the front and back of your forearms.

4. Look at your hands, including be-tween your fingers and under your fin-gernails. (Be sure to remove any nail polish from fingers and toes.)

5. Look at the front, back and sides of your legs.

6. Sit down and examine your feet, checking the soles and the spaces be-tween the toes. Also, check the nail beds of each toe.

7. Check your back, buttocks and geni-tals with a hand mirror.

8. Part your hair and examine your scalp. Use a comb or a hair dryer along with a hand mirror to help you see better. (Have a friend or loved one help with this if needed.)

Signs to watch for: If you find signs of skin cancer, see your health-care provider for a more thorough screening. *Signs vary de-pending on the type of skin cancer, but they may include…*

•**Change in an existing mole or spot.**

•**Mole or other skin mark that oozes, bleeds or becomes crusty.**

•**Mole that is painful to the touch.**

•**Sore that doesn't heal within two weeks.**

•**Shiny pink, red, pearly white or trans-lucent bump.**

•**Mole or sore with irregular borders that may bleed easily.**

Remember ABCDE: During a self-exam, be alert for signs of melanoma, the most seri-ous type of skin cancer. *An easy way to re-member the signs of melanoma is to think of "ABCDE," which stands for…*

•**Asymmetry.** The mole has an odd shape, with half of it not matching the other half.

•**Border.** The border of the mole is ragged or irregular.

•**Color.** The color of the mole is uneven.

•**Diameter.** The mole is bigger than the size of a pea or a pencil eraser.

•**Evolving.** The mole has changed in size, shape or color.

If you find signs of melanoma, see your health-care provider as soon as possible.

Also: Talk to your health-care provider for advice on the frequency of your self-checks and regular skin-cancer screening exams performed by a dermatologist. The recom-mended frequency of skin exams performed by a doctor is based on your personal risk factors, including skin type, history of sun exposure and family history, according to the American Academy of Dermatology.

Pancreatic Cancer Risk

Pancreatic inflammation, a common cause of hospitalization, can greatly increase cancer risk.

New finding: Patients with both pancreatitis and pancreatic cancer have high levels of a dangerous sugar structure known as CA19-9. Blocking the sugar could prevent pancreatitis from progressing to cancer.

Science

Catching Pancreatic Cancer Early

Diane M. Simeone, MD, an internationally recognized surgeon and scientist, the associate director for translational research at Perlmutter Cancer Center at NYU Langone Health and director of its Pancreatic Cancer Center in New York City. Her research has been widely published in leading medical journals including *Cancer Cell, Journal of Clinical Oncology* and *Cancer Discovery*.

Pancreatic cancer is a frightening disease because it's usually diagnosed only when it's reached an advanced, all-too-often lethal stage. But it doesn't have to be that way.

Everyone knows about screening guidelines for colon cancer and breast cancer, but few are aware that screening tests for pancreatic cancer also are available. Recognizing the key risk factors for this malignancy will help you and your doctor decide whether such tests are appropriate for you or a loved one.

When a pancreatic cancer is found via a screening program, there is an 80% to 90% chance that the tumor can be removed, and up to 30% to 35% of those individuals will live for five or more years.

However, when a pancreatic cancer is found in a person who has not been regularly screened and he/she has already developed symptoms (such as abdominal or back pain, weight loss, nausea and/or jaundice), there is only a 15% chance that it can be removed. This lack of early detection, along with the need for improved therapies, has resulted in a persistently low overall survival rate of 9% for pancreatic cancer patients.

Here's how to spot pancreatic cancer before it's too late...

Know Your Risk Factors

The first step to staying ahead of pancreatic cancer is knowing how to assess your risk factors. *Your risk is higher if you have any of the following...*

• **Two or more relatives with pancreatic cancer,** including one first-degree relative (parent, sibling or child).

• **A first-degree relative who developed pancreatic cancer before age 50.**

• **An inherited genetic syndrome linked to pancreatic cancer such as Lynch syndrome,** which is also associated with colorectal cancer...or BRCA mutations, which predispose a person to breast, ovarian and prostate cancers.

Note: People of Ashkenazi Jewish (Central and Eastern Europe) descent aren't the only ones who can have BRCA mutations. Though less common, individuals of Norwegian, Swedish, Italian and other ethnic groups have been found to also carry certain BRCA mutations.

Other factors that increase your risk for pancreatic cancer...

• **Long-standing type 2 diabetes (more than five years),** which increases pancreatic cancer risk by twofold.

Note: New-onset diabetes—especially when weight loss instead of weight gain appears—may be an early sign of pancreatic cancer.

• **Chronic pancreatitis,** which can be caused by heavy use of alcohol (usually four or more drinks a day), increases risk for pancreatic cancer by about threefold.

• **Personal history of another type of cancer, such as breast or colon cancer or melanoma.**

• **Smoking.** About 25% of all pancreatic cancer cases are associated with smoking.

• **Age.** Most people with pancreatic cancer are diagnosed after age 45.

• **Gender.** Men are slightly more at risk than women.

• **Obesity.** People with a body mass index (BMI) of 30 or more are 20% more likely to develop pancreatic cancer.

• **Workplace exposure to certain chemicals.** Research has found significant links between workplace exposure to chemicals, such as pesticides, asbestos, benzene and chlorinated hydrocarbons, and increased risk for pancreatic cancer.

• **Diet.** Eating a diet high in processed meats and/or red meat has been linked to increased risk for pancreatic cancer. For every 50 g of processed meat consumed daily (roughly the equivalent of one hot dog or four strips of bacon), risk for pancreatic cancer increases by 19%. The increased risk linked to red meat consumption is less significant but also present—especially in men.

Important: An easy-to-use online Pancreatic Cancer Risk Assessment tool (Go to Pan Can.org and search "Risk Assessment Test") can help determine your risk level based on your answers to a few brief questions about your personal and family medical history. You also can work with your own physician to do a thorough family history if you're more comfortable with that approach.

Next Steps

If you have any risk factors for pancreatic cancer that are controllable, take immediate action. For example, stop smoking...reduce or eliminate alcohol if you are a heavy drinker...lose weight if you're overweight...and avoid diabetes or treat it if you've already been diagnosed with this condition.

Meanwhile, if you have a family history of pancreatic cancer, talk to your doctor about getting your DNA examined through germline genetic testing, a blood test that looks for specific hereditary mutations in your cells and can help determine your risk. The cost of germline testing has plummeted in recent years, and there are validated tests that check a panel of gene mutations that can be performed for as little as $250. In individuals with a family history of pancreatic cancer, germline testing is typically covered by insurance.

Guidelines published in 2018 in *Journal of Clinical Oncology* recommend that all patients with pancreatic cancer consider having germline testing. Individuals with a strong family history of pancreatic cancer also are advised to undergo testing and screening.

At the multidisciplinary Pancreatic Cancer Center at the NYU Perlmutter Cancer Center, we found that 15% of pancreatic cancer patients have a germline mutation (also known as a "hereditary mutation") that increased the patient's risk of developing the disease, even if a strong family history wasn't present.

Knowing whether such a hereditary, or germline, mutation is present in a pancreatic cancer patient may change the treatment strategy...and have implications for testing siblings and children who might also be at higher risk.

Genetic counseling will help you understand the test results and decide whether it's appropriate to consider enrolling in a screening program run by specialists in pancreatic cancer. To locate a certified genetics counselor, consult the National Society of Genetic Counselors at NSGC.org.

If an individual is deemed to be high risk, annual imaging of the pancreas is recommended. Two types of tests are used—a pancreatic MRI/MRCP (a special type of MRI)...and an endoscopic ultrasound (EUS).

We usually start with the MRI/MRCP and then check with an EUS the next year, alternating the exams each year. The two tests are complementary and examine the pancreas in slightly different ways. Insurance should cover these tests.

The MRI is noninvasive. With EUS, an upper endoscopy is performed, passing a thin scope down the esophagus into the stomach and the first part of the small intestine after sedation is given (much like a colonoscopy, but no prep is needed). The scope has an ultrasound probe at the end, and the pancreas can be readily visualized, as it is next to the stomach.

Both tests have only very minor risks, but it's important that the screening be done in a multidisciplinary clinic where there's collaboration among various health-care providers, such as genetic counselors, gastroenterologists, pancreatic surgeons, radiologists and social workers as well as a tumor board, where this team of experts, along with oncologists, meets to discuss each patient's unique situation. Pancreatic cancer is a complicated disease, and decision-making in high-risk individuals is best done with an experienced team guiding your care.

Important: Even with a genetic mutation linked to pancreatic cancer, most people will not get the disease. But with an increased risk, it is crucial to know that screening can be an effective strategy to combat pancreatic cancer. I tell my patients, knowledge is power. As we do a better job in identifying individuals at risk, we will be much better positioned to shift the disease from the advanced state to one in which many more patients have easier-to-treat, surgically resectable disease.

With a concerted effort in early detection (and prevention), along with the development of more effective therapies and clinical trial strategies, it is likely that we will see a change in survival in pancreatic cancer patients in the coming years—and it's about time.

This is a rapidly moving field, so ask questions and seek information from doctors who are at the forefront of the research.

Getting the Best Care

The Pancreatic Cancer Action Network (Pan Can.org) is a patient-advocacy group that serves as a resource for finding a high-quality pancreatic cancer center. It's the driving force behind Precision Promise, a multi-center "adaptive" clinical trial initiative that allows multiple novel therapies to be evaluated alongside standard-of-care approaches to speed the development of new treatments.

Other excellent resources: Rolfe Pancreatic Cancer Foundation (RolfeFoundation. org), a nonprofit dedicated to early diagnosis of pancreatic cancer, research that aims to cure the disease and resources for patients and their families…and Project Purple (Project Purple.org), another nonprofit group that funds research to defeat pancreatic cancer and supports patients and their families.

Is Stomach Dysplasia the Same as Cancer?

Stephen Heller, MD, director of gastrointestinal endoscopy, Temple University Hospital, Philadelphia.

Stomach dysplasia is a precancerous condition in which cells in the lining of the stomach develop abnormal changes that can, in rare cases, lead to cancer. In the low-grade condition, it is uncommon for patients to go on to develop stomach cancer. However, in the high-grade condition, the risk increases substantially. Fortunately, though, the rates of stomach cancer have been declining in the US over the past several decades. Gastric cancer is the term doctors use to describe cancer affecting the lining of the stomach. This type of cancer has a five-year survival rate of 31% and causes more than 11,000 deaths in the US each year.

Low-grade stomach dysplasia does not require treatment. However, your doctor will probably want to monitor your condition with upper endoscopy every two to three years. In patients with known dysplasia, the doctor examines the stomach carefully for the presence of ulcers or nodules that could represent precancerous changes. The doctor also takes biopsies from normal-appearing tissue from throughout the stomach and submits these biopsies to a pathologist, who examines the tissue to look for the presence of precancerous cells. If high-grade dysplasia or even early stomach cancer is detected, treatment may include removal of the abnormal area through the endoscope without surgery.

It is unclear how much of a role genetic predisposition plays in the development of stomach dysplasia. It is known, however, that people who have a Helicobacter pylori (H. pylori) stomach infection are at increased risk for stomach dysplasia. These individuals are also at increased risk for gastritis (a condition that may lead to abdominal pain, nausea and vomiting), and they are also at elevated risk for stomach ulcers, which can potentially lead to serious problems such as bleeding or a tear in the stomach lining. Another potential risk factor for stomach dysplasia and cancer is a diet high in salty or cured foods or processed meats containing high levels of nitrates. Obesity, smoking and excessive alcohol intake are also risk factors for stomach cancer.

Anyone can reduce his risk of developing stomach cancer by eating a healthful diet that includes lots of fruits and vegetables (especially vitamin C-rich citrus fruits). Avoiding cured meats and other foods high in nitrates can help lower your risk. Exercise, quitting smoking and drinking alcohol only in moderation also help protect you. Because infection in the stomach with H. pylori is also a risk factor for stomach cancer, individuals with gastritis or stomach ulcers should ask their doctors about getting tested for this infection. If detected, the infection can be treated with a 10- to 14-day course of antibiotics. Several different antibiotics taken together are typically required to cure the infection.

Hidden Toxins Are Everywhere

Joseph Pizzorno, ND, a leading authority on science-based natural and integrative medicine. He founded and served 22 years as president of Bastyr University, the largest fully accredited university of natural medicine in the US, and is treasurer of the board of The Institute for Functional Medicine. He is author of *The Toxin Solution* and 11 other consumer books and textbooks for doctors.

Asbestos…pesticides…tobacco smoke. We do our best to steer clear of these well-known harmful substances.

But what about the toxins we haven't heard of—the ones that can be found in places we'd never suspect? The truth is, toxins are everywhere—in most rugs and paints…cleaning supplies…cosmetics and perfumes…and the fumes from a gas pump. Even most food cans and the ubiquitous pizza box, designed to hold heat and resist stains, pose risks because of chemicals that, in our bodies, alter our hormones and our immune systems.

Recent development: While most of these hidden toxins are feared for their potential to cause cancer, mounting research shows that these substances also increase risk for serious health problems, such as diabetes and asthma—and more mundane ills like fatigue, poor concentration and memory problems.

Only a few hundred of the more than 80,000 chemicals in use in the US have been adequately tested for safety. But if toxins are everywhere, how can you stay safe? The answer is to limit your "toxic load." *Here's how…*

STEP 1: **Eat organic.** A nutritious diet—lots of fruits, vegetables, whole grains, etc.—can prevent disease. But these foods aren't always as healthful as you would imagine.

Modern agriculture depends on synthetic brews of pesticides, fertilizers and herbicides. Many go-to healthy foods have been flagged by the Environmental Working Group for high pesticide levels.

My advice: I strongly advise patients to buy organic foods—both packaged foods and produce. They contain few (or none) of the most harmful chemicals.

If cost is an issue, be sure that you buy the following 12 foods identified by the Environmental Working Group as the most important to purchase as organic—strawberries, spinach, kale, nectarines, apples, grapes, peaches, cherries, pears, tomatoes, celery and potatoes.

STEP 2: **Rid your body of toxins.** Exposure to toxins increases levels of harmful bacteria in the intestines that overload the detoxifying capacity of the liver…decreases levels of beneficial probiotic organisms…and damages the intestinal lining, which allows harmful substances to pass from the gut into the bloodstream—a condition known as "leaky gut." *My advice…**

•**Take a fiber supplement** (such as Metamucil, one to two teaspoons) a half hour before or after meals. Fiber binds to toxins and harmful bacteria to accelerate their excretion in the stools.

•**Recolonize the intestine with the probiotics Lactobacillus and Bifidobacterium to help heal the intestinal walls.** Many brands contain both organisms. Take one capsule, at least one billion colony-forming units (CFUs), three times daily. I advise taking this supplement indefinitely.

STEP 3: **Take a safer painkiller.** People with arthritis or other painful conditions often take daily doses of nonsteroidal anti-inflammatory drugs (NSAIDs), such as *ibuprofen* (Motrin) or *naproxen* (Aleve)…or the pain reliever *acetaminophen* (Tylenol). But all of these drugs can impair the ability of your kidneys to remove toxins from the body.

Other choices: Take a natural pain reliever, such as the herb butterbur. It reduces inflammation and can relieve pain from headaches and other conditions. Curcumin is another excellent anti-inflammatory. Follow label instructions.

STEP 4: **Test your toxin levels.** Your doctor may suggest "target testing" if he/she suspects that you've been exposed to a certain toxin, such as lead in your drinking water. But even if you don't have symptoms (or risk factors), I advise getting a general test for toxins and repeating it every year or two.

One such test is the urinary 8-OHdG, which looks at metabolites that are released when DNA is damaged—a potential sign of elevated toxins. If your results are abnormal, work with your doctor to identify which toxin levels are elevated and their source so you can decrease your exposure as much as possible.

*Before taking any supplement, check with your doctor if you have a chronic medical condition or take medication.

Chapter 4

DIABETES AND BLOOD SUGAR BREAKTHROUGHS

The Secret Food Fix That Stops Diabetes

If you want to avoid diabetes—and who doesn't?—then choosing foods that are low in sugar and fat is probably your mantra. But there's more to the diabetes story.

Exciting research: One of the most effective—but least talked about—ways to protect against diabetes is to load up on antioxidants, those ultra-healthy substances (think vitamins C and E, beta-carotene and others), according to a growing body of scientific evidence. *Why antioxidants are such heavy hitters in preventing this increasingly widespread disease…*

Attacking the Root Cause

No doubt you have heard of antioxidants and their archenemy, free radicals. In healthy numbers, these volatile oxygen molecules roam our bodies performing useful functions such as fighting infection. But in excess numbers, these and other similar molecules can cause all kinds of damage to the body.

• **Enter antioxidants.** These substances, which are found in the highest amounts in certain vegetables and fruits and are natu-

rally produced by the body, keep the rogue oxygen molecules in check. When antioxidants run low, however, the result is oxidative stress, a condition widely known to hasten aging, heart disease and cancer.

What you may not realize: Oxidative stress has also been linked to insulin resistance, a major cause of type 2 diabetes. When insulin resistance develops, it means that the hormone insulin is not working effectively to get glucose (sugar) into the cells of your body to give them energy. This leads to too much sugar in the blood—with the result being diabetes or its precursor, known as prediabetes.

The Antioxidant Fix

If you are concerned about diabetes, you may think that the easiest solution is to take an antioxidant supplement, such as vitamin C. But the latest research shows that's not true.

In fact, research has shown that supplements are of limited or no use to most people struggling with blood sugar control—and may even cause harm. For example, vitamin

---

George L. King, MD, research director and chief scientific officer at Joslin Diabetes Center, and professor of medicine at Harvard Medical School, both in Boston. He is author, with Royce Flippin, of *Reverse Your Diabetes in 12 Weeks* and *The Diabetes Reset.*

C supplements were shown to interfere with the diabetes-fighting benefits of exercise—in part by blocking the body's production of its own natural antioxidants. The solution is as simple as choosing the right foods.

Getting the Right Foods

When choosing foods to help prevent diabetes, you want to load up on those that contain "phase 2 antioxidants," nutrients that stimulate the body's antioxidant defenses by activating a protein called nrf2 (short for nuclear factor erythroid 2-related factor 2). Nrf2 is a powerful switch that can turn on genes inside your cells, triggering the production of natural antioxidants. *Among the best nrf2 boosters…*

• **Cruciferous vegetables** such as broccoli, brussels sprouts, cauliflower and cabbage contain high levels of sulforaphane, a potent phase 2 antioxidant.

Goal: Two or more cups daily.

• **Blueberries** contain high levels of pterostilbene, an effective nrf2 activator.

Goal: One cup daily.

• **Fatty fish.** Salmon, tuna, sardines, mackerel and herring contain omega-3 fatty acids that boost nrf2.

Goal: Eat fatty fish (3 to 4 ounces per serving) three times a week.

• **Green tea** contains a wide array of antioxidants and stimulates nrf2 activity. Replace soda and juice with green tea.

Goal: Two to three cups daily.

• **Curcumin.** The active ingredient in the Indian spice turmeric is a powerful nrf2 stimulator that also has anti-inflammatory effects.

Goal: Season with curcumin instead of salt.

A Diet That Works

What does an antidiabetes diet look like? One version of this eating style is the Rural Asian Diet, developed at the Joslin Diabetes Center. The overall mix calls for 70% complex carbs (such as vegetables and whole grains)…15% fat…and 15% protein, including at least 15 g of fiber for every 1,000 calories.

Important: When it comes to limiting oxidative stress, don't forget to also exercise regularly…reduce stress…stop smoking…and get plenty of sleep.

Migraines Can Lower Diabetes Risk

Migraines may have protective effects. The intense headaches have been linked to stroke, heart attack and psychiatric disorders.

But they also seem to have some positive impact: Women with active migraines were 20% to 30% less likely to develop type 2 diabetes during a 10-year study than women with no history of migraine. And if their migraine status improved, their risk for diabetes went up.

Guy Fagherazzi, PhD, senior research scientist of diabetes epidemiology, Center of Research in Epidemiology and Population Health, University of Paris-Saclay, France, and corresponding author of a study of more than 74,000 women, published in *JAMA Neurology.*

Filtered Coffee Helps Prevent Type 2 Diabetes

An analysis of specific blood metabolites showed that people who drank two to three cups of filtered coffee daily had 60% lower diabetes risk than those having less than one cup. The study did not test French press, espresso or pods.

Rikard Landberg, PhD, professor of food science at Chalmers University of Technology, Gothenburg, Sweden, and principal investigator of the study published in *Journal of Internal Medicine.*

Seniors with Diabetes May Be in the "Danger Zone" and Not Know It

Anders L. Carlson, MD, medical director, International Diabetes Center, director, HealthPartners diabetes program, and assistant professor, University of Minnesota Medical School, Minneapolis. Research presented at The Endocrine Society Annual Meeting 2019 by the International Diabetes Center in Minneapolis.

The constant high blood sugar of diabetes damages the body, harms your health and, in the long term, shortens lives. But blood sugar that's too low is also dangerous—and can cut life short more quickly. A new study now finds that seniors being treated for type 1 diabetes may be spending more than an hour daily with low blood sugar levels—and a significant part of that time with levels low enough to put them at risk for loss of consciousness, seizures… and even death.

Researchers from 22 sites across the US that are part of the T1D Exchange tracked glucose levels in 203 patients age 60 and older with type 1 diabetes for 21 days. The patients wore a continuous glucose monitor (CGM) to record their glucose levels around the clock.

Results: On average, patients were within a healthy blood glucose target range—defined as 70 md/dL to 180 mg/dL for at least 70% of the day—for only 57% of the day (about 13.4 hours). The rest of the time was spent in a state of hyperglycemia (high blood sugar) or hypoglycemia (low blood sugar). Of particular concern was that many spent about half an hour daily with blood sugar levels low enough to be dangerous. Worse, many of the patients in the study who experienced hypoglycemia did not recognize the warning signs.

Hypoglycemia can cause falls, loss of consciousness, seizures and even death if not treated. Warning signs to look for include blurred vision, confusion, slurred speech, numbness, sweating and shaking, poor coordination, dizziness or feeling light-headed, difficulty concentrating, feeling anxious or irritable, hunger or nausea and erratic changes in behavior. People with diabetes, especially those at risk for hypoglycemia, are educated about the symptoms. However, the symptoms can be mistaken for other health issues—which can mean that hypoglycemia does not get treated.

Most people with diabetes are able to recognize early symptoms and know that they need to eat a glucose snack—such as a sugar tablet or a glass of juice. If they experience severe hypoglycemia, they may need another person to inject them with the hormone *glucagon*, which raises blood sugar levels. However, many people with diabetes do not know that using insulin, especially for many years, and also having previous episodes of hypoglycemia can cause desensitization to hypoglycemia warning signs, a condition called hypoglycemia unawareness.

Hypoglycemia unawareness is most common among people with type 1 diabetes—an estimated 40% may have the condition. But it can also affect people with type 2 diabetes. Hypoglycemia unawareness increases the risk of slipping into the hypoglycemic danger zone, becoming too confused to eat a sugary snack by themselves…or passing out. In the current study, patients who spent the most time daily with low blood sugar were hypoglycemia unaware.

Self-Protection If You Have Diabetes

If you are an older person with diabetes on insulin…

•**If you are aware of experiencing periods of hypoglycemia, don't ignore them… and let your doctor know.** You may be in the danger zone more often than you realize and may need to take additional steps to better control your blood sugar.

Likely periods of increased risk: At night while you're asleep…before lunch…after drinking alcohol…and after exercise.

• **If you find that you don't always realize when your blood sugar is low (hypoglycemic unawareness),** make family members and/or coworkers aware of the signs of hypoglycemia—and, if necessary, alert them that they may need to inject you with glucagon if you aren't able to. (It's a good idea to always carry a glucagon kit if you take insulin.)

Note: Avoiding hypoglycemia for up to four weeks can restore hypoglycemia awareness.

• **If blood sugar control continues to be problematic,** talk to your doctor about getting a continuous glucose monitoring system (CGM). A CGM sets off an alarm when glucose gets too low (or too high)…and also tracks periods of hypoglycemia and hyperglycemia so that you can tell how well you're doing.

Got Diabetes? Here's How to Do a Better Job of Tracking Your Glucose

Marwan Hamaty, MD, MBA, a board-certified specialist in endocrinology, diabetes and metabolism. Dr. Hamaty practices at the Cleveland Clinic Diabetes Center. His research has been published in leading medical journals, including *International Journal of Experimental Diabetes Research.*

C ontinuous glucose monitoring is more precise than A1C and reduces finger sticks by at least 90%.

If you have diabetes, your blood sugar (glucose) levels tend to change throughout the day. Even when you monitor your glucose often enough (typically four to five times a day), you are getting only a small portion of the whole picture.

Fortunately, a technological advancement known as continuous glucose monitoring (CGM) is now changing that.

What's more, a growing body of evidence shows that this high-tech system is poised to eclipse standard hemoglobin A1C testing, commonly known as A1C, as the gold standard for managing glucose levels.

If you or someone you love uses insulin to treat diabetes and is not using CGM, it could be time to take the plunge.

What Is CGM?

CGM relies on a tiny sensor that you insert yourself into the skin of your upper arm or belly and leave in place for several days. Because the sensor uses a tiny needle, the process is virtually painless.

The sensor continuously measures glucose in the thin layer of fluid that surrounds the cells beneath your skin—called interstitial fluid—and wirelessly sends the results to a monitor or a smartphone to record your glucose levels 24 hours a day. Results are displayed every few minutes. Retrospective data is also available to detect trends in your glucose levels.

A CGM device helps you and your doctor create a daily diabetes management plan. It could reduce the frequency (or take the place) of using a glucometer to measure your blood levels of glucose to determine your insulin needs.

CGM reduces the number of finger sticks typically needed to use a glucometer and test strips by 90%—or by close to 100% for some of the latest devices. The specifics vary among CGM devices, so be sure to discuss these details with your diabetes educator or medical provider.

An important feature of CGM devices is that they allow the information to be shared with others—for example, parents can monitor a child or adults can track how well elderly parents are controlling their diabetes.

Note: Your doctor may use a professional CGM device to see how well you're managing your diabetes. You might wear the monitor for days or weeks while trends in your glucose levels are stored in the sensor/device and can be downloaded to your doctor's computer. People with type 2 diabetes can benefit from this type of periodic monitoring even if they do not need insulin.

Beyond the A1C test

Since the 1980s, the A1C test has been uniformly used to monitor glucose levels. This simple and inexpensive blood test tells you and your doctor your average blood sugar over an eight- to 12-week period. The A1C test, which usually is performed in a doctor's office or lab, does this by measuring the percentage of your red blood cells carrying glucose.

For your glucose management to be effective in preventing complications, most diabetes guidelines recommend an A1C of 7% or less when possible. This goal needs to be personalized to each patient's circumstances, and it changes over time.

It helps to think of your A1C as a baseball batting average. It tells you how well you are hitting, but it does not tell you when you are getting lots of hits or when you are in a slump. These ups and downs are called glycemic variability.

That's where CGM shines. It shows your real-time highs and lows as well as your trends (and averages) over time. Studies show that people with diabetes who use CGM have improved A1C levels and less glycemic variability.

Why is that important? Research shows that the time you spend in hyperglycemia (glucose levels above 180 mg/dL two hours after eating) is directly related to your risk for diabetes complications, such as heart disease and stroke.

CGM also shows the time you spend in hypoglycemia (glucose below 70 mg/dL). That can be particularly useful if you have hypoglycemia at night or if you don't get warning signs of the condition, such as shakiness, dizziness and hunger.

Unrecognized hypoglycemia can progress to a dangerously low glucose level (below 50 mg/dL), which can cause confusion, heart-rhythm irregularities, blurred vision, accidents, loss of consciousness, seizures and even death.

A1C also has other weaknesses. Aiming for a reading of 7% or less does not fit everyone. This is especially true for older people who have a naturally higher A1C because they have fewer red blood cells. Forcing these individuals to lower their A1C to 7% or less can increase their risk for hypoglycemia. Additionally, when a person has anemia or other abnormalities of red blood cells, A1C may not accurately estimate the glucose average.

Who Benefits Most from CGM?

CGM, which is prescribed by a physician, is for people with type 1 diabetes or those with type 2 diabetes who use multiple daily injections of insulin. The device typically is best for those who require frequent finger sticks (at least four times daily) to control their glucose levels.

CGM can be especially beneficial for people who unknowingly experience hypoglycemia. Certain devices will warn you of a hypoglycemic trend, and some models will send you and family members a warning alarm if you dip into the danger zone.

If you use an insulin pump, you should consider a CGM device that is compatible with your insulin pump. Some CGM models and insulin pumps are integrated. Insulin delivery by the insulin pump could be automatically adjusted to prevent or reduce your chances of hypoglycemia.

When using a CGM device, you'll see in real time how your diet, activities and stress levels affect your glucose levels. With your doctor's help, you will learn how to anticipate these trends and tweak your insulin use to address them.

Getting Started with CGM

If you're interested in trying a CGM device, talk to your doctor and your diabetes educator. If they think that you'd benefit, there are many different devices on the market.

Some have more bells and whistles, such as alarms for high and low glucose levels… graphs you can download onto your computer or smartphone…and some even are connected to an insulin pump that gives you a glucose reading to use for a programmed

71

dose of insulin for your meal or to correct a high glucose level.

Not surprisingly, CGM can be pricey. Your doctor or diabetes educator can help you select the best model for your needs.* If you go with a basic CGM system and meet the required criteria, it often is covered by insurance. The out-of-pocket cost to use it may not be much more than what you would be paying for a glucometer and your test strips.

Most CGM devices still require a few finger sticks to ensure that they are accurately reflecting your glucose levels. This is called calibration. Depending on the device you choose, you may need to calibrate occasionally or every day.

Important: There is about a 15-minute delay for glucose changes in your blood (as measured by a finger stick) to show up in interstitial fluid (as measured by CGM). In certain situations, you may need to do a finger stick before making any insulin dose changes based on just your CGM. (Your doctor or diabetes educator can advise you on managing special circumstances and what's best for you.)

Once you start using CGM, the data stored on your monitor will help your doctor recommend the timing and dose you should take of a longer-acting or shorter-acting insulin…or adjust the pump setting if you're using an insulin pump.

Your job will be to follow your doctor's insulin directions and to use your readings to make any necessary adjustments to your meals and activity levels.

*To find a diabetes educator near you, go to the National Certification Board for Diabetes Care and Education at CBDCE.org.

Another Reason to Eat Real Food

A common food preservative may trigger metabolic changes linked to obesity and diabetes. In new mouse and human studies, propionate—an additive used widely in processed bread, baked goods and cheeses, among other foods—triggered complex hormonal changes that raised blood sugar and insulin levels. Mice fed regular doses for 20 weeks gained weight and became insulin-resistant—a characteristic of type 2 diabetes. Eating less cheese and processed food, including bread, will minimize exposure to propionate.

Amir Tirosh, MD, PhD, is director, division of endocrinology, at Israel's Sheba Medical Center, Tel-Aviv, and lead author of a study published in *Science Translational Medicine.*

Vinegar Can Do Wonders for Your Blood Sugar

Carol Johnston, RD, PhD, professor and assistant director of the School of Nutrition and Health Promotion at Arizona State University, Phoenix. Dr. Johnston has published various papers on the medical use of vinegar in leading medical journals.

A pple cider vinegar is a classic home remedy with traditional uses ranging from reducing age spots to easing arthritis. Only one use is scientifically proven—vinegar has a specific effect on blood sugar that is beneficial for anyone with diabetes or prediabetes. *Here's what you need to know…*

●**The scientific evidence of vinegar's blood sugar benefits is strong and consistent.** A recent statistical analysis of the 11 best studies concluded that consuming vinegar with a meal, compared with having the same meal without vinegar, reduced postmeal blood sugar spikes by an average of 40%.

Why this matters: Much of the metabolic damage caused by diabetes—and prediabetes—is caused by these spikes.

●**Any vinegar works.** Sorry, apple cider vinegar enthusiasts. It's the acetic acid—in every vinegar—that blocks absorption of carbohydrates and helps clear blood sugar from the bloodstream.

- **Raw vinegar is best.** Cooking can break down acetic acid.

- **You don't need much.** Studies suggest that two tablespoons of vinegar is a good "dose." Less isn't as effective—and more doesn't add any benefit.

- **Timing matters.** For the best effect on blood sugar, consume vinegar at or near the start of a meal.

- **Consider a premeal drink.** For the most reliable effect, dilute two tablespoons of vinegar in a glass of water and drink it with the first bites of the meal. You can sweeten it with a non-nutritive sweetener such as stevia. Or try a commercial flavored apple-cider-vinegar drink made by Bragg.

- **Make your own vinaigrette if you'd rather incorporate vinegar into a salad or vegetable dish (after the vegetables are cooked).** Why? Store-bought vinaigrettes often have more oil than vinegar. Mix your own using two parts vinegar to one part oil. Try red wine vinegar—it delivers acetic acid plus a healthy dose of cell-protecting polyphenols. Mustard counts, too—most mustards are rich in vinegar.

- **Start your next meal with a dish dressed with vinegar.** And while you don't want to be eating a lot of bread, if you do have a slice, instead of slathering it in butter, dip it in vinaigrette.

Diabetes and Depression

People with diabetes are up to three times more likely to have depression than those without the disease—and more than half go undiagnosed.

New finding: Taking an antidepressant reduced death rates by 35% in those with depression and diabetes, according to a 13-year study of more than 53,000 people.

Theory: Treating depression increases adherence to diabetes treatment.

Vincent Chin-Hung Chen, PhD, professor of psychiatry, Chang Gung University, Taoyuan, Taiwan.

Diabetes Fasting Alert

Doctors usually ask patients to fast before a blood cholesterol test.

Recent study: Nearly 20% of 525 people with diabetes experienced fasting-induced hypoglycemia (dangerously low blood-sugar levels) when they stopped eating for the recommended eight to 12 hours before a cholesterol test. The resulting dizziness and confusion are particularly dangerous when patients drive themselves to the clinic.

Also: New research suggests that eating before the test will not affect results. Discuss these findings with your doctor if you have diabetes and are told to fast.

Saleh Aldasouqi, MD, professor of medicine and chief of endocrinology, Michigan State University, East Lansing.

Ouch-Less Insulin!

People with type 2 diabetes may soon be able to forgo insulin shots.

In development: A blueberry-size oral capsule, which contains a single needle made of compressed, freeze-dried insulin that is injected into the stomach wall after it's swallowed. It appears to lower blood sugar as effectively as shots.

Massachusetts Institute of Technology

Insole May Heal Foot Ulcers

The insole, worn within a total-contact cast, contains reservoirs of oxygen to help foot ulcers heal better and faster. Each must be custom-made. The design is experimental, and it is not yet clear how much an insole will cost.

Study by researchers at Purdue University, West Lafayette, Indiana, published in *Materials Research Society Communications*.

Diabetes Medications Linked to Dangerous Cancer

Study titled "Incretin Based Drugs and Risk of Cholangiocarcinoma Among Patients with Type 2 Diabetes: Population-Based Cohort Study" led by researchers at McGill University in Canada and published in *The BMJ*.

It's hard to miss all the ads for the diabetes medications called incretin drugs (you probably know them better as Januvia, Trulicity and Victoza, among others). They promise better blood sugar control, but they may come at a potentially steep price—cancer.

Incretins are naturally occurring hormones produced in the gut in response to food. They help stimulate the production of insulin and lower blood sugar. For people with type 2 diabetes, incretin diabetes medications enhance the action of these hormones. One type of incretin drug, glucagon-like peptide-1 (GLP-1) receptor agonists such as *liraglutide* (Victoza) and *dulaglutide* (Trulicity), directly stimulate the production of these hormones. Another type, dipeptidyl peptidase-4 (DPP-4) inhibitors including *sitagliptin* (Januvia) and *saxagliptin* (Onglyza), prolong the hormones' effects.

Although these drugs benefit many people with type 2 diabetes, two early studies have suggested that they may increase the risk for a serious bile duct cancer called cholangiocarcinoma. An international team of researchers collaborated on a new, larger study to learn more about this risk—how common the bile duct cancers are among people on diabetes drugs and whether patients on incretin drugs were at higher risk for them than patients on other types of diabetes medications.

They used the Clinical Practice Research Datalink from the UK to follow more than 150,000 type 2 diabetes patients, ages 40 and over, for five years on average. Patients in the study were being treated with a DPP-4 inhibitor (21%), a GLP-1 agonist (4%) or one of seven other drugs, including insulin. (Patients with existing risk factors for bile duct cancer, such as HIV/AIDS or any gall bladder or liver disease, were excluded.)

Over the course of the study, 105 cases of bile duct cancer were diagnosed. Patients taking either a DPP-4 or a GLP-1 had double the risk for bile duct cancer compared with patients taking other drugs. However, because so few patients were taking a GLP-1 drug, the findings are not considered as significant as those for the DPP-4 drug. The overall risk for bile duct cancer was still very low—well under 1%, but because bile duct cancer is a disease with a high fatality rate, the researchers concluded that alerting the public and the medical community to the risk is important, along with urging more research.

Two possible causes are suspected for the increased cancer risk. Incretin drugs may stimulate overproduction of bile duct cells, which may start to grow out of control. Incretins also increase the risk for gallstones and inflammation, which may, in turn, increase the cancer risk.

If you're on an incretin drug or your doctor suggests starting one, have a discussion about all the risks and benefits. Along with lifestyle changes, there are many other treatment options for type 2 diabetes. Especially if you're already at higher risk for bile duct cancer because of a history of gall bladder or liver disease, an alternative to these drugs may be better for you.

Statins Users at High Risk for Diabetes

Patients prescribed statins for high cholesterol had at least double the risk of developing type 2 diabetes compared with people who did not take the drugs, according to a study of more than 4,500 men and women.

Theory: Statins cause metabolic changes and insulin resistance that can lead to diabetes.

If you take a statin: Exercise, eat a healthy diet and see your doctor regularly.

Victoria A. Zigmont, PhD, MPH, assistant professor of public health, Southern Connecticut State University, New Haven.

Why Is Low Blood Sugar So Dangerous for People with Diabetes?

Gerald Bernstein, MD, internist and endocrinologist, program director, Friedman Diabetes Program, Lenox Hill Hospital, New York City

---

If you have type 2 diabetes, you hear a lot about how important it is to keep your blood sugar from getting too high. But you also have to keep it from falling too low, a condition known as hypoglycemia. Hypoglycemia is dangerous—and can be fatal.

If you experience low blood sugar, you'll quickly learn to recognize the signs. That's because your body jumps into action when blood sugar gets low—and triggers symptoms. In very simple terms, it can be said that the whole goal of the body is to provide glucose—that is, sugar—to the brain. Glucose, which comes from the food you eat and is also produced in the liver, is the brain's only fuel.

When the supply runs low, the brain protects itself by triggering a system of hormones, including adrenaline, cortisol and glucagon, to drive the liver to make more. For most people with diabetes, an adrenaline reaction (shaking, sweating, agitation) is the first sign that their blood glucose—often referred to as "blood sugar"—is falling. Usually, they learn to recognize these signs very early and know to eat something with glucose or sugar. The body maintains the blood glucose level within a very narrow range that can be affected by many things, such as exercising without eating, even if you don't have diabetes.

When Low Blood Sugar Is Dangerous

If you forget to eat and you feel shaky because your blood sugar has dipped and then feel better after eating a small snack—that's nothing to worry about. As you learn to manage your diabetes, you'll learn how to avoid even mild low-blood-sugar episodes, especially if you also use frequent finger-stick tests to check your blood sugar.

But if blood sugar is not brought back up and the brain continues to be deprived of glucose, severe hypoglycemia results. Signs that this is happening include erratic behavior, difficulty speaking or slurred speech, confusion, convulsions—and eventually coma and death. This kind of hypoglycemia lands you in the emergency room.

When severe hypoglycemia occurs, it typically is brought on by diabetes medication. While some medications do not contribute to low blood sugar, insulin and sulphonylureas do. If you take either of these types of medications, keep glucose supplements, such as the gels or tablets available in the diabetic sections of drugstores, handy. (If you have any questions about what medications you are taking and whether there is a hypoglycemia risk, ask your doctor or your diabetes educator.)

It used to be thought that once such an episode was resolved and blood sugar was normalized again, there was nothing further to be concerned about other than to not let it happen again. But a new study from Johns Hopkins Bloomberg School of Public Health has found that having even a single episode of severe hypoglycemia raises risk for heart disease, stroke and death. The cause-and-effect isn't clear here—the researchers speculated that perhaps the increased risk could be because the people who are prone to severe hypoglycemia might be sicker in the first place. But these episodes are clearly something that you want to avoid. Again, frequent finger-stick tests can help you confirm that your blood sugar has fallen out of the healthy range.

Remember that the goal of diabetes treatment is blood glucose control and preventing complications. Achieving that depends on balancing your lifestyle, what you eat and any medications that you take, plus managing any other health conditions. Avoiding hypoglycemia, especially severe hypoglycemia, is a key goal.

Are You Addicted to Sugar?

Kathleen DesMaisons, PhD, an expert in addictive nutrition and author of an updated edition of Potatoes Not Prozac: Simple Solutions for Sugar Addiction. *She is based in Albuquerque, New Mexico, and is founder of Radiant Recovery, RadiantRecovery.com, an online community for people dealing with sugar sensitivity.*

Here's a little test: Imagine that you have just had a big lunch. You are not remotely hungry but when you come home, you find a plate of warm chocolate chip cookies, smelling delicious, on the kitchen counter. No one else is around. Do you dive into those cookies?

If you answer yes, and can't imagine why anyone would say no, you may be a sugar addict—a biochemical problem that can set the stage not only for unhealthy weight gain, but also for depression, mood swings and impulsive behavior.

To learn more, we spoke with Kathleen DesMaisons, PhD, who has spent several decades helping people with out-of-control sugar cravings.

The Roots of Sugar Addiction

There's a growing scientific consensus that too much sugar is a leading cause of America's biggest health problems, from obesity to heart disease and diabetes. But not everyone appears to have the same risk. Why?

According to theories of "addictive nutrition," some people are more sensitive than others to the brain-altering effects of sugar. People who are affected by "sugar sensitivity" are believed to have a genetic makeup that makes them especially vulnerable to the blood sugar swings that can happen after eating sweets, white bread, white pasta and other highly processed carbohydrates. The roller coaster is both emotional and physical.

But that's not all. According to this theory, you also may have chronically low levels of two key brain chemicals—serotonin and beta-endorphin. Serotonin helps regulate mood and self-control. Beta-endorphin is the body's natural opioid, capable of blunting both physical and mental pain.

Low levels of these two brain chemicals can leave you reeling, living from one soda or bowl of ice cream to the next to get your feel-good boost—and then crashing with feelings of sadness, anger and self-loathing. When you do resist your cravings, you are consumed with thoughts of your next sweet fix.

There's no blood test or formal diagnostic process to identify sugar sensitivity—and it's not the same as diabetes, which is a disease marked by high blood sugar (glucose) levels.

But if you have an insatiable sweet tooth…a history of depression…and/or past or current abuse of alcohol or drugs, sugar sensitivity may be a contributing factor.

To Tame Sugar Addiction

To help you get off this roller coaster, here's Dr. DesMaisons' seven-step plan…

STEP #1: Eat breakfast. You've heard it before…breakfast is important—but what you eat is the key. You want to avoid starting the day with a blood sugar crash, followed by a donut rescue. Even if you think you hate breakfast or don't have time, eat within one hour of getting up.

To help keep your blood sugar levels stable, don't eat just anything—build your breakfast around protein (eggs are fine, but so are beans, cottage cheese, tofu, nut butters or last night's turkey breast). You should also eat some complex carbohydrates (such as oatmeal, whole-grain toast or brown rice).

Key advice: Get one-third of your daily protein at breakfast. Aim for a half gram of protein for each pound you weigh. For example, a 150-pound person would aim for 75 g a day with 25 g being consumed at breakfast. That's roughly the amount in two eggs, two tablespoons of peanut butter and a cup of oatmeal.

Caution: If you have chronic kidney disease, speak to your doctor about your protein intake—too much can be hard on your kidneys.

Important: Be sure to master this step before moving on—even if it takes months. Take the same step-by-step approach as you go.

STEP #2: **Start a food journal.** Write down everything you eat, with dates and times. Also, your food journal should include how you are feeling physically and emotionally at any time of the day that you notice a shift. For example, you may note that you get tired every day around 2 pm when you eat a heavy lunch. The idea is to notice patterns, not beat yourself up. Use the food diary as an ongoing tool.

STEP #3: **Get enough protein at each meal.** Once you've mastered breakfast, do the same with lunch and dinner. At each meal, get one-third of the daily amount of protein you need.

Why the focus on protein? Protein not only helps stabilize blood sugar, it's also a key source of tryptophan, an amino acid your body uses to make serotonin—as mentioned earlier, the brain chemical that increases impulse control and feelings of well-being. You probably know that turkey is a good source of tryptophan, but tuna, tofu, salmon and kidney beans are as well.

Also important: To avoid blood sugar crashes, space your meals no more than six hours apart, except overnight. Ideally, you will only eat at mealtime—because that teaches you how to start and stop eating—in-

stead of grazing all day. But some people, including pregnant women and those with physically demanding jobs, need snacks.

Good choices: An apple and some cheese… or a handful of almonds and a pear.

And if you feel you need a sweet dessert, eat it right after your meal to temper the effects of the sugar. Be reasonable with dessert and don't obsess about it. Focusing on your meals rather than sweets will naturally help quiet your cravings.

STEP #4: **Try vitamins and…a nightly potato.** You should get most of your nutrients from food, but vitamin C, B-complex and zinc supplements may help balance your brain and body chemistry. Discuss this with your health-care provider.

The most surprising part of the plan—a nightly potato with the skin—has a specific purpose. The idea is to end your day with a complex carbohydrate that will raise your serotonin levels. Complex carbohydrates do this by triggering the gradual release of insulin, which, in turn, enables tryptophan to travel from the bloodstream to the brain and produce serotonin.

A potato (with a little butter, if you like) fits the bill. It can be a small red potato, a medium Yukon Gold or even a sweet potato, roasted, boiled or baked. The skin has fiber which helps curb the potato's effect on your glucose levels. Take it like medicine, three hours after dinner.

Note: If you have diabetes, consult your doctor before following this advice.

STEP #5: **Go from white to brown.** Instead of white rice and white bread, opt for brown rice and whole-grain bread. Veggies (including greens) are good, too, as well as whole grains.

STEP #6: **Cut out added sugar.** Start by saying no to cake, cookies, candy, sweet drinks and processed foods full of sugar. This might sound hard, but since it comes later in the plan, you will be shocked at what a nonevent it is.

Helpful: Don't forget to read food labels since many food products you wouldn't expect contain added sugar.

Key advice: Whole fruit, which contains natural sugars, is fine, but don't overdo it with high-sugar fruit, such as bananas, raisins or figs.

STEP #7: Get in touch with your feelings. Once you're off the sugar roller coaster, it's common to experience emotions that have been masked by your use of sugar. To better understand these new feelings, consider self-help approaches, including guided imagery or meditation, and/or talk therapy.

This plan will remove your cravings. Beyond that, use it as a life skill rather than a diet.

Chapter 5

EMOTIONAL RESCUE

Case Study: Solving the Puzzle of Sudden-Onset Depression

The patient: "Maile," a 35-year-old hotel concierge.

Why she came to see me: I had met Maile years before when she accompanied her mother to my health center, but the woman who walked into my office was hardly recognizable as the same person. Gone were the stylish clothes, the bright smile and the engaged, curious demeanor; in their place stood a disheveled, rather gaunt woman who had trouble meeting my eyes.

With some persuading, Maile revealed the following: Roughly a year earlier, she'd begun experiencing bouts of sadness that had fast-tracked from periodical to persistent. As she put it, she went from a high-functioning, organized, happ and involved woman to someone who felt "robbed of all the glitter that life held."

After missing several days of work, she'd gone to see her primary care physician at her employer's request. Maile's PCP referred her to a psychiatrist, who promptly diagnosed her with depression and prescribed Paxil.

When that failed to work, she'd shifted Maile to Zoloft. The results with both were minimal at best, and before attempting a new antidepressant or other forms of treatment, Maile wanted to explore natural options for relief. Moreover, she wanted to get to the root of her sudden, inexplicable depression.

How I evaluated her: Over the course of a lengthy discussion, it became clear that Maile's "melancholy," as she worded it, had no definable source. Her mother was now in good health, and, up until a year prior, she'd "loved" her job as a concierge at one of the hottest hotels in Waikiki, had been happily dating a restaurant manager, and had moved into an adorable, older house she kept busy decorating.

Then, out of nowhere, life turned flat. Her diet had not changed, nor her lifestyle, and yet the blues that arrived were, she said, "of the darkest sort." Her job became pure drudgery, her friends suddenly irritated her and her romantic relationship ended because she couldn't "summon enough energy for anything he suggested." Indeed, few things

Laurie Steelsmith, ND, LAc, medical director of Steelsmith Natural Health Center in Honolulu, where she has a busy private practice, and associate clinical professor at Bastyr University, America's leading center for the study of natural medicine. DrSteelsmith.com

seemed to interest her—even running on the beach, which she'd relished since she was a teenager. Away from her work, she remained isolated inside her home, doing "nothing of note." In addition to depression, she was experiencing stabbing headaches that came on suddenly—this too from an indefinable source—joint pain, muscle aches, fatigue, insomnia and inadvertent weight loss. While neither she nor her closest family members had a history of depression, she'd accepted her psychiatrist's diagnosis and took her advice to go on a SSRI, take up meditation, and go into cognitive behavioral therapy. Nothing seemed to work, however, and something inside of Maile said that something more—something physical—was amiss.

The more I inquired about Maile's medical history and personal life, the more she opened up. She came from a big, loving family and had always been healthy. Her fairly new home, she added, was located in Kaneohe.

Upon hearing this, I asked her if she'd noticed any mold in her home, as Kaneohe is situated on the Windward Side of Oahu—a region of the island that typically experiences rain or mist most days. "Now that you mention it," she said, after pausing for a moment, "I have. But it's an old house, so it's to be expected. And it's not a big deal, right?"

While I neither agreed nor disagreed, I did conduct a battery of tests to check my theory. First, I performed a full physical. Then I ordered a urine test called a MycoTOX Profile (to look for mold toxins) through The Great Plains Laboratory, Inc. I ordered a blood test to evaluate her hormone levels, as hormone imbalances can place a woman at a higher risk for depression. Lastly, I ordered a separate blood test to assess her reactions to certain antibodies in her immune system.

What my evaluation revealed: Maile's hormone test revealed what I had anticipated—they were normal for her age, even healthy. (My feeling was that she was still several years away from transitioning into menopause, when women are more vulnerable to depression.)

And yet, the question lingered…why was she depressed? While depression affects more females than males—approximately 25% of women will experience depression at some point in their lives—the illness, which can be debilitating, tends to present in one's 20s or younger. To have it appear seemingly out of nowhere at Maile's age was disconcerting.

Not for long, though: The results from her urine test and second blood test came in, and revealed that she had high levels of mold toxins in her system, and that her exposure to mold had caused a chronic inflammatory response that was impacting her brain and leading to the litany of symptoms from which she was suffering.

As I explained to Maile, molds are pervasive, toxic microorganisms that have a wide variety of species. Mold spores, which can be spread through water, insects, and air, "are found year-round both indoors and out, and survive and multiply most readily in warm, damp, shady, and humid conditions," *ABC News* reports—and Hawai'i is nothing if not humid. While mold can usually be scrubbed away, a grave mold condition can build and worsen when, say, there's serious water damage to a home—such as the older home Maile was reportedly in, on one of the rainiest parts of the island.

Generally, we associate damp, moldy homes with respiratory problems (in what's known as a mold allergy) but mounting research demonstrates that mold can also trigger depression. As psychiatrist Judy Tsafrir, MD, wrote at PsychologyToday.com, "Toxic mold based illness is a very prevalent and underdiagnosed condition that can manifest in many different ways, including with symptoms that are exclusively psychiatric, such as depression, anxiety, attentional problems, brain fog and insomnia." As she also noted, "Vulnerability to mold toxicity is only present in 25% of the population, who in most cases, have a genetic predisposition which inhibits their clearance of biotoxins." In other words, Maile's former boyfriend—who often stayed the night—didn't experience a sensitivity to the mold in her home, while Maile had an inborn vulnerability to it. The good news in all this? It was eminently treatable.

How I addressed her problem: To help Maile get her brain and body—and life— back on track, we discussed her living situation. She loved the home she was renting, but its mold was wreaking havoc on every domain of her life—her career, her relationships and, perhaps most importantly, her relationship with herself. I asked her to alert her landlords immediately and if the mold could not be eradicated, to begin searching for a different residence.

To mitigate her symptoms, I suggested she adhere to what's known as the "Shoemaker Protocol." Developed by Richie C. Shoemaker, MD—a family practice physician and author of *Mold Warriors: Fighting America's Hidden Health Threat*—the treatment requires taking nine grams of cholestyramine four times a day—a medication that binds biotoxins in the small intestine, which is then excreted in the stool. Additionally, I recommended she begin taking a broad spectrum probiotic to reestablish healthy bacteria in her gut, which would help "crowd out" the unfriendly bacteria and fungi that could be contributing to her systemic inflammation. *I also suggested she begin taking…*

• **Fish oil**—an excellent source of omega 3s that play a vital role in brain function and can positively impact mood and depression.

• **Intravenous glutathione,** a nutrient that is a potent antioxidant that can decrease systemic inflammation especially in the brain and nervous system. In addition, she took supplements to promote her own glutathione production including selenium (200 mcg), lipoic acid (600 mg), and n-acetyl cysteine (also known as NAC), 1,000 mg a day.

• **Magnesium (500 mg a day),** as research points to its ability to reduce depressive symptoms.

The patient's progress: After eight weeks of treatment, Maile returned to my office looking like the girl I'd known years before: Radiant, sparkling and energetic. The cholestyramine had made her slightly nauseous at first, but the side effects vanished within three days. At the end of the two-week cycle I prescribed, she felt "more alive" than she had in months.

She had relocated to a condo that was not only closer to her work but also closer to the ocean, which allowed her the chance to run on the beach on a daily basis. Best part yet? It was well-lit and well-ventilated, which seemed to lift her spirits even more. So much so, in fact, that work had become enjoyable again and the restaurant manager had invited her on a hike. This time, she was more than ready to join him.

Take Charge of Your Therapy Session

Ryan Howes, PhD, licensed clinical psychologist in private practice in Pasadena, California. He provides psychotherapy for adult individuals and couples. Howes writes the blog "In Therapy: A User's Guide to Psychotherapy" for *Psychology Today* and writes the "Point of View" column for *Psychotherapy Networker* magazine.

Many people enter therapy with the wrong expectations, the wrong attitude and even the wrong therapist— any of which can result in an unproductive, frustrating or disappointing experience. But you can make it a positive experience if you approach it the right way. Think of it as enrolling in a course where you are the subject matter—if you're curious, teachable and motivated, it can be one of the most rewarding classes you ever take.

Find the Right Fit

• **Take inventory of your symptoms.** Is anxiety keeping you up at night? Are you fighting with your partner? Maybe you've experienced a trauma that you can't seem to put behind you? If you've got a specific issue, look for a therapist who specializes in it—whether it's weight loss or post-traumatic stress disorder. Search for names at PsychologyToday.com or GoodTherapy.org.

Note: Think about gender preferences. If your issue is not gender-related, such as fear of flying, it won't matter. But if your issue is a controlling mother, then you might prefer a male therapist. Review bios, specialties and treatment approaches, then set up calls with a few therapists—most will offer a free initial phone consultation.

Helpful: Explain what you're dealing with, and ask the therapist how he/she might treat it. After interviewing a few therapists, trust your gut and select one to see for three or four sessions. If you feel like it's not working, move on to someone else. The type of therapist you choose—psychologist, counselor or social worker—doesn't matter as much as your relationship with that person.

• **Take ownership of your session.** You're there to talk, so take some time beforehand to think about what you want to say.

Helpful: Arrive not just on time, but early. Give yourself 10 minutes in the waiting room to reflect on where you left off last time, what's happened since then and what your priority is today. If you wait for the therapist to steer the conversation, he may never get to what you want to talk about because he doesn't know. In between sessions, keep a therapy journal.

How that helps: You can use it to jot down a few notes after each session, as well as relevant thoughts, experiences and even dreams you've had. When journaling, ask yourself, *What do I want?* and *How do I feel?* Refer to your journal before each appointment so that you can bring up the issues that are important to you.

What not to do: Don't rehash everything that happened since you last saw your therapist. Some clients do this because they don't want to deal with deeper issues, which is missing the whole point of therapy. A little conversation about an outside event is OK if something big happened that directly applies to the issue you're working on, but you need to spend more time on the thoughts and feelings that resulted from it. Otherwise, you won't make progress.

• **Don't expect answers.** Should you break up with your partner, quit your job, ground your teenager? A therapist probably is not going to answer that for you. His job is to give you the tools to answer those questions yourself. If a therapist gives you the answer, you won't be any closer to understanding yourself, and you won't be empowered to handle another situation on your own. Instead, a good therapist will help you understand what's going on inside your head and help you develop the tools and emotional strength to address challenges. He might ask, for instance, "Why do you think you feel suspicious about your partner's phone texts?" or "Why are you having trouble completing that job application?"

• **Tell your therapist if you have concerns about the sessions.** Speak up if you don't like something your therapist says, does or even the cologne he wears. If you bottle up concerns, a rift will build and you won't make progress.

Better: Address any frustrations at the beginning of the session so that you can clear the air and move on. Maybe you're upset because your therapist was late or didn't seem to get your point or his aftershave smells like the one your father wore. By telling your therapist how you feel, you're helping him understand you better. Confrontation is hard, of course, but practicing it on your therapist will help you handle it better in life, too. Start with, "I'm a little uncomfortable bringing this up…" Talking about your feelings builds trust between you and your therapist. Don't worry about hurting his feelings. Most therapists know how to handle confrontation without getting defensive. If yours doesn't, consider choosing a different therapist.

• **It's all worth mentioning.** When you're in therapy, buried or forgotten feelings get dredged up.

Example: If something about your son crosses your mind while you're discussing your childhood, tell the therapist about it. Does your sister's face pop into your head while you're describing a coworker? Say so, no matter how random or insignificant it seems. There probably is a connection to what you're talking about—it's like a gift from the psyche—that can help you and the therapist understand deeper parts of you.

• **Pick a good time for your session.** What is the best time of day for a therapy session? Maybe you're a morning person and will be more talkative then…or maybe you come to life when the sun is going down. But timing also can depend on where you have to be after the appointment. It can be tricky to go back to the office after an intense session or to meet your mother-in-law for dinner (after you were just griping about her). If you can't avoid a schedule conflict, then tell your therapist what is on your agenda, so that he can stop the more intense conversation five or 10 minutes before the session is over. The therapist can use that time to help you make an action plan and "cool down," just as you would after a workout. You also can plan your own cooldown period after the session. It helps to go for a walk or write in your journal before heading to your next appointment. This process is called "containment," and it helps you to more easily reenter the rest of the world. It's like putting your feelings on a shelf until it's time to examine them again. The idea is to let yourself regroup and collect your feelings so that you can get back to your normal routine.

Also: Take care of any housekeeping business—scheduling, payments, insurance—at the beginning of your session, not the end. It's hard to switch gears from raw emotion to a discussion of whether your therapist will take your new insurance.

• **Ask about your progress.** From the beginning, talk about the end. Ideally, that will be when all therapy goals have been met. That may be achieved in 12 sessions—or it may take six months or more than a year. If you'd like to keep to a specific time frame, let your therapist know that up front. Along the way, you need to know you're making progress. There are two clues that things are going well. The first is when you begin to "internalize" your therapist. That means when you are on your own, you start to ask yourself the same questions your therapist would. That shows you're incorporating what you've learned in therapy into daily life. The other clue is when you find yourself saying, "I've never told anyone this before." Your therapist is hearing, *This is a safe place, and this client really trusts me.* Whether it's something bad or just too embarrassing to talk about, opening up is a sign that you're healing. Talking about your progress along the way means that you will be better prepared for when therapy ends—a difficult time for some clients. It helps you tie up the loose ends, clarify takeaway points and go back out on your own with closure.

Fight Back Against Your Inner Critic

Lisa Firestone, PhD, clinical psychologist and director of research and education at The Glendon Association, a nonprofit mental health organization based in Santa Barbara, California. She is coauthor of several books about psychology, including *The Self Under Siege* and *Conquer Your Critical Inner Voice.* Glendon.org

The voice inside your head that calls you an idiot when you make even the littlest mistake could be standing in the way of your success and happiness. No one is unaffected by this voice. We all hear it—and it's incredibly negative and destructive.

Inner critics can be cruel, harshly criticizing their hosts for imaginary failings and minor faux pas. That isn't just unpleasant—it is counterproductive. Faced with frequent, heartless criticism from within, we may conclude that there's no point making an effort or taking a chance because we'll just mess it up.

Why start a new relationship when the voice in your head informs you that you're incapable of holding on to a partner? Why try to invest for the future when the voice says that you'll just mismanage the money?

This negative voice can become the filter through which you see yourself. It both drives your behavior and then later berates you for it.

Example: The voice seduces you in a friendly-sounding way, telling you to just stay home rather than go out to the party that you planned to attend. Later, the voice screams at you that you're lonely, unwanted and have no friends. In the same way, this ugly voice can drive some people all the way to drugs and alcohol, suggesting that they have another drink or hit…then later criticizing them for their stupidity and weakness in partaking.

But you are not doomed to be beaten down by this voice. *By learning where your inner critic actually comes from and ways to weaken or disregard it, you can release yourself and find happiness…*

The Roots of an Inner Critic

Your inner critic did not begin inside you—it probably traces back to criticism you heard from someone powerful who was in your life when you were a child, such as a parent, teacher, older sibling or peer. Your interactions with this person left your childhood "self" feeling inadequate. Children also learn through observation—not just words. You may have grown up hearing a parent regularly speaking harshly to himself/herself. Children internalize their parents' voices.

Example: A girl who lived with a mother and grandmother who were vocally critical of their own bodies grew up to be a woman whose inner critic said tremendously hurtful things about her own appearance. A man whose father felt like a failure grew up to view himself as one, too.

Overcoming an Inner Critic

You can't silence your inner critic by giving in to it—that just feeds it and makes it stronger. Instead, freedom lies in paying close attention to when it talks to you and then acting against it by taking some positive risks.

Example: The next time you see someone you like, ignore the voice—take a chance and ask the person out. The first time you resist the voice, it may get louder, shouting

that you'll fail…but if you persist, eventually it will fade into the background.

These five strategies can help you fight back and find a way to take risks. *You have the power to quiet that inner critic's voice and reduce its impact on your life…*

•**Separate the voice from your own thoughts.** If you had a horribly unpleasant neighbor who constantly criticized you, you wouldn't take those criticisms seriously. You would dismiss him/her with an eye roll. Your inner critic deserves similar treatment. When it raises your fears and lowers your confidence, tell yourself, *That's just my inner critic again.*

•**Give its opinion the weight it deserves—little or none.** It's a vestige of an old self. Think about it—would you run your life or make decisions based on what you thought as a child? Of course not. And yet that's what you're doing when you let your inner critic get the upper hand.

Ask yourself, *What do I really think?* Step outside yourself, and take a "third party" look at what's going on. This further separates your feelings from the inner critic's feelings. Use first person "I" sentences when considering your true opinions but not when reflecting on the inner critic's words.

Example: You miss a flight. Your inner critic tells you that you're disorganized and can't do anything right. After reflecting for a moment on this, you might respond with, *I make mistakes like anyone, but I actually get lots of stuff right. In fact, this is the first flight I've ever missed. The lines were longer than normal.*

•**Try to identify your inner critic's triggers.** When your inner critic overreacts to a seemingly minor matter, there's a good chance that it actually is reacting to a similar incident that occurred in your past. It helps to identify the root source.

Example: You hear less than full agreement when you voice an opinion at a neighborhood association meeting. Your inner critic tells you, *No one cares about your opinion—it's worthless.* Perhaps this overreaction occurred because you were the youngest child in your family and your older siblings never valued your opinions.

•**Learn self-compassion.** People who endure cruel inner critics often believe that self-criticism is a path toward self-improvement and assume that the voice is there to motivate rather than destroy. In fact, harsh self-criticism is more likely to convince you that you are not capable of self-improvement than it is to lead to growth. Self-compassion (the ability to be kind to yourself even when you are suffering and to be nonjudgmental toward yourself) is more likely to lead to self-improvement—but self-compassion is a skill that people with scathing inner critics often lack.

Strategies for developing self-compassion include positive journaling and meditation to focus your attention on where you want to go and who you want to be. With your eyes closed, take a few deep breaths and try to be mindful. Meditation strengthens your ability to stop over-identifying with negative thoughts and feelings. They don't define you.

•**Ask yourself,** *So what's my next step?* Inner critics often focus their gaze backward at their past mistakes, constantly reinforcing their shortcomings. Focusing on a single, achievable next step can kick-start positive momentum and break the cycle of negativity and rumination created by an "error."

Example: You eat a bowl of ice cream when you're supposed to be on a diet. Your inner critic says you're fat and lack the discipline to lose weight. There's no point focusing on the past—you can't "un-eat" the ice cream. Instead, ask, *What's my next step?* It might be to throw away any remaining ice cream…or to plan out all of tomorrow's eating in advance to reduce the odds of impulsive snacking.

Also: Another question that can shift focus from the unchangeable past to a more productive future is, *What would I do differently next time?*

Free Talk Therapy

If your insurance does not cover talk therapy or you are unsatisfied with in-network options, various apps offer e-mail, text, audio or video chats—some for free. *7 Cups of Tea* is a free peer-to-peer network of people trained in active listening, with licensed therapists available for a monthly fee. *Woebot* is a free chatbot, based on artificial intelligence and recommendations by psychologists at Stanford University. *BetterHelp* has therapists with a minimum of three years of experience, offers live phone-chat sessions and costs $40 to $70 per week. *Talkspace* uses therapists with at least 3,000 hours of clinical experience, who are accessible by text, audio or video, for $65 to $99 per week.

Roundup of experts on telemedical talk therapy, reported in *Men's Health.*

Are You Being "Gaslighted" by Your Spouse…or at Work?

Robin Stern, PhD, psychoanalyst in private practice for more than 30 years, cofounder and associate director, Yale Center for Emotional Intelligence, New Haven, Connecticut. She is author of *The Gaslight Effect.*

Are you in a relationship where you constantly second-guess your actions… keep apologizing profusely for everything you do…are somehow always "wrong" without understanding how that happens? You might be involved—even potentially dangerously—with a gaslighter. *Here's how to shed light on what's happening and how to protect yourself…*

"Gaslighting" describes a particularly destructive kind of psychological power struggle that is a potentially very damaging form of abuse, where one person in a relationship tries to manipulate the other person's perception of reality. The term was inspired by the 1944 movie *Gaslight.* In the movie, Gregory (played by Charles Boyer) tries to convince his wife, Paula (Ingrid Bergman), that she's going insane by manipulating events through various tricks and persuading her that the "illusions" are actual fact.

The Gaslighting Dance

In real life, typical gaslighters aren't as obvious or as malicious as the Charles Boyer character. But they do share the same craving for power and control over the other person in the relationship—and a need to always be right. Often, in order to feel more important, they also make the other person dependent on them. And being the victim of a gaslighter takes a severe toll on mental and physical health.

Gaslighters aren't only husbands...they can be a parent, partner, coworker or friend...and either gender. It's also important to recognize that gaslighting doesn't happen without the tacit agreement of the person being gaslighted. This is not a case of blaming the victim. But to stop the abuse, the "gaslightee" needs to recognize his/her own role. Gaslightees have a strong need for approval, which makes them vulnerable under the right (or wrong!) circumstances. They tend to be empathic people who can easily see the other person's point of view and accommodate the wishes of others—frequently at the expense of their own needs and comfort.

Example: Jeanne, a friendly woman, is married to Roger, who doesn't like her attention diverted away from him. He gets angry if she so much as smiles at someone else, especially another man. And because he told her that this bothers him—and told her that smiling at other men is flirting—he feels his anger is justified. Jeanne explains that she is just friendly and smiles instinctively at everyone. But Roger doesn't like it and tells her to keep her eyes on the ground when they go out.

Jeanne's first reaction to Roger's eyes-down rule is that it's crazy—and she tells him not to be ridiculous. But over time, with his continued insistence and her wanting to please him, eventually she comes to think, *Maybe he's right.*

How does someone go from recognizing behavior that's abnormal and unhealthy, even outright bizarre, to agreeing that it's acceptable? *Here's what happens...*

The Slippery Slope

Gaslighting typically goes through three stages. Progressing from one stage to the next is dependent on the persistence of the gaslighter...and the willingness of the gaslightee to accept the skewed reality.

Stage one—disbelief: Using the example above, the gaslightee starts out thinking she must have misheard or misunderstood— *You're joking that you want me to avoid all eye contact with other people when we're out, right?* Confusion and frustration are common at this stage. But although the gaslightee might argue a bit with the gaslighter, she shrugs off the behavior, hoping it was a one-off and will resolve itself.

Stage two—second-guessing: The behavior is not a one-off, however. It's part of a repeated pattern. Hearing so persistently what's "wrong" with her, the gaslightee tries to prove it's not true in order to win the gaslighter's approval. She replays conversations and events, looking for evidence that the gaslighter is wrong about his accusations. She second-guesses all her actions. They argue incessantly, with him constantly undermining her character. For instance, when Roger is furious because she had a good time laughing and talking when they're out with another couple, and claims she ignored him and enjoys being with other people more than with him, she gets defensive. She anxiously lists all the other times she can think of when she and Roger had fun together...and lies about going out for lunch with women friends.

Stage three—acceptance and depression: Stage three is powerful and intense. Because the gaslightee's strong need for approval makes arguing uncomfortable, she gives up. She realizes she can't win, anyway. She thinks the problem will be fixed if only she can get the gaslighter's approval. So she is willing to do everything the way the gaslighter wants it. She begins to accept the gaslighter's perception of her and the relationship. Not surprisingly, such extreme loss of will leads to deep depression. In its most extreme form, the hopelessness the gaslightee feels can lead to thoughts of self-harm.

Turning Off the Gas

Overcoming this dynamic power struggle isn't easy—especially if the gaslighting relationship is with a spouse or family member and/or has gone on for many years. But you can break this destructive pattern. The tools that will help are awareness, courage and the right words to use.

Becoming aware…

• **Listen to friends.** Your buddies might see things more clearly than you can. For instance, if your date accused you of being overly sensitive, your friend can offer a reality check: *Maybe you are sensitive. But that has nothing to do with the fact that he left when you were 10 minutes late without even calling you—and then told you that you're upset because you're too sensitive.*

• **Write it down.** Write down the conversations you have with your gaslighter. Looking at who said what as though it were a script between two characters in a play can help you spot gaslighting patterns. Notice where the conversation veers off to be comments about you and your "flaws," not a response to what you just said. *Using the example above…*

You: "Hey, I know I was a few minutes late—sorry about that—but we agreed to meet for the movie in line. Why didn't you wait…or call?"

Gaslighter: "Wow, you have trouble keeping track of time, and you're blaming me for leaving—and now you feel bad? You are way too sensitive!"

Blaming his behavior (not doing what was agreed to, not calling) on you, and your (perfectly normal) reaction on your "character flaw" (sensitivity) is classic gaslighting.

• **Talk to a therapist.** A trained professional can distinguish distortion from fact and also can be more objective than you. Maybe you are sensitive. But that doesn't mean you have to put up with abusive behavior.

Finding Courage…

• **Be ready to walk.** Unless your gaslighter is willing to change, the only solution may be to leave. Being clear that you are ready to do that makes an unarguable statement that the gaslighting behavior is unacceptable—but you need to stick to your position, or there are no consequences for your gaslighter and no reason to change.

Note: Be prepared for changes in your behavior to cause your gaslighter to react by expressing even less approval of you. Sometimes, the abuse (name calling, etc.) may ramp up to the point where you need to leave. If at any time you feel frightened or unsafe, leave immediately. Even if the steps you need to take impact you financially or socially, keeping yourself safe is your first priority.

The Right Words…

• **Go-to phrases that help.** Having specific words and phrases to use when you feel yourself losing the power struggle can keep you from getting pulled back into the manipulative vortex. *Phrases to memorize…*

• "I'm not going to talk to you while you're yelling at me."

• "I don't want to have this conversation while emotions are so heated. Let's pick it up later."

• "I'm going to go have a cup of tea right now. This conversation isn't feeling fair/respectful."

• "I won't continue this conversation when you are telling me what's wrong with me."

• "We will have to agree to disagree—I just don't see it that way."

Of course, what you say to your boss or to your parent will be very different from what you say to your partner. How easy it might be to leave also will be different. *Examples*…

Your dad: "Haven't heard from you in weeks. Just like your mother, you're all about yourself." (*Reality*: You called him this week and had a conversation…the statement about your mother is gratuitous meanness and not true of you or your mother.)

You: "Dad, we don't agree about how often I call you—we will have to agree to disagree. I'm getting a cup of coffee now. Would you like one?" (Avoid defending yourself, ignore the insult and "leave" the power struggle.)

Your boss: "We need to wrap up this project—are you clueless about that? Where is the document you promised to revise?" (*Reality*: He didn't ask for it, and you didn't promise it.)

You: "I didn't know you needed it this week. I will have it for you tomorrow. We had agreed that deadlines would be in writing, which I think will be very helpful. Will that be possible next time?" (Ignore the insult, bring the conversation back to the topic.)

Your boss: "We never agreed to that. You're so forgetful! Are you going through menopause?" (*Reality*: You are, but you know you hadn't agreed on a deadline—and he is again deflecting the conversation.)

You: "I will take responsibility for sending you an e-mail after our meetings about what work needs to be done and when. In the meantime, I will go back to my office and get you what you need." (Avoid his bait and the temptation to defend yourself and keep the conversation on the topic.)

• **Finally, forget about right or wrong.** While it's possible for a gaslighter to change a long-standing pattern of manipulation, control—and especially abuse—is hard to give up without professional help, something the gaslighter will need to want. But if your gaslighter is committed to changing and you do stay in the relationship, focus on healing…taking responsibility for what you say and do…and being honest. You will need to be disciplined around hot-button issues so that you don't slip back into old patterns.

And you will need to apply the compassion you so easily extend to others to yourself as well.

Things You Can Say to Opt Out of a Power Struggle

If you're involved with a "gaslighter"—a spouse, coworker, family member or friend who tries to control you by manipulating your perception of reality—the following 16 phrases can help keep you out of his/her destructive vortex. Memorize the phrases that seem most useful for your own situation so that you can pull them out when you need them.

• **"You're right, but I don't want to keep arguing about this."**

• **"You're right, but I don't want to be talked to that way."**

• **"I'm happy to continue this conversation without name-calling."**

• **"I'm not comfortable with where this conversation is going.** Let's revisit it later."

• **"I think this conversation has gone as far as it can go."**

• **"I don't think I can be constructive right now.** Let's talk about this at another time."

• **"I think we have to agree to disagree."**

• **"I don't want to continue this argument."**

• **"I don't want to continue this conversation right now."**

• **"I hear you, and I'm going to think about that.** But I don't want to keep talking about it right now."

• **"I'd really like to continue this conversation,** but I'm not willing to do so unless we can do it in a more pleasant tone."

• **"I don't like the way I'm feeling right now, and I'm not willing to continue this conversation."**

• **"You may not be aware of it, but you're telling me that I don't know what reality is.** And respectfully, I don't agree. I love you, but I won't talk to you about this."

- **"I love having intimate conversations with you,** but not when you're putting me down."

- **"It may not be your intention to put me down,** but I feel put down, and I'm not going to continue the conversation."

- **"This is not a good time for me to talk about this.** Let's agree on another time that works for both of us."

Source: Above list excerpted from *The Gaslight Effect: How to Spot and Survive the Hidden Manipulation Others Use to Control Your Life* by Robin Stern, PhD, cofounder and associate director, Yale Center for Emotional Intelligence, New Haven, Connecticut.

How Capable Is Your Gaslighter of Relating to You?

If you're involved with a "gaslighter"—a spouse, coworker, family member or friend who tries to control you by manipulating your perception of reality—you need to decide whether to leave the relationship or stay and fix it. A critical factor in that decision is whether your gaslighter wants to change…and is able to. *Here are positive signs to look for…*

Does he/she…

…seem capable of understanding and respecting your point of view?

…at least occasionally key in to your feelings and needs?

…at least occasionally put your feelings and needs ahead of his/her own?

…feel remorse about the times he hurts you—in a way that leads him to change his own behavior?

…show interest in changing for his own reasons, not simply to please you or to prove what a good guy he is?

Source: Excerpted from The Gaslight Effect: How to Spot and Survive the Hidden Manipulation Others Use to Control Your Life by Robin Stern, PhD, cofounder and associate director, Yale Center for Emotional Intelligence, New Haven, Connecticut.

The Brain Fix for Digestive Problems

Sarah Kinsinger, PhD, a board-certified health psychologist, associate professor of gastroenterology and nutrition and director of Behavioral Medicine for the Digestive Health Program at Loyola University Medical Center in Maywood, Illinois.

Digestive problems—whether it's an upset stomach, diarrhea, constipation or abdominal pain—can make life miserable.

Until recently, doctors have treated these problems by focusing on the gut—approximately 30 feet of tubes and organs through which food is ingested, digested and excreted. Now an increasing body of scientific evidence shows that a new target—the brain—is a missing link in finding relief.

What most people don't realize: Your gut contains more than 100 million nerves, more than what's found in your spinal cord. This "enteric nervous system," connecting the gut and brain, is in constant two-way communication.

For example, signals from the brain play a key role in the day-to-day, moment-to-moment function of digestion. By the same token, feelings like fear, anger and depression are now being increasingly recognized for their effect on digestive functions.

Given the strength of the brain-gut connection, it should be no surprise that top-down treatment with a psychologist (or "brain-gut therapy," as it's come to be called) can help—and in some cases is more effective than conventional medical care, including many medications. *What you need to know…*

The Brain-Gut Axis in Action

While many details of this "upstairs-downstairs" interaction have yet to be worked out, we know that signals from the brain—via neurotransmitters and nerve signals—control the muscular contractions that move digested food through the digestive tract, regulate secretions such as stomach acid and enzymes that break down food and influence pain sensitivity in the gut.

Because your brain and gut are in such close and constant communication, stress and troubling emotions that alter brain function readily disrupt the smooth workings of your digestive system. These effects are most clearly seen in disorders of brain-gut interaction, where there is no evidence of physiological abnormalities with testing.

•**Irritable bowel syndrome (IBS),** a chronic condition involving abdominal pain accompanied by symptoms like diarrhea, constipation and bloating, is the most common of these. Others include functional dyspepsia (stomach pain, bloating and nausea following meals) and certain cases of heartburn.

But the brain also can contribute to worsening symptoms of organic digestive disorders, such as Crohn's disease or ulcerative colitis, where symptoms are the result of an autoimmune disorder causing inflammation in the gut. In some cases, patients with these disorders continue to experience abdominal pain or diarrhea even when inflammation is well controlled by medication.

The back-and-forth interaction between the brain and gut can create a vicious cycle. When planning to travel, attend a concert or party or simply appear in public, many people with chronic bowel conditions fear that they will pass gas or have an urgent need for a bathroom or sudden, severe pain.

These fears can trigger physiological arousal in the body (the "fight or flight" response) and amplify awareness of sensations that might otherwise be ignored. This stress response can trigger contractions in the intestines and intensify pain sensations. These symptoms and associated anxiety can prevent individuals from enjoying social situations and enjoying life to the fullest.

What Brain-Gut Therapy Can Do

The brain-gut connection is more than theoretical. There's research showing that when we change how the brain works—the goal of all psychotherapy—it can have profound effects on gastrointestinal symptoms.

•**Cognitive behavioral therapy (CBT),** which changes patterns of thinking and behavior, has the most research support, with at least 20 randomized trials showing its effectiveness in curbing gut-related symptoms. In these studies, typically 60% to 70% of patients are "treatment responders," meaning that they report significant reductions in abdominal pain and improved bowel habits following CBT treatment.

•**Gut-directed hypnotherapy** is the second most researched psychological treatment for IBS and has been validated by several randomized clinical trials. One of the largest observational studies of hypnotherapy for IBS involved 1,000 patients with severe symptoms that had failed to respond to prior medical treatment.

Result: With hypnotherapy, 76% of patients reported clinically significant reductions in IBS symptoms.

While pain reduction is the most prominent benefit, patients also report improvements in bowel habits (more regular bowel movements and improvements in stool consistency) and relief from "non-colonic" symptoms such as fatigue, backaches, headaches and body aches.

Why these treatments confer such benefits is unclear. They may reprogram the brain to tune out or dial down the perception of sensations coming from the gut and help normalize muscular contractions and secretions in digestive organs.

CBT helps patients become aware of the connection between thinking patterns, behaviors and physical sensations in the body and learn to reframe unhelpful thinking patterns.

For example, a patient who gets anxious about travel or parties days before may be encouraged to consider the real probability of an ill-timed episode and the coping strategies he/she might use should one occur. CBT often includes training in relaxation practices, such as mindfulness or diaphragmatic breathing, to reduce physiological stress and empower patients to manage symptoms.

With gut-directed hypnotherapy, patients achieve a deeply relaxed, focused and receptive mental state, where suggestions like a sensation of warmth in the abdominal area can soothe pain and reduce awareness of pain symptoms. Hypnotic suggestions also may modulate nerve function to prevent muscle spasm...or recalibrate the brain's response to signals coming from the gut, easing hypersensitivity to normal sensations.

Both treatments are relatively short-term, typically involving about seven to 12 sessions over the course of three months. But the benefits are often long-lasting. A number of studies show that improvements are maintained for a year or more, and in one trial of hypnotherapy, these benefits were maintained for up to five years. Health insurers often cover these treatments.

Is Brain-Gut Therapy for You?

Brain-gut therapy has been shown to work for men, women and children with irritable bowel syndrome (IBS). The most important question is, are you open to it and willing to become actively engaged? Both cognitive behavioral therapy (CBT) and hypnotherapy are a kind of brain training, which demands regular practice—that is, homework—to be effective.

Patients most often consider brain-gut therapy after standard medical treatment (such as laxative or antidiarrheal medications) and lifestyle modifications (such as exercise and diet changes) haven't given them the results they want.

People who prefer a drug-free approach may turn to brain-gut therapy earlier. The ideal situation is when a therapist and medical doctor are in regular communication and work together to help the patient. It's best not to wait too long to seek treatment. The more unsuccessful treatment experiences you have, the more stressful the condition becomes.

Your gastroenterologist may know of a mental health provider offering these treatments. Otherwise, look for a provider specializing in CBT or hypnotherapy who is also experienced working with patients with chronic health conditions.

Best resources: The Rome Foundation, a nonprofit organization that researches and educates the public about functional gastrointestinal disorders, has a searchable directory of gastrointestinal mental health providers nationwide, RomeGIPsych.org. The website IBShypnosis.com lists providers who specialize in hypnosis for IBS.

The Art of Doing Nothing

Sandi Mann, PhD, senior lecturer in the School of Psychology, University of Central Lancashire, UK. She is lead author of the study "Does Being Bored Make Us More Creative?" and author of *The Science of Boredom: The Upside (And Downside) of Downtime.* MindTrainingClinic.com

There's a simple activity that spurs creativity, boosts problem-solving abilities and calms anxieties. This activity might sound like it's really something, but actually it's really...nothing. Just a few minutes spent doing nothing could turn out to be among the most productive parts of your day.

Thanks in large part to smartphones, even the briefest breaks in the day are now filled with checking messages, surfing the Internet, listening to podcasts and playing games. As a result, standing around doing nothing seems wasteful, and many people fear it makes them appear unimportant.

But researchers are discovering that banishing boredom and inactivity does not actually make life better. Studies have shown that brief stretches of mindless activity tend to boost people's creativity and problem-solving abilities.

Example: A study published in *Creativity Research Journal* found that participants did better on the creative task of coming up with as many uses as possible for a pair of plastic cups if they first had engaged in an activity that let their minds wander—the bor-

91

ing task of reading mindlessly from a phone book.

Daydream Believer

Why does doing nothing improve creativity and problem-solving skills? Because your brain isn't actually doing nothing when you do nothing—it's daydreaming. And though daydreaming carries negative associations, it's actually time well spent.

When researchers conducted MRI scans on the brains of people who were daydreaming, they found that multiple parts of their brains were highly active—including the "executive network," which is associated with complex problem solving—according to a study published in *Proceedings of the National Academy of Sciences*.

You likely have had the experience of waking from a deep sleep to discover that your dreaming brain has thought up a useful idea. This is the same concept behind daydreaming—but with less risk that you'll forget the idea.

Harnessing the Power of Doing Nothing

The secret to getting something out of doing nothing is to allow your mind to wander without exercising any control over where it goes during this time.

Some people can achieve this dreamy let-your-mind-wander state almost anywhere—if you often catch yourself staring into space in noisy, busy places such as coffee shops or on train platforms, you probably don't need to take any special steps to daydream. You just need to put away your phone or your book and let it happen. Other people may have to actively seek out conditions that are conducive to purposeful daydreaming.

Even people who don't daydream can get in on the action if they try daydreaming while…

•**Standing in line.** Supermarket and airport lines once were prime daydreaming time before the advent of smartphones with all their distractions. Boring queues can be

that again. Direct your eyes up toward a spot high on a wall or in a distant corner of the ceiling to reduce the odds that you'll make eye contact with other people or spot other things that grab your attention. Daydreaming in lines can be an effective anxiety-control strategy, too—when you feel frustration about the length of a line, tell yourself to instead be thankful for the opportunity to daydream. It feels better to know that the downtime actually is a good use of your time.

•**Enjoying quiet time during drives.** Turn off your car's radio, and just let your mind wander during your commute or other drives. Make sure you're still paying attention to the road, of course.

•**Sitting in a spot with a pleasant but not dramatic view.** Gaze out a window at a tree…look into a fireplace with a fire burning…or focus on a pond in a park. Just watch the fire…the water…the wind blowing the leaves…or the clouds floating by.

•**Strolling with or without your dog.** Going for a walk is a good way to get away from the potential distractions of home and the workplace. Walking amid trees or fields tends to be more conducive to daydreaming than walking through neighborhoods or cities because nature provides fewer distractions and irritating noises.

•**Swimming.** Swimming isn't doing nothing—it's great exercise. But some people find that it's an ideal opportunity for musing on things. The water cuts down on outside distractions, and the rhythm of the strokes can be hypnotic.

•**Engaging in an activity that occupies your hands but barely engages your mind.** Knit…doodle…bounce a ball against a wall…or color in coloring books. These sorts of activities can encourage people who find it frustrating and unpleasant to be unoccupied. The activity occupies the hands and mind enough to stave off that frustration, at least for a while, but requires such a minimal amount of brainpower that it doesn't prevent you from getting lost in thought.

Three Do-Nothing No-Nos

Yes, it is possible to go wrong when your goal is to do nothing more than daydream…

● **Meditation and yoga are not conducive to daydreaming.** When people meditate or do yoga, they typically try to focus their attention on a single concept or action. This does have benefits, but it's very different from letting the mind wander.

● **Killing time by browsing the Internet or watching mindless TV is not the right sort of doing nothing.** These activities are doing nothing in the sense that you're accomplishing nothing—but staring at a phone, computer or TV screen tends to inhibit your thoughts from wandering freely.

● **Focused problem-solving is not daydreaming.** If you consciously steer your mind to seek a solution to a specific problem, you will undercut the creative power of daydreaming. Instead, let your thoughts drift wherever they take you. Trust that your mind is aware of the big problem you face and is working on that problem even when you're not directing it to do so. —Sandi Mann, PhD

Letting your mind wander for even just a few minutes can be useful, if that's all the time you have. But it's best if you can try to find at least a few times each week for extended bouts of daydreaming—target 30 minutes, if you can manage that without frustration setting in. Once frustration starts, productive daydreaming becomes unlikely.

Beat the Not-Working Blues

Leaving the workplace can cost retirees (and those who have been laid off) their identity, purpose, sense of self-worth and so-

cial circle—all of which can have emotional health benefits. Working just one day a week provides the same psychological benefits as working full time, so a paid part-time job can be a solution.

Brendan Burchell, PhD, director of graduate education in the department of sociology at University of Cambridge, UK, and coauthor of a study of 70,000 people, published in *Social Science & Medicine*.

Procrastinators: It's Not (Completely) Your Fault!

Study titled "Genetic variation in dopamine availability modulates the self-reported level of action control in a sex-dependent manner," by researchers at Ruhr-University Bochum, Germany, published in *Social Cognitive and Affective Neuroscience*.

Whether you live or work with a procrastinator (or you're one yourself) the last thing you'd think these chronic stallers need is another excuse. However, new research may give procrastinators a break—especially women. It turns out that as much as 46% of the reason for stalling rather than knuckling down to tasks has to do with anatomy and genes.

Procrastinators hear the well-known proverb *Don't put off until tomorrow what you can do today* more times than they'd probably like. But what keeps procrastinators from getting things done is not laziness but cognitive flexibility—jumping from thought to thought because they're so easily distracted. Now research is finding clues for why and how this happens. *To better understand, here's some background on procrastination and the brain…*

The Science of Procrastination

One of the things that determines impulsivity is brain levels of the messenger chemical dopamine, which stimulates the parts of the brain that are responsible for impulsive thoughts. High levels of dopamine make it harder to focus on goal-directed, action-oriented decisions—and, in fact, are associated with higher scores on psychological tests for procrastination.

Dopamine levels vary by individual...and by gender. The hormone estrogen stimulates the release of dopamine, and also stimulates the brain cells (neurons) that bind to dopamine. It is well-known from studies going back 20 years that estrogen increases the number of neurons that are sensitive to dopamine. Both men and women have estrogen in their bodies, but women have it in higher amounts—and have a slightly higher response to dopamine.

Dopamine production is also controlled by a gene. The higher-expression variant of the gene causes the body to produce more dopamine...while the lower-expression variant causes the body to produce less dopamine.

A 2014 study of procrastination from University of Colorado Boulder that compared fraternal twins with identical twins found that both procrastination and impulsivity were about 46% and 49% respectively the result of inherited genetic traits. (Because all twins share the same environment, but only identical twins share the same genes, comparing results between the two kinds of twins allowed researchers to calculate what could be attributed to environment versus to genes.)

The Procrastinating Brain

More recently, researchers from Ruhr-University Bochum in Germany conducted a study in 2018 that found that an area of the brain involved with processing emotion—the amygdala—was larger in people who scored high on a test for procrastination. The researchers then wondered whether the larger amygdala in procrastinators was linked to having the higher-dopamine-expression gene. So they conducted another study.

For the newest study, 278 healthy adults, ages 18 to 37 and fairly equally divided between men and women, were asked to fill out questionnaire tests for procrastination.

The students also had gene tests to determine their type of dopamine-expression gene...and brain scans of their amygdalas.

Genetic testing found that 113 students had the lower-expression gene and 163 students had the higher-expression gene, evenly split between men and women. *Results also found...*

For women, having the high-expression gene was associated with a significantly higher procrastination test score—about two points higher on a scale of 0 to 12. No difference in score was found for men with the higher-expression gene.

Brain scans of both men and women with higher procrastination scores did confirm that they had bigger amygdalas, as found in the earlier research—but a larger amygdala was not linked to either variant of the dopamine-expression gene.

The Takeaway

This is the first study to suggest that at least part of the reason some people are prone to procrastination may have to do with genetics and anatomy. The researchers suspect that the high-dopamine-expression gene combined with higher levels of estrogen in the young women accounted for their higher procrastination scores—and explains why the same effect wasn't seen in men. The researchers are planning further research into the roles of estrogen and also norepinephrine, another chemical brain messenger controlled by the dopamine-expression gene, which may shed more light on what drives procrastination.

In the meantime, you may be tempted—especially if you're a woman—to say that it's not your fault that you do everything at the last minute...or late (or never). But as with other conditions influenced by genetic tendencies, you're not a prisoner of your DNA. It may take more effort to knuckle down and get going—but it's not impossible!

What You Can Do to Help a Loved One at Risk for Suicide

Daniel J. Reidenberg, PsyD, executive director of Suicide Awareness Voices of Education (SAVE), managing director of the National Council for Suicide Prevention and general secretary of the International Association for Suicide Prevention. Based in Minneapolis, he also is the former chair of the American Psychotherapy Association. SAVE.org

Kate Spade. Anthony Bourdain. Jeremy Richman (father of a Sandy Hook victim). These tragic, high-profile deaths shine a light on the frightening, rising trend of suicides. According to the Centers for Disease Control and Prevention (CDC), the rate of suicide in the US has increased by 35% between 1999 and 2018, with more than 48,000 people taking their own lives in 2018. For men it increased 28%, and for women a shocking 55%.

More sobering statistics: The suicide rate for females is highest among those ages 45 to 64, and the highest increase in suicide is in men who are age 50 and over. We don't have any definitive reasons why middle age is such a vulnerable time, but multiple factors likely play a role—excessive stress at midlife, financial challenges and better reporting of suicide numbers.

Losing a loved one is always devastating, but in the case of suicide it's even more so because it theoretically didn't have to happen. Survivors of suicide—the partners, family members and friends left behind—often are tormented by guilt about what they might or should have done: *If I had seen the signs more clearly, acted faster, would he/she still be alive?* The answer may be no—suicides can and do occur without warning—but in many cases, there are red flags. And there are steps you can take to keep someone from suicide.

Risk Factors in Plain Sight

Not surprisingly, some estimates suggest that up to 90% of suicides occur in people suffering from psychiatric issues. They may have bipolar disorder, schizophrenia, dementia, anxiety disorder or post-traumatic stress disorder or they may abuse substances, particularly alcohol. If you know a loved one who suffers from any of these, you likely already understand the importance of watchfulness. Likewise, if someone you know suddenly becomes overwhelmed by a death, job loss or a chronic or terminal illness, you should be on alert for trouble.

But what about those problems you can't see? Many psychiatric issues are undiagnosed—it's estimated that only half of Americans experiencing major depression receive treatment, yet research consistently shows a strong link between depression and suicide. There are many other risk factors, as well, that may be hidden from your view. *Examples…*

• **Being a victim of trauma or abuse—experiences some people may never share—increases the odds of suicide.**

• **Taking a medication—one that you don't know someone is on or that you are not familiar with—that puts a person at risk.** More than 200 commonly used prescription medications have been linked to increased suicide risk.

According to a recent study, more than one-third of Americans take medications that may increase their risk for depression, and close to one-quarter take drugs that list suicidal symptoms as a side effect. As you might expect, medications to treat mental health issues, such as some types of antidepressants and sedatives, can fall into this category. But so do some birth control pills, steroids, beta-blockers, anticonvulsants, proton pump inhibitors, some antibiotics (including fluoroquinolones) and medications for acne, asthma, allergy and smoking cessation.

Before someone you love starts a new drug, have him/her ask the doctor about risks or side effects and double-check with the pharmacist. If suicide is a potential side effect, have a discussion with the doctor about getting a different prescription. If suicidal thoughts are a possibility, be on the lookout for out-of-character behavior, including withdrawing from routine activities or changes in sleeping and eating patterns.

Watch for Red Flags

When someone is suicidal, it's unusual if there aren't any warning signs, but it can be difficult to see them. Everyone is busy with his own life and may not pick up on red flags. It may be months between visits with a friend, sibling or college-age child, making it hard to see a trend. The person considering suicide also is likely to hide his thoughts because of the stigma and shame associated with them. Someone who commits suicide may even have seemed "fine" the day before.

That's why it's important to recognize clues that are a cry for help. The consensus-based list of warning signs, according to *Suicidal Awareness Voices of Education* are (in order of risk)…

- **Talking about wanting to die or to kill oneself**
- **Looking for a way to kill oneself**
- **Talking about feeling hopeless or having no purpose**
- **Talking about feeling trapped or being in unbearable pain**
- **Talking about being a burden to others**
- **Increasing the use of alcohol or drugs**
- **Acting anxious, agitated or reckless**
- **Sleeping too little or too much**
- **Withdrawing or feeling isolated**
- **Showing rage or talking about seeking revenge**
- **Displaying extreme mood swings.**

The Conversation You Must Have

If you see any of the red flags listed, you're going to need to talk with the person. A common misconception is that just mentioning suicide can put the idea into someone's head, but that couldn't be further from the truth. Your willingness to talk actually can prevent a death. It's certainly not an easy conversation to have, but providing support and connectedness with others during a difficult time are what therapists call "protective factors" because they make someone less likely to engage in suicidal behaviors. *Still, what you say and how you say it can help or hurt the situation…*

- **Avoid making the person feel guilty about his thoughts.** Saying, "You wouldn't be thinking about hurting yourself, would you?" sends the message that you really don't want to hear what's going on with that person, and his response likely will be to shut down. Nor should you minimize what the person is going through by referring to it as a "rough patch" or saying "Things aren't that bad" or "You have everything to live for." These statements reinforce the idea that the person is weak, increase feelings of guilt and hopelessness and make him think that he can't tell anyone how he feels.

- **Bring up your concerns honestly and openly.** Say, "I'm genuinely worried about you. Can we talk?" Start by asking, "Do you feel so bad that you think about committing suicide?" If the answer is "yes" or "sometimes," follow that with, "Do you have a plan to kill yourself?" With each successive "yes" or "maybe," gather as much information as you can while keeping the conversation going—"Have you thought about what method you would use?" "When are you thinking about doing this?"

Note: Even though it may be uncomfortable, it's important to use the word "suicide" in the conversation. This person's brain is focused on death and dying, and that's what you need to connect with. Talking about it in a nonjudgmental, nonconfrontational way is more likely to make him accept help.

Surely, you'll be frightened if presented with affirmative answers or actual plans. *Know, however, that there are immediate steps you can take to help…*

- **Acknowledge what the person has said to you.** Say, "I'm glad you shared that with me."

Other helpful statements: "You don't have to go through this alone" or "Treatment does work."

• **Ask who else he has talked to.** If your loved one has not already reached out to a doctor or a crisis hotline, suggest doing it together—"I'm worried about what you're saying. Let's call the National Suicide Prevention Lifeline at 800-273-TALK (8255) right now."

• **Do some research together.** Go online and look at the suicide warning signs together, just as you would do for any sort of ache or pain, to help minimize the stigma of mental illness. Hopefully, this exercise will convince the person that it's time to get help.

• **Make an appointment.** If the person doesn't seem to be in imminent danger, reassure him that suicidal feelings are treatable. Together, call and set up a time for the person to see a mental health professional as soon as possible. Be tenacious about following up. If necessary, make the appointment yourself, and go to the appointment with him.

• **Recognize an emergency situation.** If you suspect imminent danger, call 911 or take your loved one to a hospital emergency room. Don't leave someone alone if he seems to be at high risk. If he storms out or locks himself in a room, you may have to call for help.

Important to know: Firearms are the most commonly used method of suicide among men in the US, and poisoning (including pills) is the most common method among women in the US, so also explain that you are removing access to these—or another method the person might have told you about.

Inserting yourself into someone else's life this way is difficult, but—when it comes to suicide prevention—it's necessary. Never worry about being intrusive or overbearing. Finding support, staying connected and limiting isolation can help save a life.

The Healing Power of a Good Chat

Rebecca Shannonhouse, editor-in-chief, health content, Bottom Line Inc.

Smoking and obesity would top anyone's list of serious health risks. But did you know that research has shown loneliness to be on par with those dangers? It has been linked to high blood pressure, diabetes and cancer. Loneliness also increases one's odds of dying early by 26% and is considered a risk factor for Alzheimer's disease. It's estimated that about 42 million American adults suffer from loneliness.

England, where loneliness also has been identified as a health threat, has been at the forefront of addressing this problem by connecting people to local social groups. Now a new initiative known as "chat benches" in local parks is taking hold there. To promote conversation, a small sign is posted on random park benches, indicating that people sitting there are "happy to chat." This simple idea is scientifically sound. There's strong evidence that face-to-face conversation is particularly powerful in helping people overcome loneliness. *In lieu of a chat bench, you can…*

• **Nurture your existing relationships.** This includes your spouse (if you have one), friends, neighbors, etc. Call them regularly and make concrete plans to get together.

• **Put "friendship reminders" on your calendar.** Remind yourself to take steps to meet new people. Seek out groups of people with similar interests—a class at a community college, a choir group, a political action organization, etc.

• **Pick up the phone.** If you're feeling lonely and don't have anyone to talk to, call 800-971-0016. Someone on the Friendship Line, sponsored by the not-for-profit Institute on Aging, will be happy to chat!

15-Minute Vacation

Meditation is as effective as a vacation for stress reduction and increasing positive emotions. Fifteen minutes of meditation per day brings about as much improvement in these areas as a day of vacation.

Study by researchers at University College Groningen, the Netherlands, published in *Journal of Positive Psychology*.

Cope with the Death of a Pet

Mary Craig, DVM, CHPV (certified hospice and palliative care), owner of Gentle Goodbye Veterinary Palliative Care & At-Home Euthanasia, serving Westchester County, New York, and Fairfield County, Connecticut. GentleGoodbye.org

It can be difficult to deal with the death of a pet. Our furry companions ask so little of us and give us so much, yet the social "rules of grieving" are different for pets versus people. So when you have to say goodbye to one, you may not know what to do. And although it may seem like you'll never heal, you can work through your pain.

• **Acknowledge what you're feeling.** Emotions run the gamut from anger (*Why didn't I get a diagnosis sooner?*) to denial (*How can this be happening?*) to guilt (*Did I choose euthanasia too soon? Not soon enough?*). Or you may be deeply sad or simply feel relief that your pet is no longer suffering. All of these feelings are natural, and you may experience some or all of them. Let yourself feel them fully.

• **Expect the unexpected.** Sometimes the death of a pet stirs up memories of past losses—maybe your mother who passed away years ago loved to play a game with your dog, for example. If you have other pets, they actually will mourn in their own ways. You may notice them having less energy and/or appetite. Maybe they'll want to be alone more than usual or be more clingy than usual. Give them extra love, and allow them their time to grieve, too.

• **Memorialize your pet.** Part of the reason our grief seems overwhelming is that there are no set mourning rituals for pets, as there are when a person dies. Many people find it tremendously comforting to hold a memorial service for a pet...scatter the animal's ashes in a favorite spot in the yard...plant a tree in the pet's memory...make a photo book...or donate to a rescue organization. It also may help to share memories in a pet-bereavement chat room or through a pet-loss hotline. There is a list of links to pet-loss websites and chat rooms on my site GentleGoodbye.org under "Grief Resources."

• **Be patient.** You may feel this grief for longer than you expect. Just as with human loss, feelings mellow and the pain becomes softer as time goes on. But if you feel "stuck" or can't function, seek the support of a mental health professional. Don't let anyone make you feel bad for what you are going through.

• **Listen to your heart when it comes to getting a new companion.** There's no right or wrong decision or right or wrong time to adopt another animal. Accept that your lost pet will continue to have a special place in your heart, but that there's always room for more love.

Pretend You're an Extrovert

Acting like an extrovert boosts happiness, says Sonja Lyubomirsky, PhD.

Recent study: Researchers instructed 123 college students, who were a mix of introverts and extroverts, to act talkative, assertive and spontaneous (all extrovert traits) for one week and then be deliberate, quiet and reserved (introvert traits) another week.

Result: Well-being scores were significantly higher for participants during the extrovert week and decreased during the introvert week.

Surprising: When "faking" being extroverted, the introverts reported no discomfort.

Sonja Lyubomirsky, PhD, professor of psychology, University of California, Riverside.

Binge Drinking Worse for Women

Binge drinking may be worse for women.

Recent study: Female rats were more sensitive to alcohol and had higher levels of alcoholic liver injury than comparable male rats. A protein that enables tumor growth and cancer increased 20% in male rats given alcohol equivalent to the amounts binge-drinking humans take in…but the protein level went up 95% in female rats.

Reason: Unknown—further research is necessary.

Shivendra D. Shukla, PhD, Margaret Proctor Mulligan Professor of medical research, University of Missouri School of Medicine, Columbia, and leader of a study published in *The Journal of Pharmacology and Experimental Therapeutics*.

Drinking Too Much? Answer These Questions to Find Out

Excerpted from "Alcohol Use Disorder" by the National Institutes of Health/National Institute on Alcohol Abuse and Alcoholism.

Problem drinking that becomes severe is given the medical diagnosis of alcohol use disorder (AUD). An estimated 16 million people in the US have AUD. It is characterized by compulsive alcohol use, loss of control over alcohol intake and a negative emotional state when not drinking alcohol.

To be diagnosed with AUD, you must meet criteria outlined in the *Diagnostic and Sta-*

tistical Manual of Mental Disorders (DSM). Anyone meeting any two of the 11 criteria below during the same 12-month period is diagnosed with AUD, according to the DSM-5, the current version of the DSM. The severity of AUD—mild, moderate or severe—is based on the number of criteria met.

To assess whether you or a loved one may have AUD, here are some questions to ask. *In the past year, have you…*

•**Had times when you ended up drinking more or longer than you intended?**

•**More than once wanted to cut down or stop drinking, or tried to, but couldn't?**

•**Spent a lot of time drinking?** Or being sick or getting over the aftereffects?

•**Experienced craving—a strong need, or urge, to drink?**

•**Found that drinking—or being sick from drinking—often interfered with taking care of your home or family?** Or caused job troubles? Or school problems?

•**Continued to drink even though it was causing trouble with your family or friends?**

•**Given up or cut back on activities that were important or interesting to you, or gave you pleasure, in order to drink?**

•**More than once gotten into situations while or after drinking that increased your chances of getting hurt** (such as driving, swimming, using machinery, walking in a dangerous area or having unsafe sex)?

•**Continued to drink even though it was making you feel depressed or anxious or adding to another health problem?** Or after having had a memory blackout?

•**Had to drink much more than you once did to get the effect you want?** Or found that your usual number of drinks had much less effect than before?

•**Found that when the effects of alcohol were wearing off, you had withdrawal symptoms,** such as trouble sleeping, shakiness, irritability, anxiety, depression, restlessness, nausea or sweating? Or sensed things that were not there?

If you have any of these symptoms, your drinking may already be a cause for concern. The more symptoms you have, the more urgent the need for change. To see if AUD is present, visit a health professional so a formal assessment of your symptoms can be done.

Dark Chocolate vs. Depression

In a recent study, people who ate dark chocolate daily in any amount were 70% less likely to report symptoms of depression than people who did not eat dark chocolate. Other forms of chocolate were not linked to lower depression prevalence.

Lin Yang, PhD, an epidemiologist in the department of cancer epidemiology, Alberta Health Services, Calgary, Canada, and coauthor of a study of more than 13,000 people, published in *Depression & Anxiety*. CEPR.ca

Is Stress Getting the Best of You?

Jacob Teitelbaum, MD, nationally recognized expert in the fields of pain, sleep, chronic fatigue syndrome and fibromyalgia. Based in Kailu Kona, Hawaii, he is author of numerous books, including the newly updated *Real Cause, Real Cure* and *From Fatigued to Fantastic!* (available at BottomLineStore. com), and the free iPhone and Android app *Cures A-Z*. He serves on the Science and Education Advisory Board for EuroPharma, donating the fees for that service to charity.

If you get overwhelmed by daily stress and often feel more tired than you think you should, you're not alone. But don't be too quick to simply shrug off these symptoms as the price we pay for today's fast-paced world.

You may be suffering from adrenal fatigue. While feeling stressed out and exhausted could point to a variety of conditions ranging from sleep apnea and anemia to heart problems and depression, adrenal fatigue should definitely be on your radar as your doctor investigates your symptoms.

There is no test for adrenal fatigue, so it's a controversial diagnosis and some doctors don't believe that the condition is "real." But based on my clinical experience with thousands of patients, I am convinced that it is real—and treatable.

What Is Adrenal Fatigue?

To understand adrenal fatigue, it's important to review the function of your adrenal glands. Located above each kidney, these walnut-sized glands pump out adrenaline, the fight-or-flight hormone that speeds your heart, boosts your blood pressure and shunts blood from your gut to your muscles—readying you for instant action. If your stress levels don't let up day after day, then your body's endocrine system kicks into even higher gear, triggering a hormonal cascade that includes the release of the "stress hormone" cortisol, followed by the hormone glucagon, which raises your blood sugar to supply your brain and muscles with more energy to cope with the extended physiological demands.

The problem is that your hunter-gatherer body hasn't yet evolved to adapt to the chronic stress of 21st-century living. After years of nonstop stress—marked by cortisol levels so chronically high that they eventually get depleted to chronically low levels—the adrenal glands become literally exhausted...the hallmark of adrenal fatigue.

Red Flags for Adrenal Fatigue

If your doctor has taken your medical history and ordered blood tests but hasn't found a cause for your symptoms, check to see if you have these red flags for adrenal fatigue. *Beyond feeling overwhelmed by stress and tired all the time, do you...*

• **Feel irritable when you're hungry?** Exhausted adrenal glands can't pump out enough cortisol to trigger glucagon production, so your blood sugar levels are often low, which starves the brain, causing sugar cravings and irritability—aka "hangry."

•**Have frequent infections?** These may include sore throats and colds that take longer than normal to clear up. Both high and low cortisol levels weaken the immune system.

•**Ache all over?** My patients tend to have constantly tense, achy muscles when their adrenal cortisol levels are unable to supply steady levels of blood sugar for energy after prolonged stress.

•**Feel dizzy sometimes when you stand up?** Cortisol controls blood pressure, and a deficit can result in low blood pressure.

•**Have a chronic disease?** Cortisol interferes with the action of insulin, the hormone that balances blood sugar. This can set you up for chronic ailments such as type 2 diabetes, obesity, heart disease, Alzheimer's disease and certain cancers.

If these symptoms apply to you, consider seeing an MD who specializes in holistic/functional medicine (consult The Institute for Functional Medicine, IFM.org)…or a naturopathic doctor (check with the American Association of Naturopathic Physicians, Naturopathic.org).

Note: Your doctor can treat you based on your symptoms and results from a salivary cortisol test. Because there is no specific diagnostic test, insurance is unlikely to cover this treatment, but it may help to have your doctor write a letter to your insurer if you respond positively to treatment.

When I identify adrenal fatigue in a patient, I recommend this three-step plan, which typically improves symptoms within one to two weeks…

STEP #1: Tweak your diet.

To ease stress on your adrenal glands, avoid…

•**Sweets.** Sugary foods and beverages cause blood sugar levels to repeatedly rise and fall, exhausting your glucose-controlling adrenal glands.

•**Coffee.** Like sugar, excessive caffeine forces the adrenal glands into action—and eventual exhaustion. Limit yourself to one cup of coffee in the morning and have decaf the rest of the day.

Smart alternative: Green tea has components that stop its caffeine from stimulating your adrenal glands, and it contains theanine, an amino acid that promotes calmness and concentration.

For adrenal gland support, focus on…

•**Protein.** Consume protein-rich foods at every meal, such as fish, eggs, beans and occasional modest portions of meat. These foods help stabilize blood sugar levels. Also include plenty of vegetables with your protein, particularly leafy greens, which help nourish and repair adrenals.

•**Water and salt.** Your adrenal glands regulate blood volume and blood pressure, tasks that require plenty of water and salt. But if you have weakened adrenal glands, your body doesn't adequately retain water and salt. Telltale signs of adrenal burnout are feeling thirsty and urinating more often… and craving salt.

To overcome this imbalance, drink water when you are thirsty. If you crave salt, let your taste buds guide how much you add to your foods.

Important: If you have high blood pressure or heart failure, don't increase your salt intake without consulting your physician.

•**Small meals.** To stabilize fluctuating blood sugar levels, go for five (or even six) smaller, high-protein, low-sugar meals daily.

STEP #2: Use supplements.

Supplements can help strengthen your exhausted adrenal glands and normalize your blood sugar levels.*

•**Adrenal extracts,** taken from the adrenal gland of a cow or pig, supply exhausted adrenal glands with the raw material needed for rejuvenation.

*Take these only under your doctor's supervision.

• **Chromium** is a mineral that helps normalize blood sugar levels.

• **Licorice extract** slows the breakdown of your body's cortisol.

• **Vitamin B-5** (pantothenic acid) promotes cortisol production.

• **Tyrosine** is an amino acid that your body uses to make the neurotransmitters norepinephrine and dopamine.

Helpful: Instead of taking multiple supplements, consider an adrenal supplement such as Adrenaplex from EuroPharma's Terry Naturally or Adrenal Stress End from Nature's Way—both of which contain adrenal extracts and licorice.

Note: If you have high blood pressure or diabetes, check blood pressure and glucose levels after two to four weeks to ensure that the licorice extract is not affecting these conditions.

STEP #3: Adopt healing attitudes.

If you have adrenal exhaustion, viewing life as a constant crisis—and you as its victim—will further exhaust your adrenal glands. *To reduce stress…*

• **Ask yourself,** *Am I in imminent danger?* The answer almost always will be no, which can help you turn off your fight-or-flight reflex

• **Think twice.** If you're having negative thoughts—worried, irritated or sad—focus instead on a positive thought, such as a pet or a hobby you love. Soon, this "switching" process will become second nature.

• **Practice gratitude.** Take a moment to remember what you're grateful for—the sunny day, a planned vacation, etc.

Smart strategy: Make a gratitude list—and when you feel stressed, take three deep breaths, read your list…and relax.

Reduce Stress with Forms of Focused Breathing

S *low breathing* can relieve anxiety. Inhale through your nose for three to five seconds, then exhale at the same rate through your nose or mouth. *Box breathing* can help you refocus. Exhale all air, hold for a count of four, breathe in through your nose for a count of four, hold for a count of four, then breathe out through your nose for a count of four. *Nighttime breathing* is good for unwinding before sleep. Inhale deeply to fill your chest and rib cage for a slow count of five…hold for a count of three…slowly release for a count of five. *Controlled breathing plus visualizing* helps with relaxation anytime. Create a detailed, relaxing mental picture while using any comfortable breathing rhythm and count.

Laura McDonald, American Council on Exercise–certified personal and group fitness trainer and yoga instructor, writing at BHG.com.

Night Owls: Read This

N ight owls who reset their body clocks reduce stress and improve performance. In a three-week study at universities in the UK and Australia, participants with bedtimes after 2 am reported lower rates of depression and stress and performed better on cognitive and physical tests after shifting their schedules by two hours…getting to sleep and waking earlier…maximizing exposure to sunlight in the morning…and limiting screen time and light before bed.

Elise Facer-Childs, PhD, Transitional Fellow in Industry at Monash University's Sleep and Circadian Rhythms Program, Notting Hill, Australia, and lead author of a study published in *Sleep Medicine*.

The Simplest Sleep Trick Ever

Rebecca Shannonhouse, editor-in-chief, health content, Bottom Line Inc.

A h, the joy of a good night's sleep! Like most people, I treasure those precious hours of slumber. So when I recently had trouble sleeping several nights a week, I knew I needed help.

Knowing that sleeping pills have been found to add less than 35 minutes of sleep each night...and have potential side effects, including dizziness, daytime drowsiness and even sleepwalking, I wanted to try a safer option. That's when I opted for a sleep mask. When I tried one, I was pleasantly surprised by how much my sleep improved within a matter of days.

How could something so simple help? Even when we turn out the lights, our blinking and backlit gizmos—cell phones, cable-TV boxes, clock radios, smoke alarms, etc.—often allow light to enter our bedrooms. This is a problem because melatonin, a hormone that regulates both sleepiness and the quality of sleep, is highly sensitive to light. A study reported in *The Journal of Clinical Endocrinology & Metabolism* found that light exposure during normal sleeping hours reduced melatonin production by more than 50%.

The beauty of a sleep mask is that it blocks ambient light—even if it's just a sliver of light from a streetlamp that slips through your bedroom curtains.

Poor sleep is no small matter. It has been linked to heart disease, depression, accidents and even diabetes. Even though some people may need medication, a sleep mask could be worth trying first. For me, it was the best $10 I could have spent.

Negative Response to Stress Harms Health

P eople who felt lingering negative emotions after being exposed to everyday stress-producing events were more likely to report chronic illness and functional limitations a decade later, compared with people who experienced stress but were able to let go of their negative response to it. The stressors did not have to be major—just everyday events. The association was not found with the stress itself or with negative responses to it. What mattered was the speed with which people could overcome their reactions.

Analysis of data from the "Midlife in the United States Survey" by researchers at University of California, Irvine, published in *Psychological Science*.

Hope Aids Recovery from Mental Disorders

A mong people undergoing cognitive behavioral therapy (CBT) for social anxiety disorder, panic disorder, generalized anxiety disorder or obsessive-compulsive disorder, those who experienced increased hope during CBT had improved anxiety symptoms and were better able to move toward recovery. The study defined hope as the capacity of patients to identify strategies or pathways to achieve goals—and the motivation to pursue those strategies or paths.

Matthew Gallagher, PhD, associate professor of psychology, University of Houston, and leader of a study of 223 adults, published in *Behavior Therapy*.

Surprising Way to Reduce Negative Emotions

T hink of bad thoughts as if they were people. For instance, if you are feeling sad, imagine sadness as a person and write down a description of what the person looks like. One group of volunteers did that in a recent study, which was inspired by the Pixar film *Inside Out*, in which a child's emotions are portrayed as humanized characters in her mind. Another group in the study wrote about the emotion itself and how it affects them. The group that imagined sadness as a person reported less sadness when recalling an unhappy time in their lives—possibly because imagining sadness as a person made it possible to think of it as being somewhat distanced and detached from them.

Caution: The same technique was also found to reduce the impact of positive emotions, such as happiness. So it is best tried only with negative feelings.

Fangyuan Chen, PhD, assistant professor, department of management and marketing, Hong Kong Polytechnic University, Hong Kong, and leader of a study published in *Journal of Consumer Psychology*.

Negative Moods May Signal Poor Health

People who feel sad or angry have higher levels of inflammation—part of the body's response to infections and wounds. Clinical depression and hostility were already known to be associated with inflammatory biomarkers. Now it appears that even lower-level bad moods may increase inflammation—which, if it becomes chronic, can contribute to heart disease, diabetes and some cancers.

Jennifer Graham-Engeland, PhD, associate professor of biobehavioral health, Penn State University, State College, Pennsylvania, and leader of a study published in *Brain, Behavior, and Immunity*.

New Fast-Acting Antidepressant

Esketamine (Spravato), chemically similar to the anesthetic drug *ketamine*, is approved as a nasal spray in combination with an oral antidepressant in people who have not responded adequately to two antidepressant treatments. Found to improve depression more quickly than antidepressants now in use, esketamine's side effects include dizziness, nausea and sedation.

James Greenblatt, MD, chief medical officer, Walden Behavioral Care, Waltham, Massachusetts, and clinical faculty member, Tufts University School of Medicine, Boston.

Bothered by Noise

Murray Grossan, MD, Tower Ear, Nose & Throat/Cedars-Sinai Medical Center, Los Angeles. Grossan Institute.com

Sensitivity to noise is not typically due to aging. The condition is called hyperacusis, and it's characterized by an exaggerated response to ordinary sounds that are tolerated well by others.

Often the most disturbing sounds are sudden high-pitched noises, such as alarms, which annoy most people but could cause an extreme reaction in those with hyperacusis.

Other examples: Children's screams, the clanging of silverware and dishes and clapping. The intensity of symptoms can vary widely—from mild decreased sound tolerance...to a strong sensitivity to specific sounds, like someone chewing gum...to a fear of sound.

Hyperacusis may be a symptom of another condition including depression or anxiety...PTSD...Lyme disease...Ménière's disease...noise-induced hearing loss...tinnitus...head injury...or migraine headaches. But it also can occur with no underlying condition.

Symptoms accompanying hyperacusis can include difficulty concentrating, relaxing and sleeping...and anger, irritability, anxiety and depression.

If you're concerned, see an audiologist for the diagnosis, assessment and management of hyperacusis. You may be referred to an otolaryngologist, psychologist or another specialist.

Treatment should include help for any underlying condition, which may solve the problem, but also may include counseling to help relieve stress, which only makes the condition worse. Acoustic therapy can decrease a patient's sensitivity to sounds. In one approach, the patient wears a hearing aid–like device, which makes steady, gentle sounds. The hope is that the auditory nerves and brain centers will become desensitized and able to tolerate normal sounds again.

Helpful: Practice listening to sounds that bother you at a low volume, then gradually increase the volume and duration over time… and/or add some white noise—a fan or a white noise machine—to your environment.

Note: Sometimes hyperacusis resolves on its own without treatment.

When Anxiety Steals Your Joy

Debra Kissen, PhD, MHSA, clinical fellow, Anxiety and Depression Association of America (ADAA), cochair, ADAA's Public Education Committee, and executive director, Light on Anxiety CBT Treatment Center of Chicago.

Not everyone who suffers from anxiety looks like they're suffering. Some anxiety sufferers might seem outwardly calm, deal competently with whatever life throws at them—and even be quite successful. Yet inside, they're just barely keeping a grip on their fears and worries.

These people have high-functioning anxiety. Their suffering is not as obvious as the paralyzing version—but it's just as damaging. The term "high-functioning anxiety" is relatively new and not currently recognized as a mental-health diagnosis. One reason may be that a diagnosis of anxiety disorder has to meet the criteria that symptoms (such as fear, worry, sleep problems, stress) impair functioning at work, at school or in other critical areas of life.

People with high-functioning anxiety are functioning fine—even brilliantly. But their functioning is at great cost. Constantly suppressing their inner turmoil takes a toll on joy. And the stresses that might stay suppressed (at least for a while) in one area, such as work, tend to pop up somewhere else, such as with family and friends. Also, not dealing with it now can turn anxiety into a full-fledged disorder down the road…and even increase risk for other health issues, such as dementia and heart disease.

How to Find Your Zen

If you or someone you know fits the description of high-functioning anxiety, here are the strategies that can help…

•**Cognitive behavioral therapy (CBT).** This form of psychotherapy is effective for breaking the cycle of negative thoughts that leads to anxious feelings. Treatment is usually short-term and focuses on learning self-calming skills that challenge negative thoughts.

•**Belly breathing.** Slowing your breathing tells your brain that you're safe. Inhale slowly through your nose, letting the air move down into your abdomen so that your belly expands with your breath. Then let your belly deflate as you exhale slowly through your mouth.

•**Mindfulness meditation.** Mindfulness meditation combines belly breathing with focusing thoughts on the present—rather than dwelling on problems from the past or worries about the future. Mindfulness meditation has been shown to relieve not just anxiety but also depression and pain.

•**Muscle relaxation.** Physical tension is a hallmark of anxiety. Tensing and then relaxing specific muscle groups trains you to notice when your muscles are tight—and how to release the tension in your muscles, which releases mental tension as well.

•**Yoga.** An ancient mind-body practice that combines deep breathing, physical movement and meditation, yoga stretches and strengthens muscles while improving mental well-being.

•**Healthy lifestyle.** Don't underestimate the anxiety-reducing benefits of regular exercise, proper sleep, limiting caffeine and alcohol, and eating a healthful, balanced diet.

•**Medication.** If the above steps don't give you relief, you may benefit from medication. Certain drugs, such as selective serotonin reuptake inhibitor (SSRI) antidepressants, including *fluoxetine* (Prozac) and *sertraline* (Zoloft), can help ease anxiety.

Finally, bear in mind that some anxiety can be good—if it's not excessive, it can spur you to reach a desired goal!

Have a Better Day

As soon as you put your feet on the floor in the morning, say, "This is going to be a great day." It's a very small thing that can have a big impact on how happy and satisfied you feel in your life.

BJ Fogg, PhD, founder and director of the Behavior Design Lab at Stanford University, California, and author of *Tiny Habits: The Small Changes That Change Everything.*

Green Is Good!

Merely having a view of a park or other green space from your home (along with access to gardens) has been shown to reduce cravings for alcohol, cigarettes or unhealthy foods—yet another good reason for cities to invest in healthy natural environments.

Health & Place

Contact with Nature

Just 20 minutes spent sitting or strolling in a place that lets people feel more closely in touch with nature significantly reduces the body's production of the stress hormone cortisol. Regular contact with natural surroundings can be a low-cost solution to the stress-inducing effects of urbanization and indoor lifestyles filled with screen viewing. The time of day does not matter as long as nature exposure occurs during daylight. The study's participants also were asked to avoid aerobic exercise, use of social media, the Internet, phone calls, texts, conversation and reading during their nature experiences.

MaryCarol Hunter, PhD, associate professor, School for Environment and Sustainability, University of Michigan, Ann Arbor, and leader of a study published in *Frontiers in Psychology.*

Chapter 6

FOOD, DIET AND FITNESS

The Healthiest Diet

The best nutrition advice sounds surprisingly simple—eat whole foods, preferably plants. But it gets tricky...once you consider that some whole foods are better than others when it comes to fighting major killers such as heart disease, cancer, diabetes and infections. For example, did you know that blueberries and blackberries far outperform other fruits as sources of antioxidants—substances that protect your cells from all sorts of damage?

Here's the clincher: Before you assume that your diet is "good enough," consider this—the number-one cause of death in the US is the Standard American Diet (SAD), according to research published in *JAMA*. For most leading causes of death, your genes account for only 10% to 20%. So getting your diet in optimal shape should be at the top of your priority list. Of course, fitting in all the nutrients backed by strong scientific evidence can be challenging. But it's doable—if you build your diet around a few key foods.

To keep it simple, nutrition expert Michael Greger, MD, FACLM, has spent more than a decade combing through the evidence to create his daily list of must-have foods...

• **Beans are a go-to source** for healthy **protein but also offer iron, zinc, fiber and potassium.**

What they do: Help lower cholesterol and high blood pressure and play a role in the prevention of colon cancer and stroke.

Which kinds to eat: Try a variety, including black beans, black-eyed peas, lentils, split peas and chickpeas. Canned beans are fine as long as you choose low-sodium varieties or simply rinse them well before using.

Daily dose: Three servings. A serving is one-quarter cup of hummus or bean dip or one-half cup of cooked beans.

Note: I recommend legumes over meat because they are loaded with nutrients—and are naturally low in saturated fat and sodium and free of cholesterol.

• **Berries are the fruits with** extra bragging rights.

What they do: Studies show that berries protect your brain, heart and liver, boost immunity and offer potential cancer protection.

Michael Greger, MD, FACLM, founder of the website NutritionFacts.org and author of *How Not to Die: Discover the Foods Scientifically Proven to Prevent and Reverse Disease.* He is also author of *How Not to Diet: The Groundbreaking Science of Healthy, Permanent Weight Loss.*

Which kinds to eat: Blueberries and blackberries have the highest levels of antioxidants, as noted earlier, but others, including goji berries and cranberries, also pack nutritional punches.

Helpful: Frozen berries retain most nutrients—if not more than fresh.

Daily dose: One serving. That's one-half cup of fresh or frozen berries.

• **Other fruits shouldn't scare you off because of their natural sugar.** As long as you eat your fruit whole or blended, with its fiber intact, the sugar is not a health problem.

What they do: Studies show that people who eats lots of whole fruits lower their risk for type 2 diabetes.

Which kinds to eat: Everything from apples and watermelon to avocados.

Daily dose: Three servings. A serving is one medium-sized fruit or one cup of cut fruit.

• **Cruciferous vegetables are nutritional powerhouses that produce a chemical called sulforaphane,** which is linked to a wide variety of health benefits.

What they do: These vegetables may help fight cancer, boost liver function, manage type 2 diabetes and protect your brain and eyesight.

Which kinds to eat: The category includes broccoli, kale, cabbage and cauliflower but also arugula, bok choy, collard greens and even horseradish.

Important tip: Frozen versions will not produce sulforaphane—unless you sprinkle them with mustard powder, which contains the necessary enzyme destroyed in the freezing process.

Daily dose: One serving. That's one-half cup of chopped vegetables, one-quarter cup of broccoli sprouts or one tablespoon of horseradish.

• **Greens.** Dark green, leafy vegetables pack the most nutrition per calorie of any food.

What they do: In research conducted at Harvard and published in *JAMA* and *Annals of Internal Medicine*, each additional daily serving of greens was linked to a 20% reduction in risk for heart attack and stroke.

Which kinds to eat: The list includes many cruciferous vegetables, such as kale, collard greens and arugula, but also extends to other leafy greens such as spinach and mesclun salad mix.

Helpful: If you find greens bitter, try mixing them with lightly sweetened dressings or fruits, such as fresh figs or grated apples.

Daily dose: Two servings. A serving is one cup raw or one-half cup cooked.

• **Other vegetables should be included to get the "rainbow" effect of a bountiful veggie diet.**

What they do: People who eat a variety of vegetables (and fruits) show decreased signs of inflammation and lower rates of type 2 diabetes.

Which kinds to eat: Get a colorful mix including artichokes, zucchini, asparagus, yams, beets and squash. Don't forget onions, garlic and mushrooms (technically fungi). Plain white button mushrooms may offer the greatest health benefits.

Daily dose: Two servings. A serving is one cup raw or one-half cup cooked.

Good rule of thumb: Fill half of every plate you eat with vegetables—ideally, including breakfast.

• **Flaxseeds are potent sources of lignans,** plant estrogens that can dampen the sometimes harmful effects of the body's own estrogens.

What they do: Flaxseeds help fight breast cancer, high blood pressure and prostate enlargement.

What kinds to eat: Grind whole seeds or buy them pre-ground to help ensure that you'll absorb the nutrients. The powder lasts about four months at room temperature and up to six months in the freezer. Sprinkle on oatmeal, salads, soups and other foods.

Daily dose: One serving—one tablespoon ground.

• **Nuts and seeds are a perfect snack food.**

What they do: Nut eaters are less likely to die from cancer and heart and respiratory diseases, studies show. Nuts also can provide the fat that aids the absorption of plant nutrients.

Which kinds to eat: Almonds, Brazil nuts, cashews, chia seeds, pistachios, pumpkin seeds and sunflower seeds are all good, but the evidence is strongest for walnuts, which are high in omega-3 fats and antioxidants.

Daily dose: One serving. That's one-quarter cup of nuts or seeds or two tablespoons of nut or seed butter.

• **Herbs and spices add flavor, color and antioxidants.**

What they do: Herbs and spices help control blood pressure when they are used in place of salt. One standout, turmeric, contains a pigment, curcumin, which is particularly beneficial for brain health. Turmeric is linked to reduced inflammation and anticancer effects.

Which kinds to eat: Grate fresh turmeric root to use in cooking or add a raw slice to a smoothie. Sprinkle turmeric powder onto sweet potatoes or roasted cauliflower. Use other spices, from basil to thyme, to flavor everything. Spices make a great substitute for salt.

Daily dose: One-quarter teaspoon of turmeric powder (or one-quarter inch raw), plus any other salt-free herbs and spices you like.

• **Whole grains including bread, rice, cereal and even pasta can be part of a healthy diet**—as long as they come in whole-grain form.

What they do: Reduce risks for heart disease, type 2 diabetes and stroke.

Which kinds to eat: Branch out beyond wheat, oat and corn to quinoa, amaranth, millet, buckwheat and sorghum. Labels should list whole grains. The best products are high in fiber (at least 5 g per serving) and contain little or no added sugar.

Daily dose: Three servings. A serving is one-half cup of hot cereal or pasta, one tortilla or slice of bread or three cups of popped popcorn.

7 Surprising Foods That Beat Disease

William W. Li, MD, president of Angiogenesis Foundation, Cambridge, Massachusetts. He has served on the faculties at Harvard University, Tufts University and Dartmouth Medical School and is author of *Eat to Beat Disease: The New Science of How Your Body Can Heal Itself.*

There are more than 200 foods that can intercept or even reverse certain diseases by boosting our health defenses. Of course, other foods that can damage our health have been shown to suppress the same systems, leaving us vulnerable to disease.

You may be thinking that you already know that barley, broccoli and dark leafy greens are good for you. You may be comfortable with your food choices, but challenging yourself to add the surprising foods identified here is well worth the effort. All are backed by extraordinary science...and none are in that "yuck, health food" category. You can easily add them to your meals to enrich and diversify your diet.

• **Chicken thighs.** Did you think white meat was the healthiest choice? Surprise!

Why it's so good for you: Dark chicken meat contains vitamin K-2 (also known as menaquinone), which has been shown to help control angiogenesis, one of our five defense systems. Angiogenesis is the process our bodies use to form and grow blood vessels. A healthy angiogenesis system regulates when and where blood vessels should grow and can prevent tumors from getting the blood they need to thrive.

Research at University of Illinois and Hiroshima University in Japan has found that vitamin K-2 can directly attack prostate cancer and colon cancer cells. Vitamin K also has been associated with a reduced risk for lung cancer. (See the section on Gouda cheese, page 110.)

Keep in mind: Chicken thighs often are attached to chunks of fat, so trim off the fat before cooking.

• **Mangoes.** I call the mango a grand-slammer food because, from a health standpoint, it activates all five defense systems at once, hitting a home run for your health.

Why they're so good for you: Mangoes contain the bioactive compound mangiferin. Bioactive compounds modulate metabolic processes in the body. Mangiferin improves blood-sugar control and can prevent tumors from forming, according to research from several leading Chinese hospitals and universities.

Keep in mind: If you can't find fresh mangoes, frozen ones are just as nutritious. Even though they can help your metabolism, remember that mangoes are high in natural sugar, so people with diabetes or others who are limiting their sugar intake should ask their doctors about the recommended amount to eat.

• **Purple potatoes.** These strikingly hued potatoes are becoming more available and often are seen on restaurant menus.

Why they're so good for you: Research has shown that purple potatoes can kill colon cancer stem cells and reduce the number of tumors. Scientists at Penn State University fed the equivalent of one purple potato a day for a week to mice that were at high risk for colon cancer, and they found that they had 50% fewer tumors than mice not fed the potatoes. That is similar to the effect seen in prescription drug recipients.

Note: Ask at your grocery store if it carries the Purple Majesty variety—the kind used in the research. Purple potatoes can be prepared in different ways and still offer a health benefit.

• **Sourdough bread.** Remarkably, the element that gives sourdough bread its mildly sour taste is also what makes it healthful.

Why it's so good for you: The probiotics. Sourdough bread starter uses a natural, healthy bacteria called *Lactobacillus reuteri*, which has been shown in the lab to improve immunity, suppress tumor development, slow weight gain and speed up wound healing.

The bacteria even can stimulate the brain to release oxytocin, the feel-good hormone. Scientists had long assumed that the health benefits of Lactobacillus reuteri were destroyed in the heat of an oven, but researchers at Massachusetts Institute of Technology found that even the fragments of killed bacteria can deliver the same benefits.

Keep in mind: Some sourdough bread does not actually use the right bacteria and is just flavored to taste tangy. Buy at bakeries where you can ask about the process. Eating bread loads you up with calories, so don't go overboard eating sourdough.

• **Gouda cheese.** It's surprising that cheese has health benefits, but it is indeed true when it comes to certain hard cheeses, such as Gouda.

Why it's so good for you: Just like chicken thighs, Gouda is high in vitamin K-2. Landmark research from Germany (the EPIC–Heidelberg study) examined the link between K-2 and cancer and found that eating between one and three slices (about one to three ounces) of hard cheese each day was associated with a 62% drop in risk for lung cancer. And eating the equivalent of two slices per day led to a 35% decrease in the risk for prostate cancer.

Keep in mind: Cheese is a source of saturated fat and high sodium, so less is more.

• **Kiwifruit.** This fruit—which is actually a large berry—came from China, where it was known for its benefits for digestion.

Why it's so good for you: Researchers at National University of Singapore showed that kiwi makes it easier for your gut microbiome to grow healthy bacteria, which can improve the state of your immune system. Meanwhile, scientists in Scotland found that kiwi can help prevent and repair damage to our DNA that is caused by the environment and linked to many serious diseases, including cancer.

Keep in mind: Eating one kiwifruit a day is beneficial, but even more benefits were seen by researchers with three kiwifruits per day.

•**Concord grape juice.** OK, technically this is a beverage. But it's a powerhouse nonetheless.

Why it's so good for you: Besides being good for the heart as reported in previous studies, grape juice boosts your immune system, according to a study from University of Florida. Drinking one and a half cups of Concord grape juice every day for nine weeks was found to increase the level of T-cells, which play an important role in immunity and fighting cancer.

Keep in mind: Like all fruit juice, grape juice contains natural sugar, so if you need to control your blood sugar for any reason, check with your doctor before adding this to your diet. Also avoid juices with added sugars or artificial sweeteners.

Exotic Foods You Should Be Eating...But Probably Aren't

Sharon Palmer, MSFS, RDN, a registered dietitian nutritionist and author of *The Plant-Powered Diet.* She also holds a master of science degree in sustainable food systems and is nutrition editor for *Today's Dietitian.* Read her blog at "The Plant-Powered Dietitian" at SharonPalmer.com.

There are an estimated 50,000 edible plant species—from apples to zucchinis—on this big, beautiful planet. Yet only a few hundred species contribute significantly to what humans consume.

That means you're probably missing out on a veritable cornucopia of luscious fruits and vegetables—each with its own color, flavor, texture and aroma...not to mention unique nutritional benefits. And you're probably walking right past these items in your grocery store. *Five lesser known fruits and vegetables that will enrich your diet...*

Celeriac

Also known as celery root, the gnarled, hairy celeriac may not be the prettiest of the pack, but it delivers a powerful punch of flavor and nutrition. Celeriac is a type of celery, which is in the same family as parsley and parsnips, but it's grown for its underground root rather than its stalks.

Beneath its rough skin, you'll find crisp white flesh with a hint of celery flavor that you can use in a variety of dishes.

Why it's good for you: Celeriac provides a trove of nutrients, such as fiber...vitamins C, B-6 and K...phosphorus...manganese...and potassium. This means that the root is particularly good for your bones, heart and blood pressure.

How to enjoy it: Add grated raw celeriac to salads or slice it into sticks and dip into hummus. You also can cook and purée it for soups...or mash or roast it as a side dish.

Dragon Fruit

This prickly plant with a bright fuchsia peel and greenish scales and horns may resemble a dragon, but its fruit is delicately sweet and tender. Dragon fruit thrives in warm regions, including Southeast Asia, Mexico and the Caribbean.

Why it's good for you: Dragon fruit is rich in antioxidant compounds and fiber, offering benefits such as a reduced risk for certain types of cancer. Even the seeds contain essential fatty acids, which may help lower cholesterol.

How to enjoy it: Simply slice it in half and discover the tender white flesh studded with black edible seeds—scoop it out with a spoon and enjoy this delicately sweet fruit that has a kiwilike taste. You also can slice the fruit into wedges and add it to a tropical fruit platter or dice it to top off a bowl of granola or liven up a deep green salad.

Jackfruit

A versatile staple native to India and Southeast Asia, jackfruit is in the mulberry family and grows on trees to gigantic proportions—reaching up to 80 pounds. It is sweet when ripe, so it's often used in jams, juice and desserts.

When the fruit is unripe, it yields a stringy, chewy texture and red color, similar to that of pulled meat. Jackfruit can serve as a meat alternative when marinated in flavorful sauces.

Why it's good for you: Jackfruit is a good source of fiber…vitamins A and C…riboflavin…and minerals, such as magnesium and potassium. The fruit is also rich in phytochemicals, including carotenoids, which have been linked to cancer protection, heart health and reduced risk for age-related eye problems, according to research published in 2019 in *International Journal of Food Science*.

How to enjoy it: Jackfruit can be found as a whole fruit (ripe and unripe) or canned (unripe) at most specialty Asian or natural-food markets. Enjoy sweet jackfruit in desserts or as a spread over toast. Try simmering unripe jackfruit in flavorful sauces, such as curry or barbecue. For a meat alternative, serve this simmered, saucy version of jackfruit with steamed whole grains, such as quinoa or couscous.

Persimmon

This intensely sweet, flavorful fruit is delicious served fresh and when used in cooking. While there are hundreds of varieties of persimmons, the Japanese persimmon is what we usually see in the US—the acorn-shaped Hachiya is the most common of this variety.

Like many persimmons, Hachiya is astringent, so it must be fully ripened to a very soft flesh before you can eat it. The tomato-shaped, nonastringent Fuyu persimmon, on the other hand, can be eaten when it is crisp and firm.

Why it's good for you: The persimmon is rich in beta-carotene, as well as manganese, fiber and tannins, plant compounds linked to reduced blood cholesterol levels. Preliminary research also has found that persimmon may help guard against thyroid cancer, according to a study published in *British Journal of Nutrition*.

How to enjoy it: The persimmon is best enjoyed as a fresh, seasonal whole fruit, but you also can add it to baked goods, such as breads, cookies and muffins. Or for a tasty, colorful treat, toss some sliced persimmon into your oatmeal, yogurt bowl or a hearty salad.

Pomelo

At first sight, you might suspect that a pomelo is really an enormous grapefruit. Indeed, it is closely related. Pomelo is the largest of the citrus fruits and one of the original citrus species, originating from China and Southeast Asia. Like grapefruit, pomelos can vary in color (green or yellow) but unlike their cousins, they can grow to the size of a small bowling ball.

When comparing tastes, the pomelo's flavors range from sweet and sour to tangy and tart, which makes this fruit wonderfully adaptable. The pomelo is considered a symbol of prosperity for the Chinese New Year, and it's easy to see why—when you dig through its fragrant skin and thick membrane, you uncover a fresh, jewel-like fruit treasure.

Why it's good for you: Pomelo is an excellent source of vitamin C, potassium, fiber and beta-carotene. Citrus fruits, like pomelo, are beneficial for heart, bone and brain health, as well as cancer protection.

How to enjoy it: Pomelo is extremely versatile, due to its unique flavor and texture. It pairs well with herbs, such as mint, cilantro and basil…fruits, such as pineapple, coconut and mango…and spring vegetables, including carrots and radishes. Heat can make pomelo bitter, but you can add this fruit to hot dishes at the end of cooking. Pomelo is delicious in salads, fruit platters and breakfast bowls. You also can try pomelo juice in recipes that usually call for lemon, such as pasta, roasted vegetables and salads.

That Sounds Delicious

Good-for-you-foods that sound indulgent are more likely to be eaten. According to research done at Stanford University and other US institutions, simply knowing that a healthy food is good for you isn't enough to make people choose it. "Taste-focused" descriptions that feature specific flavors and textures excite your taste buds.

Example: The next time you want your family to eat baked squash, tell them it's "herb-crusted roasted squash."

Bradley P. Turnwald, PhD, postdoctoral scholar in the department of psychology at Stanford University, California, and coauthor of a study published in *Psychological Science.*

Too Little Sleep Linked to Unhealthy Eating

Thorsten Kahnt, PhD, assistant professor of neurology at Northwestern University Feinberg School of Medicine, Chicago. Northwestern.edu

People are more likely to indulge in unhealthy foods that are high in fat or sugar when they haven't had enough sleep. In a recent study published in eLife, participants partook more heavily of an array of unhealthy foods including doughnut holes, chocolate chip cookies and potato chips following nights when they got only four hours of sleep than when allowed a full eight hours of sleep.

Smell, not exhaustion, seems to be at the root of the increased snacking. Brain scans revealed that when someone is sleep-deprived, her piriform cortex, a region of the brain that processes odor, experiences a heightened ability to identify food smells...while its ability to communicate with the insula, a region that processes signals associated with food intake, is diminished.

Net result: Tired people are more likely to succumb to the smell of high-calorie foods, such as doughnuts and potato chips—not just their mere presence.

It's possible (though not yet proven) that sleep-deprived brains intentionally steer people toward high-calorie foods when they're fatigued as a survival strategy. For much of humankind's history, packing on a few extra pounds during stressful times when sleep was in short supply was a prudent precaution. In the past, the problem that was costing someone sleep might make food hard to come by the next day.

What to do: Try to avoid the smell of fatty or sugary foods following nights when you didn't get sufficient sleep. If you can't avoid those tasty smells, remind yourself that you are especially likely to be tempted by these foods when you are tired. This awareness can boost your ability to resist. If you're trying to lose weight, include "get sufficient sleep" as part of your diet plan.

4 Healthy Nighttime Snacks

Janet Bond Brill, PhD, RDN, FAND, a registered dietitian nutritionist, a fellow of the Academy of Nutrition and Dietetics and a nationally recognized nutrition, health and fitness expert who specializes in cardiovascular disease prevention. Based in Allentown, Pennsylvania, Dr. Brill is author of *Blood Pressure DOWN, Cholesterol DOWN* and *Prevent a Second Heart Attack.* DrJanet.com

Let's be honest—most people love to nosh a bit if they become engrossed in a new TV series or a big-screen film they can finally watch at home. But is it possible to snack healthfully? Yes, it is.

As a nutritionist who has done her own share of late-night snacking, here are my four favorite yummy treats—each under 200 calories...

• **Dark-chocolate covered banana.** Get your potassium from the banana and a heart-healthy dose of dark chocolate with this sinfully delicious dessert treat. Cut a ripe banana into slices and place them on a plate. Melt a tablespoon of dark chocolate baking chips in the microwave and drizzle over the banana slices. Top with a tablespoon of fat-free whipped topping—all for just 190 calories.

• **Pumpkin pie Greek yogurt.** Pumpkin is packed with disease-fighting antioxidants and a generous punch of protein. Plus, it's low in calories and it's filling. A six-ounce serving of plain 0% Greek yogurt contains no fat, about 15 g to 20 g of protein (equivalent to two to three ounces of meat) and 20% of your daily recommended calcium intake.

Directions: Take one small container of 0% fat plain Greek yogurt, add in two tablespoons of pure canned pumpkin…sweetener of choice (to taste)…and one-half teaspoon of pumpkin pie spice. Mix together and top with fat-free whipped cream and one tablespoon of diced walnuts for an approximately 170-calorie sweet treat.

• **Red bell pepper slices with a zesty dip.** Red bell peppers are packed with nutrients such as folate, potassium and vitamins A, B-6, C, E and K. And all this for a mere 30 calories per pepper. Dip the slices in honey mustard for added zip (two tablespoons has 140 calories)…or salsa (nutrient-rich, no fat and about 10 calories in two tablespoons).

• **Cinnamon apple chips.** For a sweet and healthy, high-fiber snack, grab some nutritious apples, add some cinnamon and a touch of sugar.

Ingredients:
3 small Red Delicious apples, cored
1 teaspoon cinnamon
2 Tablespoons sugar (*Optional:* To reduce the sugar and carbohydrate count, substitute one tablespoon of Truvia Baking Blend or Splenda Sugar Blend for the sugar.)

Directions: Preheat your oven to 200°F, and line two baking sheets with parchment paper. Using a sharp knife, slice the apples as thin as possible (leave the nutrition-packed peels on the apples). Place the apple slices on the parchment paper in one layer. Mix the cinnamon and sugar, and sprinkle half of it onto the sliced apples. Bake for 40 to 50 minutes, flip the apples, add the rest of

the cinnamon/sugar mix to the other side and bake for another 40 to 50 minutes. The apples will be a golden brown. Remove from the oven and let the chips cool. The chips are best eaten within a couple hours of cooling. Makes two servings (each less than 200 calories).

Don't Sleep with the TV On

Sleeping with the TV on may lead to weight gain.

Recent finding: Women who slept with TV or other lights on were 17% more likely to gain at least 11 pounds over five years than women who slept in darkness. And those women were 30% more likely to become obese.

Self-defense: If you watch TV in bed, set a timer to turn it off automatically.

Dale P. Sandler, PhD, chief of epidemiology branch at National Institute of Environmental Health Sciences, Durham, North Carolina, and lead author of a study published in *JAMA Internal Medicine*.

The Best Protein Powders

Tod Cooperman, MD, president, founder and editor in chief of ConsumerLab.com, a subscription-based website ($47.40 annually) that evaluates consumer products relating to health, wellness and nutrition. ConsumerLab.com recently completed an extensive product review of protein powders, shakes and drinks.

There was a time when bodybuilders and the elderly were just about the only people to use protein supplements. No more!

Now: There's an ever-increasing selection of protein powders available not just in health-food stores but also on the shelves of most US supermarkets and drugstores.

Why We Need Protein

Our bodies need protein to build and maintain our muscles, bones and skin. Protein also helps keep our energy levels high and promotes weight loss in those who want to drop unwanted pounds.

Protein is especially important as we grow older. With each decade after age 30, we lose as much as 3% to 5% of our muscle mass, leading to weakness that also increases our risk for falls and broken bones. A recent report suggests that people with pronounced muscle loss, a condition known as sarcopenia, face more than twice the risk for a fall-related fracture.

Adults should get 0.36 g of protein per pound, according to the recommended dietary allowance. For example, someone weighing 150 pounds would need to get 54 g of protein daily. But research published in 2019 in *The Journal of Nutrition, Health & Aging* found that 30% of men and 45% of women ages 51 to 60 failed to meet this basic threshold...and 37% of men and 48% of women fell short during their next decade of life.

While foods (such as meat, seafood, dairy, legumes and nuts) should be our main sources of this vital nutrient, more and more people are turning to protein powders and drinks to help them get adequate levels in their diets. Such products are not only convenient, but also are free of the saturated fat and cholesterol that are often found in protein-rich foods.

Caveat: Protein—whether it's from food or a supplement—is not a miracle fix. Regular resistance exercise, such as lifting weights or using weight machines, is also necessary. As part of an overall fitness program, older adults should do strength training two to three times a week. Strength-training regimens may include squats, wall push-ups and exercises, such as biceps curls, that use hand weights.

The Changing Face of Protein

The proteins found in powders and drinks are no longer your run-of-the-mill dairy-based products, derived from whey or casein. There's a recent push for more plant-based sources, including pea, hemp, rice, soy or other nondairy ingredients, which work well for people who are lactose intolerant.

So which products contain the highest-quality ingredients at the best prices? For four top picks, we spoke with Tod Cooperman, MD, president and founder of Consumer Lab.com, which identifies the best health and nutritional products through independent testing.

ConsumerLab.com approves protein supplements based on their quality, value, taste and mixability. The products below also did not exceed contamination limits for lead, cadmium, arsenic or mercury.

Important: Because high protein intake can impair kidney function in people with kidney disease, they should talk to their doctors about how much and what types of protein they should consume. Some doctors advise increasing overall fluid intake when consuming a high-protein diet or protein supplements to help protect the kidneys, but this is probably not necessary if you have normal kidney function. Before adding a protein supplement to your diet, check with your doctor if you have any concerns. *Among the top low-sugar powders tested by ConsumerLab.com...*

•**MyProtein Impact Whey Isolate**
Protein source: Whey.
Price: 52 cents per 20 g of protein.
Why it's a top pick: Low in carbs and virtually fat-free, this whey isolate (it contains only 0.31 g of lactose per serving) has a slight powdered-milk taste and blends well into drinks. It provides 22 g of protein per serving and 12% of an adult's daily value for calcium. It's gluten-free.

•**NOW Sports Pea Protein, Natural Unflavored**
Protein source: Pea.
Price: 37 cents per 20 g of protein.
Why it's a top pick: Mixing easily and smoothly into liquids, this product enhances the taste of vegetable smoothies and pro-

vides 24 g of protein per serving. At 330 mg of sodium per serving, it's slightly higher in sodium than most protein powders but is gluten- and lactose-free.

•**Nutiva Organic Hemp Protein**

Protein source: Hemp.

Price: $1.04 per 20 g of protein.

Why it's a top pick: With a bountiful 8 g of fiber per scoop—one of hemp's big benefits—this unsweetened supplement also has naturally high levels of potassium, iron, magnesium and zinc. Its complex but pleasant vegetable flavor is offset by a somewhat gritty texture that makes it less suitable for mixing with plain water but terrific in a smoothie. This powder provides 15 g of protein per serving. It has no measurable lactose but is not gluten-free.

•**Garden of Life Sport Organic Plant-Based Protein, Vanilla**

Protein source: Mixed.

Price: $1.35 per 20 g of protein.

Why it's a top pick: Primarily pea-based but also containing navy, lentil and garbanzo beans as well as cranberry protein, this powder mixes easily and evenly into water and other thin beverages. It provides 15 g of protein per serving and has a clean vegetable flavor with only a slight artificial-sugar sweetness despite its stevia content. This gluten-free powder has no measurable lactose.

Use Some "Flour Power" to Get More Nutrition

Janet Bond Brill, PhD, RDN, FAND, a registered dietitian nutritionist, a fellow of the Academy of Nutrition and Dietetics and a nationally recognized nutrition, health and fitness expert who specializes in cardiovascular disease prevention. Based in Allentown, Pennsylvania, Dr. Brill is author of *Blood Pressure DOWN, Cholesterol DOWN* and *Prevent a Second Heart Attack.* DrJanet.com

When it comes to baking, the go-to ingredient for generations of Americans has been all-purpose flour, which is made from wheat. But if you're looking for some variety in taste, an extra boost of nutrition and even some gluten-free options, other flours should be on your radar. Most grocery stores now stock these "alternative" flours, but if yours doesn't, check your local health-food store or shop online. *My four favorites…*

•**Rye flour.** Rye is a very healthy whole grain that's popular in Scandinavia, where their dense, fiber-filled black bread is made of 100% pure rye flour. Here in the US, rye bread is made from a mixture of rye flour and wheat flour. Rye grains are highly nutritious, filled with soluble fiber, vitamin E, calcium, iron, magnesium and potassium. The high levels of magnesium and potassium help lower blood pressure, and the soluble fiber lowers cholesterol. Rye also has been shown to promote weight loss and elimination and to help prevent type 2 diabetes. Rye, which tastes sweet and malty, is sometimes used in baked goods such as piecrusts or crackers.

Note: Rye does contain gluten, albeit less than what's found in all-purpose flour. To bake with rye flour, mix with all-purpose flour—use up to 40% of light rye or about 20% of dark rye/pumpernickel flour.

•**Chickpea flour.** Chickpeas (also known as garbanzo beans) are a legume—not a grain—so this flour is gluten-free. Packed with plant protein, iron, fiber, vitamins and minerals (especially the blood pressure–lowering mineral potassium), chickpea flour is highly nutritious. With a subtle flavor, chickpea flour is a versatile ingredient for use in the kitchen. Chickpea flour, which adds a nutty taste and gives a nice protein boost over wheat, can be used for baked goods such as batter to coat fritters for frying and as a thickener for soups. If you choose to substitute chickpea flour for all-purpose flour, use three-quarters cup of chickpea flour for each cup of all-purpose flour.

•**Almond flour.** Ground almonds are a wonderful way to get your daily dose of heart-healthy nuts. High in protein, insoluble fiber, vitamins, minerals and monounsaturated fat, almond flour gives baked goods a rich flavor and makes them more tender and moist. If you substitute one-to-one for all-purpose flour, use more egg to offset almond flour's density.

- **Oat flour.** One of the healthiest grains on Earth, oats are filled with vital nutrients such as plant protein, vitamins (especially B vitamins) and minerals (especially iron and zinc). Oats also contain two unique disease-fighting substances—a group of antioxidants known as avenanthramides and the powerful cholesterol-lowering soluble fiber called beta-glucan. Unlike all-purpose flour, oat flour is gluten-free. (Just be sure to buy a product labeled as such if you are gluten-free, since contamination can occur during processing.) Oat and wheat flours have a similar taste profile, except that oat flour is sweeter and more dense. Due to the lack of gluten, oat flour will need more yeast for baked goods that rise. Oat flour is best for baking quick breads, pancakes and cookies, which allow for a one-to-one substitution for all-purpose flour.

Why Healthy Poke Bowls Are All the Rage

Janet Bond Brill, PhD, RDN, FAND, a registered dietitian nutritionist, a fellow of the Academy of Nutrition and Dietetics and a nationally recognized nutrition, health and fitness expert specializing in cardiovascular disease prevention. Based in Allentown, Pennsylvania, Dr. Brill is author of *Blood Pressure DOWN, Cholesterol DOWN* and *Prevent a Second Heart Attack*. DrJanet.com

"Poke Bowl" mania is everywhere—on social media…in your local grocery store…and even at a nearby poke bar. So what are these one-dish wonders? In case you're not quite sure, poke (pronounced "POH-kay") is the ubiquitous rice bowl filled with super-fresh raw fish and other vibrantly colored toppings. *It's not too late to learn how to make your own poke bowl creations…*

A Customized One-Dish Meal

Poke is a traditional Hawaiian dish that dates back centuries. Today's poke bowl is a delicate dish of fresh, diced raw fish (often marinated) and served cold over rice. The rice and fish are seasoned and topped with vegetables and sauces packed with savory umami (the so-called "fifth" taste—after sweet, salty, sour and bitter—that imparts a meaty-type richness).

All ingredients are sliced and diced into bite-size portions. The beauty of a poke bowl is that it is an easily customizable dish, so you can change up the ingredients to your liking. Think of it as the next generation of fast-food sushi, where you can have a complete, nutritious meal ready to eat in minutes, no rolling required. And even if you're a vegetarian, you can create your own fish-free poke bowl.

Make Your Own Healthy Poke Bowl

At the most basic level, a poke bowl is made up of…

- **The base.** This is typically white rice. To make it healthier, choose brown rice, quinoa, farro or fresh dark leafy greens instead. Arugula is especially healthful, as it is a cancer-fighting cruciferous vegetable.

- **The protein.** Cubed, sushi-grade raw salmon or ahi tuna (yellowfin tuna) is the standard protein. However, if you're worried about eating ahi tuna due to overfishing and/or its high mercury level, choose the salmon sashimi instead. If you don't like raw fish, then cook it to your liking. It will take only a few minutes.

Note: Be sure that you do not marinate the fish in soy sauce or you'll add too much sodium. Remember, you can always opt for some other lean protein, such as hamachi (Japanese amberjack or yellowtail fish)…cooked shrimp, chicken, crab or octopus…scrambled egg…or tofu (as a vegetarian option).

- **The veggies.** Healthy choices include cubed avocado, seaweed, shaved radish, shredded carrots, shredded Napa cabbage, cubed cucumber and edamame.

• **Seasonings.** Instead of high-sodium soy sauce, try a plain (but flavorful) rice vinegar, which has no sodium and is low calorie, with sesame oil. For spice, try sliced jalapeños, sriracha sauce (which contains capsaicin, a chili pepper derivative good for metabolism) or wasabi. A sprinkle or two of Eden Shake Furikake Sesame and Sea Vegetable Seasoning (a Japanese seasoning mixture of sesame seeds, chopped seaweed and salt—one tablespoon has 150 mg of sodium) is another healthy option.

• **The toppings.** Cubed mango, sliced pears, scallions, pickled ginger and onions, chopped nuts and sesame seeds are nutrition-packed options for toppings. To keep it healthy, stay away from the fried stuff (such as onions or wonton strips)!

"Grass-Fed" Beef Labeling Can Be Deceptive

Mark Hyman, MD, practicing family physician and founder and director of The UltraWellness Center, Lenox, Massachusetts. His most recent book is *Food Fix: How to Save Our Health, Our Economy, Our Communities, and Our Planet—One Bite at a Time.* DrHyman.com

Grass-fed beef has assorted health benefits vs. its grain-fed and fattened cousins. It has higher levels of vitamins, antioxidants and other nutrients, including more anti-inflammatory omega-3s and conjugated linoleic acid and fewer pro-inflammatory omega-6s. Also, grazing helps restore natural pasture ecosystems, leading to less reliance on chemical pesticides and herbicides. And since antibiotics are not used, grass-fed beef is significantly less likely to harbor drug-resistant bacteria. A 2015 study found that 18% of conventional beef samples were contaminated with "superbug" bacteria resistant to several classes of antibiotics, compared with 9% of sustainably raised (including grass-fed) samples.

Problem: There are no federal government standards for grass-fed beef nor for grass-fed beef labeling—meat companies can label meat "grass-fed" even if grass was only a minor part of the animals' feed.

Potentially misleading label: "Grass fed, grain finished" typically means that the animal ate grass much of its life but was fed a grain-rich diet to boost its weight in its final months. This is less than ideal even if the animal truly was grass-fed for most of its life—altering diet in these final months leads to changes in the nutritional composition of its meat.

What to look for on the label: A label identifying beef as grass-fed can be trusted if it's certified by a reliable third-party verifier such as the American Grassfed Association (AmericanGrassfed.org) or the Food Alliance (FoodAlliance.org). In order to be certified grass-fed beef by these organizations, the animal must have lived on pasture and eaten an exclusively grass (and/or other "forage," such as hay) diet throughout its life. Whole Foods uses the term "pasture-raised," and its beef is third-party verified. Another option is to purchase beef from a local farm, perhaps at a local farmer's market.

Antibiotics and Pesticides in Milk

A study of four brands of organic milk and four brands of conventional milk found no such residues in organic samples but some level of them in 26% to 60% of samples of conventional milk. Residue levels were above federal guidelines for amoxicillin in one sample and for sulfamethazine and sulfathiazole—two common antibacterial agents—in several samples.

Unknown: Whether residues at the levels found have any impact on human health.

Jean A. Welsh, PhD, associate professor, department of pediatrics, Emory University, Atlanta, and leader of a study published in *Public Health Nutrition.*

Fun New Fruit Salad Flavors

Make your fruit bowl even brighter with traditional flavorings used in untraditional ways...

Balsamic glaze: Buy a bottle of a sweet and tangy balsamic reduction, and use it as a delicious drizzle over fresh fruit. It's especially luscious over berries, cherries and peaches. The thick syrupy texture of the reduction is far better on fruit than straight balsamic vinegar, which is thinner and more acidic.

Chili and lime: Liven up tropical fruit such as mango and pineapple. Toss three cups of cut fruit with a dressing of one tablespoon of lime juice whisked with one tablespoon of honey plus a generous pinch of ancho chili powder.

Creamy lemon-poppyseed: Swirl one tablespoon of lemon juice, lemon zest and a touch of honey into a cup of plain yogurt, then stir in a teaspoon of poppy seed. Add the dressing to your cut fruit for a creamy treat that really pops.

Ellie Krieger, RD, author of *Whole in One: Complete, Healthy Meals in a Single Pot, Sheet Pan or Skillet*. EllieKrieger.com

Celery: The Stealth Health Food Worth Getting More of

Janet Bond Brill, PhD, RDN, FAND, a registered dietitian nutritionist, a fellow of the Academy of Nutrition and Dietetics and a nationally recognized nutrition, health and fitness expert who specializes in cardiovascular disease prevention. Based in Allentown, Pennsylvania, Dr. Brill is author of *Blood Pressure DOWN, Cholesterol DOWN* and *Prevent a Second Heart Attack*. DrJanet.com

You might think that celery is just one of those plain-Jane foods that you find on a veggie platter or sticking out of your Bloody Mary. And because celery is emblematic of dieting, you probably wouldn't be surprised to learn that a five-inch stalk has just three calories. But did you know that for those three calories, you also get a whole lot of nutrition? High in fiber, bulked up with lots of zero-calorie water plus a nice dose of disease-fighting antioxidant phytonutrients, vitamins K, C and A, folate and potassium, this fabulous, crunchy, super-low-calorie food deserves a second look—even if you're not dieting. Research suggests that the powerful antioxidants in celery help the body fight off heart disease (by lowering blood pressure)...boost immune function...and lower inflammation.

Some other little-known nuggets about celery...

***FACT #1:* Calories do count.** Some people claim that celery is a "negative-calorie food"—a term that means you will burn more calories digesting celery than it contains, for a net loss. This sounds plausible—in theory—but in reality, even the lowest calorie foods, such as celery, grapefruit and cucumber, still contain more calories than it takes to break down and absorb them in the body.

***FACT #2:* Celery juice is not a cure-all.** Search social media for #celeryjuice, and you will be inundated with gorgeous photos of what is often touted as a miracle green elixir, a drink capable of curing everything from eczema and infertility to cancer and even mental illness. The problem is, there is no scientific data supporting these claims. Plus, when you juice a lot of celery, you concentrate the vegetable, so it's going to be higher in sugars, carbohydrates and calories. With the juicing process, you also strip away the beneficial fiber—the very substance that helps you feel fuller longer, improves your intestinal health and feeds the healthy bacteria in your gut.

***FACT #3:* Raw is best.** Celery often is eaten raw—and for good reason. Blanching or boiling celery causes a significant loss of antioxidants, according to research. When eaten raw (or steamed), celery retains almost all the antioxidants.

It's time to get creative: Celery makes a great addition to almost all salads, and it definitely adds some crunch and pizzazz to the mouthwatering salad recipe below!

Couscous, Orange, Grape and Celery Salad

1 cup uncooked couscous

1 small orange

2 Tablespoons extra-virgin olive oil

1 Tablespoon white wine vinegar

Dash of sea salt

Dash of freshly ground black pepper

3 approximately 5-inch celery stalks plus ½ cup celery leaves, chopped

½ pound red seedless grapes, halved

Directions: Cook couscous according to package directions. Remove from heat and let cool. Zest the orange peel, and juice the orange. In a small bowl, whisk together one tablespoon orange zest, juice from the orange, extra-virgin olive oil, white wine vinegar, salt and pepper for the dressing. In a salad bowl, mix together the couscous, celery and grapes. Toss in the dressing and serve. Makes two servings.

Nutritional information per serving: Calories, 250…fat, 15 g…cholesterol, 0 mg… carbohydrates, 46 g…dietary fiber, 2 g… total sugars, 21 g…added sugars, 0 g…protein, 6 g…sodium, 35 mg.

Avocados Can Help You Eat Less

People who ate a meal that included half an avocado felt fuller and more satisfied after six hours than people who ate a low-fat, high-carbohydrate meal. Researchers believe this may be due to the fat and fiber in avo-

---

Keep Food Separate

Don't let different foods touch one another on your plate. This will help you to more clearly see how much you're eating and practice better portion control.

Joel Harper, celebrity trainer and author *of Mind Your Body: 4 Weeks to a Leaner, Healthier Life.*

---

cados—half of one avocado has about five grams of fiber.

Study by researchers at Center for Nutrition Research, Illinois Institute of Technology, Chicago, reported in *Nutrition.*

Food Addiction Is Real

Ashley N. Gearhardt, PhD, associate professor of psychology at University of Michigan and director of its Food and Addiction Science and Treatment Lab, both in Ann Arbor. One of the preeminent researchers in the field, she was principal developer of the Yale Food Addiction Scale. FastLab.psych.lsa.umich.edu

A lot of people love their junk food— candy bars, potato chips, donuts and greasy french fries, to name just a few. They know all these foods are bad for them, but they just can't help themselves. Are these people "addicted"—the way that others are hooked on alcohol or opioids?

The concept of "food addiction" has been kicked around since the 19th century, but only recently—as obesity has reached epidemic proportions in the US—have doctors and scientists taken it seriously.

Now: With mounting scientific evidence showing that certain patterns of food consumption do have much in common with drug and alcohol addictions, many of the mysteries of out-of-control eating patterns are finally being unraveled.

Are you—or someone you know—a food addict? *What you need to know…*

Doctors diagnose an addiction when the use of a substance, such as drugs or alcohol, or a behavior like gambling is beyond a person's control. When it takes hold, you can't stop your addiction—despite the toll it's taking on your health, work and personal relationships.

Satisfying your "appetite" for the substance or behavior consumes considerable time and energy. You may experience intense cravings for the object of your addiction and suffer physical and emotional pains of withdrawal without it.

On a biological level, the brains of individuals who are addicted to a substance or behavior are different from other people's brains. Circuits that process reward are overstimulated, and those that regulate self-control are less active. In other words, in addiction the strong desire for the drug is coupled with weaker brakes, which makes it hard to stop the behavior even when it is getting you into trouble.

Recent scientific evidence: Using brain imaging and other analyses, researchers have seen similar biological patterns in people whose food consumption fits the "addictive" pattern, according to research published in 2018 in *Nutrients*.

Still, the diagnosis of food addiction remains controversial. Unlike alcohol or painkillers, food can't be an "addictive" substance, some argue, because we need it to survive.

There's some truth to that argument because people don't become addicted to food in general, but almost always to certain highly processed products—typically salty snacks like potato chips and food products that are high in fats and refined carbohydrates, particularly added sugar, and low in protein and fiber. Junk food, in other words.

The simple carbs of these highly addictive edibles hit the bloodstream rapidly to spike blood sugar, and the oral pleasure of high-fat or salty foods further amps up the brain's reward system. Whole foods—or those that are less processed—affect blood sugar levels and the brain much more gradually.

Contrary to what many people assume, not all addicts are obese or overweight. In fact, 11% of people whose weight is normal have significant symptoms of food addiction, according to a systematic review published in *Nutrients*.

However, the more you weigh, the greater the risk—among obese individuals, the rate of food addiction is 25%. At the same time, as these figures show, many obese—even morbidly obese—people are not addicts.

As scientists investigate the connection between body weight and food addiction, it appears that being overweight can be a cause—as well as a consequence—of this addiction. There is evidence that obesity changes how the brain's reward system operates, making it necessary to have more food to get the same emotional charge—you need two slices of pizza where one used to do.

Food addiction affects both men and women, although some studies suggest that rates are a bit higher in women. Middle-aged women (ages 45 to 64) are more likely to have food addiction than older women, according to research published in *The American Journal of Clinical Nutrition*. It appears to run in families—children of food-addicted parents are more likely to develop the problem themselves, possibly reflecting the influence of both upbringing and genetics.

While the US isn't the only country plagued by food addiction, surveys show that the problem is significantly less common in other countries. Americans live in what many call a "toxic" food environment—junk food is cheap, always available and relentlessly advertised.

What's more, many of these foods are designed to be addictive. So-called "Big Food"—the major food manufacturers—invest heavily in research to develop products that have precisely the effects on the brain and body that lead to their compulsive consumption.

The harmful effects of food addiction are, not surprisingly, mainly those that occur with obesity—increased risk for heart disease, diabetes, orthopedic problems and certain cancers. But there is also evidence that the surplus of fat and refined carbs of addictive foods raises cholesterol and the risk for diabetes even if you're not overweight.

Regardless of your body weight, as the continuous urge to overeat addictive foods robs your energy and time, more wholesome activities are neglected, and the out-of-control feeling damages self-esteem. It's common for food addiction to also lead to isolation and depression.

You can take steps on your own to improve your relationship to food—especially if your addiction symptoms are not significantly interfering with your daily life. *What to do…*

•**Keep a journal to identify foods that trigger compulsive eating or craving.** Note the situations in which you struggle for control—are you stressed, angry, frustrated or bored?

•**Find nonaddicting foods that you enjoy**—clementines, unsalted nuts, baby carrots, air-popped popcorn and hummus, for example—and keep them handy. Whole foods are good choices because they do not have the amped-up reward levels of junk food.

•**Don't miss meals or deprive yourself to make up for yesterday's bingeing.** When we are hungry, it tells our brain's reward system to be extra responsive to food. That's why being really hungry can make us more vulnerable to addictive foods.

•**Be alert for signs of stress and/or boredom, and use nonfood remedies**—take a short walk or listen to your favorite music. When you're hit with a craving, distract yourself. Research shows that even intense cravings often subside quickly on their own.

•**Get professional help.** If preoccupation with food stays out of control and interferes with your life despite your efforts to curb your addiction symptoms, you need more help than you can give yourself. See your doctor for a physical exam—problems like a malfunctioning thyroid can amplify the drive for food.

The field is new, so there are few clinicians who treat food addiction. Your best bet is a therapist who uses cognitive behavioral therapy (CBT) for eating disorders and can adapt it to addiction. To find a CBT professional near you, consult the Association for Behavioral and Cognitive Therapies at ABCT.org.

There is little scientific evidence that 12-step programs, such as Overeaters Anonymous, help with food addiction, but such a program may be worth considering if other options have failed.

Get a Grip on Junk Food

Make a plan for how many treats you will allow yourself weekly—sticking to the plan will create a reward in itself to help balance the short-term reward of eating a doughnut or piece of cake. Chew slowly and enjoy the taste of whatever you eat—paying attention will make you appreciate the food more and can lead to consuming fewer calories. Eat junk food when you are almost full, never on an empty stomach—your self-control is lower when you are hungry so you are more likely to overindulge.

Teresa Fung, ScD, professor of nutrition, Simmons University, Boston, writing at Medium.com/popular-science.

Lots of Coffee Is OK

Even heavy coffee drinking is good for health. People who drank one to eight cups of coffee a day—or even more—were less likely to die from any cause over a 10-year study period than people who did not drink coffee. The protective effect applied to ground and instant coffee, caffeinated or decaffeinated.

Study of nearly 400,000 UK coffee drinkers by researchers at National Cancer Institute, Rockville, Maryland, published in *JAMA Internal Medicine*.

Unusual Caffeine Drinks

Robert S. McCaleb, president and founder of the Herb Research Foundation, a nonprofit research and educational organization based in Boulder, Colorado. He designed the herbal tea component of the World Tea Academy's Certified Tea Professional program.

D o you ever wish you could get a little dose of caffeine but you don't like coffee and are bored with the same old teas? If you're looking for something a little different as far as your caffeination requirements go, you may want to consider yerba maté, guayusa and yaupon.

Made from assorted species of the holly plant, these beverages have been enjoyed by indigenous peoples in South America and Central America and the lower US for thousands of years. In addition to caffeine, they all have lots of vitamins, minerals, antioxidants and amino acids, so you can feel good about indulging in them.

The caffeine levels for these drinks typically are somewhere between those of green and black tea but below coffee. Many people find the energy boost they produce less jittery than coffee, even when comparable amounts of caffeine are consumed.

Yerba maté, guayusa and yaupon are sometimes roasted after harvesting, giving them deeper earthy, toasty, woody tones—something that might remind you a bit of a black tea. And sometimes they're simply dried rather than roasted, resulting in flavors that are similar to green tea—grassy and almost spinachy rather than earthy.

Here are a few options if you're interested in exploring these drinks…

•**Yerba maté is a very popular tradition-al beverage in Argentina, Paraguay, Uruguay and other parts of Central America and South America.** It's probably the caffeinated holly drink that is easiest to find in supermarkets and tea stores.

Examples: Guayaki Traditional Organic Maté ($18 for 75 tea bags)…and Numi Maté Lemon, which combines yerba maté, green tea and lemon myrtle ($6.35 for 18 tea bags).

•**Guayusa grows mainly in the Amazon rain forest of Ecuador.**

Examples: RUNA Organic Guayusa Tea ($19.98 for one pound of loose-leaf tea)…Celestial Seasonings Organic Mint Guayusa ($5.39 for 20 tea bags).

•**Yaupon is made from the only caffeinated plant native to North America.** The yaupon plant grows wild around the Gulf Coast. It has slightly more caffeine than the other beverages listed here, though still only about as much as a cup of black tea. Yaupon was regarded as an unwanted weed in modern times. It was only rediscovered as a beverage in the past decade when a small Texas company called CatSpring began harvesting, processing and selling wild yaupon.

Examples: CatSpring Marfa Dark Roast Black Yaupon or Pedernales Green Yaupon (both $10.99 for 16 tea bags).

Exercise Creates Better Food Habits

Young adults who exercised for 30 minutes three times a week at a relatively high intensity—after previously exercising for no more than 30 minutes a week—were more likely to choose lean meats, fruits and vegetables and less likely to opt for unhealthful options. The change happened even though researchers told participants not to alter their diets.

Molly Bray, PhD, chair of the department of nutritional sciences, University of Texas at Austin, and corresponding author of a study published in *International Journal of Obesity*.

Get Fit Together!

John S. Raglin, PhD, sports psychology researcher, professor in the department of kinesiology and director of graduate studies at the School of Public Health at Indiana University–Bloomington. He is author of a published paper titled "Factors in Exercise Adherence: Influence of Spouse Participation" and dozens of other studies on sports psychology.

Y ou know all about the motivational advantages to working out with an exercise buddy, but are they the same when the buddy is your spouse or life partner? The answer is yes and perhaps more so. Working out with your spouse or partner can strengthen your relationship along with your muscles. *Here's how to start off on the right foot…*

Commit to an Exercise Plan

Sticking with an exercise program isn't easy. The average dropout rate is 50%, most often after just a few months. But exercising with your significant other can change that. I studied married people who joined a fitness program by themselves and as a couple. After 12 months, the couples had a better-than-90% adherence rate—that's remarkably high when you consider average adherence is about 50% after 12 months for people joining without their spouse. Most interesting was that they didn't need to be doing the exact same exercise program, provided they went to the gym together, so the issue of "he's stronger than I am" or "I don't like the same machines" doesn't matter. You don't have to work out side by side—you just have to make the commitment to exercise at the same time and place.

For busy working couples, it even can create date-night closeness. It's a terrific alternative to sitting silently in a movie.

Keys for Exercise Success

• **Account for your differences.** Most couples have different fitness levels, and you need to create a plan that accounts for those.

If you're working out with machines in a gym, it's easy to simply go together for a set period of time or go to a class together. But if you want to go running or biking together and one of you can handle a greater pace and distance than the other, you'll have to make accommodations.

Try this: Agree to separate distance goals. Start off together at the same speed, but pick a point where the person with less stamina will stop and allow the other to continue or where the one who is in front will pause and wait for his/her partner.

Hint: Make your route a repetitive loop that goes past your car or your home to make it convenient for one person to stop if needed. Don't put yourselves in the position of having to navigate differences on the fly when one of you suddenly runs out of gas at the midway point of the route.

• **Introduce your partner to the workouts you like.** If you are already in a class and want your partner to join (kickboxing, for example), make sure he will feel comfortable joining. If your partner thinks of the activity as being for the opposite sex, don't force it. On the other hand, if your spouse is open to trying it, help him avoid feeling awkward with the activity itself. Do this with a preview—demonstrate how to do key moves and use any equipment. It's like hosting friends in an unfamiliar city—you make the right introductions and give them the lay of the land so that they'll be more comfortable and confident.

• **Create a backup plan.** People drop out of fitness programs for many reasons—from a brief illness to changes in work schedules. To avoid getting derailed, preemptively take steps to create work-arounds should speed bumps occur.

Example: If one spouse has to miss a week of exercise for a business trip, agree that the other will do it alone rather than sit it out—it's easier for one partner to rejoin activities than for two people to both do a reboot. And if one continues on his own, the other will be more likely to jump back into the routine. Have a list of alternate activities in case neither of you can get to a scheduled class. Switch to an after-dinner walk, for example.

• **Set and reset goals.** Initially, your shared aim might be to exercise a certain number of times a week for a certain length of time. After a while, each partner might add individualized goals. Maybe one wants to build more muscle, while the other wants to boost cardiovascular fitness. That's all OK. In fact, it gives each partner an additional opportunity to be supportive—cheer each other on and celebrate as you reach personal goals. ("Show me your muscles!") Just remember that if you get to your goal first, take time to reinforce all the progress your spouse has made, too. Being at different fitness levels becomes a problem only if one partner feels inadequate or believes that he is falling too far behind. Note that classes in gentle disciplines such as yoga and tai chi will have you both going at the same steady pace, no matter what your respective fitness levels are. Spin and Pilates also allow for different levels in the same class.

• **Consider a personal trainer.** If you're having trouble coming up with a fitness plan, consider signing up with a professional trainer who can take each partner's skill set into account, as well as make adjustments so that you're both doing the same type of program but at your own pace.

Important: Shop around for a trainer who has experience working with couples—ask friends, the manager at your gym and coaches at your local schools for recommendations.

• **Train together for an event.** When you set a competitive goal, such as running a 5K, you train harder and more regularly, and you can revel in the accomplishment of the goal. This can be very exciting for both partners. If you won't be side by side during the actual event, you still will be able to support each other before and after the event.

Breast Size Affects Workout

About half the women with larger breasts say that their breast size affects the amount and level of their fitness activity—only 7% of women with small breasts said the same thing. On average, women with the largest breasts spend 37% less time exercising per week than women with small breasts.

Self-defense: Find the right sports bra. It should have separate nonstretch cups and adjustable, wide shoulder straps. Some women find wearing two bras at once gives extra support and comfort.

Study by researchers at University of Wollongong, Australia, reported in Shape.com.

5 Pilates Moves You Can Do from a Chair

Stefanie Gordon, Pilates Method Alliance–certified Pilates teacher (PMA-CPT), National Academy of Sports Medicine–certified personal trainer, corrective exercise specialist and STOTT Pilates certified instructor, based in Short Hills, New Jersey. Ms. Gordon is also a pre/postnatal Pilates specialist with The Center for Women's Fitness in Chicago.

It seems like everyone, including fitness gurus, celebrities, professional athletes—and probably some of your friends—can't say enough about the core-strengthening, flexibility-building benefits of Pilates. If you haven't tried it yet, maybe it's time! No need to sign up for a class or buy equipment—just get a steady chair (one that doesn't roll) without arms.

While Pilates might seem like a "new" trend, it actually was developed in the 1920s and gained popularity in this country during the 1960s and '70s. Designed as a complete mind-body regimen, Pilates incorporates breath and alignment principles into a full-body workout that strengthens the abdominal, back and pelvic muscles needed for nearly all body movements. Pilates also increases flex-ibility and helps make your movements more efficient, protecting you from injury as you go about your daily activities.

Pilates—especially more advanced moves—can seem intimidating. But many moves are perfect for beginners.

The following routine is suitable for old-er people who may have less flexibility or anyone who has been sedentary and is just starting Pilates.* Except for the last move, each exercise starts in a seated position with feet flat on the floor, spine neutral (maintain the natural curve of your lower spine) and knees hip-width apart. For the most benefit, do the whole routine two to three times a week.

•**Seated Rotation.** Works the transverse abdominis (the deepest layer of front abdomi-

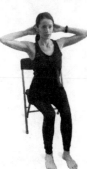

nal muscles—beneath your "six-pack" muscles) and obliques (side abdominals), helps pelvic stability and mid-back (thoracic) flexibility.

What to do: Clasp your hands behind your head and slowly exhale as you ro-tate your upper body to the right…and slowly inhale, pulling in your abdominals, as you rotate back to center. Then exhale as you rotate to the left…and inhale as you ro-tate back to center. Keep your buttocks stable on the seat of the chair. Repeat (center-right-center-left-center) eight times.

•**Seated Leg Lifts.** Also works the trans-verse abdominis, as well as strengthens hip flexors.

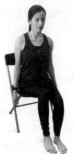

What to do: Keeping your hips stable, inhale as you slowly lift one foot two inches straight up from the floor (your knee should stay bent)…and exhale as you slowly lower your foot back to the floor. Then do the same with the other foot.

*Consult your doctor before starting this (or any new) exercise program.

Important: Tighten your abdominal mus-cles and feel the lift coming from your abs, not your leg muscles. Repeat the move (alter-nately lifting each foot) 10 times.

•**Seated Saw.** Encourages mid-back rota-tion, core engagement and stretches the up-per body.

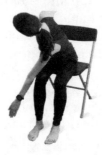

What to do: Start with arms raised straight out to your sides, making a "T" with your torso. In a smooth move, rotate your torso to the right, bending forward to reach down with your left arm to touch your left pinky finger to the outside of your right foot…then straighten back to the starting position…and rotate to the left, bending forward to touch your right pinky finger to the outside of your left foot… and return to the starting position. Repeat the whole move five times.

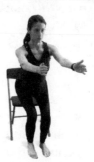

•**Sit-to-Stand.** Targets the transverse abdominis mus-cles and the major muscles of the legs—quads (front thigh), glutes (buttocks) and hamstrings (rear thigh).

What to do: Sit with arms held straight out in front. Take a breath and exhale slowly as you stand up. Then take another breath and exhale slowly as you slowly sit back down.

Note: Don't crash down onto the chair. If you do, you're not using your muscles enough! Repeat 10 times.

•**Hamstring Stretch.** Stretches the lower back, hamstrings and calf muscles.

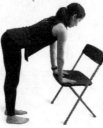
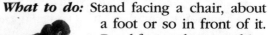

What to do: Stand facing a chair, about a foot or so in front of it. Bend forward at your hips and place your hands flat on the chair seat with your arms straight but elbows not locked. Keep your up-per back flat (not rounded) with your pelvis neutral (that is, maintain the natural curvature of your lower spine) and your legs straight but knees not locked. Take a deep, slow breath in…and then exhale slowly. Repeat the breath pattern for a total of five times.

Alternative: If you can't straighten your legs while leaning on your hands on the chair seat, raise the height of the seat with a couple of large books.

Get a Full-Body Workout with This Modified Plank

A bear plank is an extra-challenging but stationary full-body exercise. Start on all fours with your shoulders lined up with your wrists and your knees at a 90-degree angle. Keep your back flat. Lift your knees so they hover a few inches off the floor. Flex your core and hold the position for up to a minute—be sure to keep breathing regularly. Slowly bring your knees back down to the floor. Rest for 10 seconds and repeat.

Tehrene Firman, fitness blogger writing at MSN. com.

Supercharge Your Workout with a Weighted Vest

Wayne L. Westcott, PhD, a professor of exercise science at Quincy College in Quincy, Massachusetts, and a strength-training consultant for the American Council on Exercise and the American Senior Fitness Association. He is also coauthor of several books, including *Strength Training Past 50.*

This underused piece of exercise paraphernalia is designed to add some heft to a variety of workouts.

Bonus: Even if you're just a casual exerciser, a weighted vest can make your muscles stronger, help you burn more calories and crank up the benefits of your cardio workout.

Important: To make sure that a weighted vest and the workouts described here are right for you, check with your doctor. Use of a weighted vest may not be appropriate for those with osteoporosis, pregnant women, obese individuals and people with orthopedic injuries, especially those affecting the spinal column.

Once you get your physician's go-ahead, a weighted vest can help you…

• **Build lean mass.** A weighted vest is a great tool to combat the age-related loss of muscle mass and strength known as sarcopenia and to preserve your ability to complete activities of daily living, such as climbing stairs and carrying groceries.

• **Burn more calories.** Strap on a weighted vest that equals 15% of your body weight and walk at an easy 2.5-mph pace, and you'll burn 12% more calories than a person not wearing a vest, according to research. Wearing a weighted vest has also been shown to feel less taxing than adding intensity by other means, such as increasing speed or walking on an incline.

• **Retain bone mineral density.** In a Canadian study, researchers found that a weighted vest helped reduce bone turnover (a physiological process that fuels bone loss) while reducing body fat and increasing muscle mass in postmenopausal women.

• **Improve walking ability.** Wearing a weighted vest can improve walking ability in people with gait problems caused by conditions such as Parkinson's disease and certain types of palsy.

The Right Vest for You

To choose a weighted vest that's right for you, first look for a formfitting vest that covers your chest. If it extends down toward the waist, even better. This will better distribute the weight of the vest without affecting your hip movements when walking. Wide shoulder straps are a plus—they don't interfere with your range-of-motion and put less stress on the shoulders than narrow straps. Also look for a vest that offers a relatively even weight distribution for the front and back.

When determining the weight of your vest, start with 5% to 10% of your body weight. For example, if you weigh 120 pounds, look for a vest with a starting weight of six to 12 pounds. Most vests also have pockets that allow you to add weight packets as you get stronger, but don't exceed 15% to 20% of your body weight.

Helpful: Always add weight gradually—for example, by two-pound increments, adding a one-pound weight to both the front and rear vest pockets to prevent injuries.

3 Easy Ways to Use Your Vest

If a weighted vest is new to you, it's smart to incorporate it into your existing exercise plan. Consider starting with 15-minute endurance training sessions and progressing gradually by five-minute increments to 45-minute sessions. *You can use a vest for…*

•**Warm-ups.** This will help you quickly engage muscle fibers and raise your core body temperature. Walking at a slow pace with the vest on is the perfect warm-up for weighted-vest walking at a brisk pace. While you shouldn't run with a weighted vest (it creates too much landing force), a pre-run weighted-vest walk can serve as an effective running warm-up.

•**Walking.** You can create a cross training–like program by wearing your weighted vest every other day—go at a slower pace for 20 minutes on the days with it and at a faster pace for 30 minutes on the days without it.

Bonus: On the "off" days, you'll feel lighter and find it easier to increase your pace, which is great for motivation.

Note: Weighted vests may be used in other weight-bearing exercise, such as elliptical training, but should not be used in exercises such as running, as mentioned above, and rope jumping that produce large landing forces.

•**Strength training.** Wear your weighted vest to increase resistance for standing exercises done with a straight torso, such as squats and stationary lunges.

However: To avoid overstressing your back, don't wear a weighted vest for exercises that involve bending your trunk forward or backward or that require horizontal body positions, such as planks and push-ups.

A standard strength-training protocol while wearing a weighted vest is to complete a total of three sets of eight to 12 reps with two minutes of rest between each set. Start with just the vest. You should be able to do at least eight reps in good form. Once you're able to complete 12 reps for each of the three sets, you can add weight to the vest.

Important: The additional muscle stress associated with wearing a weighted vest requires at least 48 hours recovery time between successive strength-training workouts. Although endurance training usually requires less recovery time, an every-other-day protocol is recommended to avoid overtraining syndromes.

10,000 Step "Rule" Revisited

When about 17,000 women (average age 72) wore an activity tracker for seven days as they went about their day-to-day lives, those who took an average of 4,400 steps each day were 41% less likely to die during the four-year follow-up period than women who took fewer than 2,700 steps, regardless of how fast they walked. Longevity continued to improve with more steps taken…up to 7,500 steps per day. There was no further reduction in the risk for death when additional steps were taken.

I-Min Lee, MD, ScD, professor of medicine, Harvard Medical School, Boston.

Move Your Trunk for Better Health

Karen Erickson, DC, chiropractor, Erickson Healing Arts, an integrative chiropractic practice in New York City. She is a fellow of the American College of Chiropractic, and on the inaugural leadership team for the American Chiropractic Association's Council on Women's Health.

Remember the 1960s dance called the Twist? All the millions of people twisting to Chubby Checker and The Beatles' version of *Twist & Shout* very likely weren't focused on improving their health. But it turns out that moving your trunk, as the gyrations of the Twist did so well, actually is very good for you. So come on, come on, come on—let's do some trunk twisting!

Your trunk, the part of your body from your shoulders to your hips, doesn't get much of a workout doing daily activities. For one thing, we spend a lot of time sitting—12 hours a day, on average. But even if you're one of the 33% of Americans who have a gym membership and actually use it, most exercises don't involve moving your trunk either. When your trunk stays mostly static, it reduces the ability of your rib cage, diaphragm and lungs to expand. This can diminish lymph and blood circulation to the muscles and organs of the trunk. Lack of trunk movement also weakens core muscles, leading to poor posture and raising risk for tension and injury to the back, shoulders and hips.

You can reverse all that by stretching your trunk and strengthening your core muscles. It's not difficult, and doing it daily pays off big. Right away, you'll notice improved posture and increased flexibility. You may even feel less winded, because your diaphragm, the principle breathing muscle, will work better, too.

Simple Trunk-Toning Moves

One of the easiest ways to get some trunk movement into your day is to walk while swinging your arms. Do this empty-handed so that your arms can swing freely. Try for 20 to 30 minutes daily.

Three more easy moves that do wonders for flexibility, circulation and general well-being...

Plank

There are many variations on the Plank, which engages your abdominal muscles and helps build core strength. For basic Plank, get into a push-up position, with hands directly below the shoulders and arms straight. Hold the position for 10 to 30 seconds to start, building up to one minute. Do once a day.

Variation: Once you can hold the position for one minute, try a three-legged plank—lift one foot slightly off the floor for 30 seconds, then lower it back to the floor. Switch feet and repeat.

Bridge

The Bridge exercise engages your glutes and tones your entire torso. Start by lying on your back, arms at your sides, with your knees bent and your feet flat and close to your buttocks. (You should be able to touch your heels with your fingertips.) Next, raise your hips as high as you can, resting your weight on your head and upper back. Ideally, your body will be in a straight line from your shoulders to your knees. Hold the position for 15 seconds, working up to one minute. Then slowly lower your hips back to the floor. Repeat four times.

Tip: Remember to breathe naturally during the exercise—don't hold your breath.

Trunk Twist Series

This three-part exercise stretches your entire core and helps counteract leaning forward to read, text, etc.—plus it feels great!

Step 1: Stand with your legs shoulder-width apart. Place your hands on your shoulders, and slowly twist to your right...then to your left. Repeat the left-to-right twist two times.

Step 2: With your hands still on your shoulders, bend your torso sideways as far as comfortable without straining your low back and hold for several seconds...then bend to the opposite side and hold for several seconds. Repeat two times.

Step 3: With your hands clasped behind your head, slowly bend backward by lifting your chest toward the ceiling. Hold the stretch for a few seconds, then slowly straighten up. Repeat two times.

Caution: Only bend as far as is comfortable, keep your chin tucked and don't let your head flop back. Stop if you feel a strain in your neck or lower back.

Finish: End by gently bending your head and upper torso forward to balance the stretches you just did.

8 Simple and Surprising Ways to Improve Your Posture

Joel Harper, celebrity trainer and author of *Mind Your Body: 4 Weeks to a Leaner, Healthier Life* and the Bottom Line blog "Your Personal Mind-Body Coach." JoelHarperFitness.com

Your posture is not only important for your physical and emotional health—it also sends a message to others about who you are and how you feel about yourself. People unconsciously notice your posture when speaking to you or simply seeing you. Slumped shoulders or a tilted head sends all sorts of negative messages. It says, *I'm tired...I'm not confident...I'm grumpy...I'm not approachable...I'm worn out.* Beyond inadvertently projecting these messages to others, you also are internalizing these messages yourself. Your posture affects your thoughts, your words and your overall energy.

Luckily, there are simple things you can do every day to improve both your posture and the messages that it sends to your mind and spirit...

•**Use a "mental mirror."** Look at all the people around you, and ask yourself, *When someone looks at me, how do I look?* Seeing yourself in this mental mirror helps you automatically sit up a little straighter, pull your stomach in, drive your shoulders back and raise the top of your head.

•**Look up.** When you walk, do you look down? Most people do. The problem is that when you look down, your shoulders immediately roll forward, putting tremendous pressure on your neck. Whenever you're walking, look straight ahead instead. A lot of people think, *Oh, I'm going to trip.* But you won't because you have peripheral vision that keeps you from tripping and you certainly don't need to look at your feet to know what they're supposed to do. When you look straight ahead, it reduces strain on your neck. If you must look down, do so with your eyes—not with your whole head.

•**Clasp your hands behind your back.** When standing, interweave your hands behind your tailbone with elbows slightly bent. If you have to move your shoulders to do that, then your shoulders were rolled forward. Ideally, if you put your hands behind you, your shoulders shouldn't move at all. This exercise reminds you to get in the habit of thinking about your posture and standing up a little straighter. It's a simple trick that will make a big difference.

•**Find out how tight your neck muscles are.** Put your hands in front of your face with your palms facing you and pinkies linked together. Then put your hands up on top of your head, and gently drop your chin toward your chest using just the weight of your arms. There are certain stretches you shouldn't feel at all. This is one of them. If you do feel it, that's a sign your neck and shoulder muscles are too tight. Do this stretch daily for five deep inhales, and the stretch will get easier. This move allows you to get rid of the tension in your neck and shoulders. If tightness continues, consider getting a massage.

Warning: Stiffness also may be a sign that you are dehydrated. Most people don't drink enough water. You can improve your posture just by drinking more water. To determine how many ounces you should drink through the course of each day, cut your body weight in half and use that number.

• **Put an hourglass on your desk or set an alarm to remind you to move.** This way, you have a visual reminder of when an hour has gone by. A lot of people get lost in their work, and the next thing they know, they've been sitting at a desk for three hours. The hourglass makes you a little bit more accountable for getting up and walking for at least a minute or two—whether it's just to get some water or walk some papers over to another desk.

Make sure all your stretches are balanced. Many people think they should stretch both sides equally, but if one side of your body is tighter than the other, you need to adjust for that and stretch the tighter section more. Be mindful of this imbalance. The goal is that both sides should feel similar when done stretching. Give each stretch a number from zero to 10. Zero means you don't feel it, while 10 means you feel it a lot. If one side is a four and the other is a six, go back to the six side again and stretch until it feels closer to the four. Work gradually, and open up that area so that it's equivalent to the other side.

• **Be aware of what good posture feels like.** Put your back against a wall with your butt flush against it. Position your heels about one inch away from the wall, and keeping your shoulders back, try to pull your stomach back toward the wall as much as you can. Everybody's different. The size of your butt and the arch in your back will determine how close your lower back will be to the wall. While in this position, try to put the back of your head against the wall behind you with your chin straight. A lot of people can't do it because they're so hunchbacked. If you do this move over and over again, it will help you become aware of the right posture and improve it. Once this posture starts to feel more comfortable, it means that the muscle balance in your chest and your back are equal.

• **Start each day more mindful of your posture.** Every morning, before you get going for the day, lie on your back—either in bed or on the floor. Interweave your fingers and put your hands behind your head with your elbows flared to the side. Bend your knees, and with your feet flat on the bed or the ground, drop both knees to the left side. Place your right knee over your left so that your right knee can ultimately go all the way down to the bed or floor, and just relax there. This is a passive stretch. Passive stretching means that you're letting gravity do the work and you're not pressing it, you're not pulling and you're not forcing it. Then switch sides and drop both knees to the right. You want to do this every day to free your back muscles and allow good posture habits.

The Single Best Stretch

Bad posture often starts in the hips. When your hips are out of line, it throws off your back. And if your back bothers you, you tend to compensate with your shoulders and neck.

Try this stretch, which you should feel in your outer hip…

While sitting up straight in a chair, place your right ankle on top of your left knee, and gently press your right knee down, holding for three deep inhales. Do this on one side, then the other side, and then come back and do the tighter side again.

Important: Be aware of which side is tighter. Work gradually, and open up that area so that it's equivalent to the other side.

Don't Let Cold Weather Sabotage Your Fitness!

Denise Austin, an influential fitness and health professional for 40 years. Known for her at-home workouts, Denise hosted the longest-running TV fitness show in history. She is author of 12 books on fitness, including *Fit and Fabulous After 40*. Denise Austin.com

Even though it can be tempting to curl up under a cozy blanket on the couch and hibernate on those cold winter days, you know that will undermine your fitness—and your overall health.

Good news: It takes only a few tweaks to your daily routines (both outdoors and indoors) to stay active during the winter...and even—dare we say it?—make it fun. *What you need to know...*

Why You Need Winter Exercise

Physical activity is crucial no matter what the season, but wintertime exercise offers unique benefits...

• **Increased immunity.** Research published in *British Journal of Sports Medicine* found that adults (ages 18 to 85) who got about 20 minutes of aerobic exercise (done intensely enough to break a sweat) at least five days a week for 12 weeks had only about half as many colds as those who were sedentary.

• **Reduced risk for lethargy, low mood and irritability.** These are telltale symptoms of seasonal affective disorder (SAD), but getting natural light outdoors helps guard against it.

• **More vitamin D.** Sunshine accounts for up to 90% of our annual intake of vitamin D—a key nutrient for bone health, muscle strength and other vital functions. Even though you'll get more winter sunshine in some southern and western states, exercising outdoors—no matter where you live—allows you to get more vitamin D than you would if you stayed indoors.

The Joys of Outdoor Exercise

If you live in an area where the mercury plummets during the winter, there's something undeniably invigorating about crisp outdoor air. Classic winter sports, such as skiing and ice skating, are great heart-pumping, muscle-strengthening forms of exercise.

But if you're not keen on hitting the ski slope or ice rink, there's an alternative that works for most people, regardless of their fitness level. You guessed it...good old-fashioned walking. It's a convenient way to get both a cardio workout and weight-bearing exercise for stronger bones.

My advice: During winter, walk at least 20 minutes a day to promote circulation and burn fat.

Note: To warm up your muscles, do your favorite stretches and light arm pumping and walking inside your house, or march in place, for three to five minutes, before going outdoors.

Helpful: Listen to your favorite music if you like, but stay alert to your surroundings. I like upbeat songs like "Walking on Sunshine."

If walking doesn't excite you, liven it up by grabbing a neighbor or friend to join you for a brisk jaunt. Or if solitude is more your thing, head for a state park, where the beauty of a recent snowfall or the glint of winter sunlight can enrich the experience.

Stay Safe Outdoors

While outdoor exercise has undeniable benefits, it can be dangerous if you don't do it correctly. If you have any lung problem (such as asthma), heart disease, diabetes or any other chronic condition, check with your doctor before exercising outdoors in cold weather. *In addition...*

• **Wear moisture-wicking fabrics closest to the skin when layering your clothing.**

Also: Forgo cotton—it stays wet if you perspire.

• **Avoid tight clothing.** It can inhibit blood flow and lead to loss of body heat.

• **Cover your head, ears and fingers.** Your body focuses on keeping your core warm, so your extremities are vulnerable. Also, you never want to walk with your hands in your pockets—that can throw off your balance. And don't forget sunglasses—especially in snow, which reflects more UV rays.

• **Opt for bright colors so that you stand out in cloudy, gray or dim surroundings.** Fluorescent yellow-green is the safest choice for daytime exercise.

• **Don't wear sneakers made of "summer" fabrics (such as mesh material).** Instead, choose sneakers made of heavy, heat-trapping material with rugged soles for traction.

• **Moisturize exposed skin (such as on the face and lips) to prevent chapping, and don't forget sunscreen.**

Sneak in Some Indoor Activity

Don't miss opportunities for indoor activities, too. *If you're tired of the usual options, such as gym workouts, yoga, dance classes or even mall-walking, try these moves (several times a day)…*

• **Do leg squats for a minute or so while brushing your teeth or blow-drying your hair.** If you have bad knees, do mini-squats while gripping a counter.

• **Do push-ups against the kitchen counter while waiting for your coffee to brew.** Aim for 15. If you have wrist problems, try arm scissors—extend your arms in front of your body and parallel to the floor. Then, scissor your arms horizontally. Aim for 30.

• **Lift hand weights while talking on the speaker mode of your phone or watching TV.** Work your triceps (hold one hand weight with both hands behind your head with your elbows bent at 90 degrees, then straighten your arms to bring the weight over your head)…and biceps (hold a hand weight in each hand down at your sides with your palms facing up, then curl both weights to shoulder height). Repeat each exercise for at least one minute.

Helpful: Start with light hand weights and work up to a weight that's comfortable for you.

• **Do the stairs.** Instead of walking up (or down) your stairs once, go up and down four times. If you're concerned about your balance, use a handrail.

A Little Bit of Exercise Could Save Your Life

Regularly participating in running—even once a week—is associated with up to a 27% reduced risk for death from any cause…up to a 30% lower risk for death from cardiovascular illness…and up to a 23% reduced risk for death from cancer. The percentages were those of runners from an analysis of 14 previous studies, comparing their death rates with the death rates of people who did no running.

Željko Pedisic, PhD, associate professor of public health, Victoria University, Melbourne, Australia, and leader of a meta-analysis of studies involving 232,149 people, published in *BMJ*.

Stretches for Body Parts You Didn't Know Needed It!

Jessica Matthews, DBH (doctor of behavioral health), a certified yoga teacher, professor of kinesiology at Point Loma Nazarene University in San Diego and 2017 IDEA Fitness Instructor of the Year. She is author of *Stretching to Stay Young: Simple Workouts to Keep You Flexible, Energized, and Pain-Free.*

Regular stretching enhances flexibility and range of motion in joints, which helps the body move with greater ease when doing other kinds of exercise as well as during daily activities, while also helping to prevent injuries such as muscle strains and falls. Stretching also can help to reduce pain and stiffness. And when paired with mindful breathing, stretching can help mitigate stress and reduce mental tension.

However, most people tend to leave some muscles out of stretching routines because they're not aware of them, such as the quadratus lumborum and the tibialis anterior…and other muscles they may exercise to strengthen but not know they also need to be stretched, such as the biceps and obliques.

The American College of Sports Medicine recommends that flexibility exercises be performed at least two to three days per week, with daily stretching being most effective. The following passive static stretches should be held to the point of mild tension or slight discomfort to enhance joint range of motion, but never to the point of pain. Each stretch should be held for 15 to 30 seconds per repetition. *Some commonly ignored muscles and the stretches that keep them limber…*

• **Biceps stretch.** The biceps brachii is located at the front of the upper arm and is the primary muscle involved in flexing the elbow

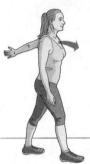

and moving the forearm. Biceps exercises tend to focus on concentrically engaging (shortening) the muscles in order to build them up. Even when followed by lengthening motion, the lengthening is created by tension and doesn't really stretch the muscles. Stretching the biceps helps maintain their ideal length and range of motion and minimizes risk for injury.

Bonus: Biceps stretches may support improved posture, countering a rounded shoulder position by also stretching the shoulders and pectoral muscles.

How to do it: Stand facing a wall, as close as you can get to it. Extend your left arm along the wall straight out to shoulder height and place your palm flat against the wall, thumb pointing up. Keep your right arm relaxed at your side. Keeping your left palm on the wall, rotate your body clockwise (to the right) by pivoting on your feet to assume a position with shoulders and hips perpendicular to the wall and your right foot slightly ahead of your left foot. Complete the stretch by rotating your hips and shoulders away from the wall while your feet stay firmly in position. Hold the stretch for three to five breaths (approximately 30 seconds). Switch sides and repeat. Complete two repetitions per side.

• **Quadratus lumborum and obliques stretch ("standing crescent moon").** The quadratus lumborum (QL) is a deep abdominal muscle that connects your lower spine to your pelvis. The QL gets taxed by extended periods of sitting, poor posture and also strain from repetitive day-to-day movements,

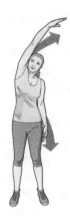

leading to tightness and pain in the lower back. The obliques—internal and external—are muscles found on the sides of the rectus abdominis (the "six-pack" muscles) and run from hips to rib cage. They help stabilize the spine and aid in flexion (the ability of the spine to bend), lateral flexion (bend to the side) and rotation (twist). Tight obliques can pull the spine out of alignment and lead to poor posture. Research also shows that when lateral flexion is restricted, it increases risk for low-back pain. Lateral flexion of the spine is often neglected in daily exercise routines.

How to do it: Stand with feet hip-width apart, arms at your sides. Keeping your left arm relaxed at your side, inhale and sweep your right arm out to the side and up, fingers pointing toward the ceiling and your palm facing to the left. Next, exhale while reaching your right arm over your head toward your left side, keeping your fingertips pointed out, as you lean your torso to the left to stretch the right side of your body. Hold the stretch for three to five breaths (approximately 30 seconds). Switch sides and repeat. Complete two repetitions per side.

• **Tibialis anterior stretch.** Your tibialis anterior is located on your outer shin and is

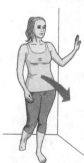

involved in moving the foot and ankle, specifically pointing your foot up. You're probably familiar with tight tibialis anterior muscles—commonly called "shin splints." Lengthening the muscle helps avoid this potential pain. Exercises that stretch the backs of the legs, such as runners do to warm up, put the foot and ankle in a position that tightens the tibialis anterior. To stretch this muscle, you need to do the opposite—point your toes forward, a move that is not part of many exercises.

How to do it: Stand barefoot next to a wall or chair on your left side with your feet together. Bracing your left hand on the wall or holding a chair for support, bend your right knee and extend your right leg back, pointing the toes of your right foot so that you can place the tops of your tucked-under toes on the floor behind you. Keeping the tops of your toes on the floor, shift your weight slightly forward to create a stretch in the front lower part of your leg (shin). Hold this stretch for three to five breaths (approximately 30 seconds). Switch sides and repeat with your left leg. Complete two repetitions per side.

Illustrations of stretching figures: Copyright © Christian Papazoglakis/Illozoo

Walkers: Try This 100-Step Trick

Exercise guidelines call for 150 minutes of aerobic exercise per week at "moderate" intensity or 75 minutes at "vigorous" intensity.

But how do you know if you have reached your desired intensity of exercise?

New finding: In a study of 76 adults, researchers found that counting steps walked per minute (called walking cadence) is the key to knowing how hard you are exercising.

What to do: Wear a watch with a second hand (or set the timer on your smartwatch) and go for a walk. Simply count the number of steps you take in 15 seconds, then multiply that number by four.

Moderate intensity begins at about 100 steps per minute, while vigorous intensity kicks in at around 130 steps per minute.

Note: While the study was conducted on adults ages 21 to 40, preliminary data on older adults suggest the findings will be similar.

Catrine Tudor-Locke, PhD, professor of kinesiology, University of Massachusetts at Amherst.

Get One Hour of Fitness in 5 Minutes

Tom Holland, exercise physiologist and certified strength and conditioning specialist based in Darien, Connecticut. He is author of *Beat the Gym: Personal Trainer Secrets—Without the Personal Trainer Price Tag.* TeamHolland.com

If you're like most people, finding the time for exercise can be as challenging as the exercise itself. But you don't have to carve an hour out of your schedule—a five-minute workout one or more times per day can lead to noticeable improvements in your physical strength and cardiovascular fitness.

You don't need fancy equipment. *These very basic and well-known moves will work all the major muscle groups…*

1. Do a one-minute warm-up. You can jog in place or do jumping jacks to increase your heart rate and blood flow, raise your body temperature and improve your muscle elasticity. This will prepare your body for more vigorous exercise.

2. Do 30 seconds of squats. From a standing start, bend your knees, as if you're about to sit on an imaginary chair. Do not go any lower than a 90-degree angle where your thighs are parallel with the floor and your heels are down. Then return to a full standing posture. Hold your arms out in front of you for balance as needed. Repeat as many times as possible.

Beginner strategy: If you can't do deep squats, do more shallow squats—lower your body only a few inches. Then increase this depth as the days pass and you get stronger.

3. Do 30 seconds of push-ups. You probably already know how to do push-ups—with your hands positioned slightly more than shoulder width apart.

Beware of pitfalls: Keep your body straight, butt in line, and your neck in a neutral position. Repeat this exercise as many times as possible in 30 seconds.

Beginner strategy: If you are not yet strong enough for a traditional push-up, do "knee push-ups," where your knees are on the ground instead of your toes.

4. Do a 30-second plank. Position yourself in the push-up position—body perfectly straight, supported by your toes and hands with arms extended, hands below your shoulders. Contract your abs, and hold this position for 30 seconds.

Beginner strategy: Support yourself on your toes and forearms rather than on your toes and hands…and/or try to hold the plank for less than 30 seconds.

5. Repeat steps two through four. Perform a second round of the three exercises above.

6. Do a one-minute cool-down. Jog in place for 30 seconds, then do 30 seconds of stretches. Stretch your quads by holding one foot up behind your backside for a few seconds (grasp a chair for balance if necessary), then repeat with the other foot. Stretch your shoulders by grasping your right elbow with your left hand and pulling your right arm across your body (keep your right shoulder down), then repeat on the left arm. If any other parts of your body feel tight, go ahead and stretch those, too.

One Strong Workout Hikes Metabolism for Days

A recent study showed that metabolism-influencing brain neurons stay active for up to two days after a single workout. And those changes lasted longer with more training. The neurons are associated with reducing appetite, lowering blood glucose levels and burning more energy. This means that taking a day or two off from exercise does not harm long-term fitness routines, as long as the workout before the time off is sufficiently intensive.

Study by researchers at UT Southwestern Medical Center, Dallas, reported in *Molecular Metabolism*.

Chapter 7

GET THE CARE YOU NEED

Get the Attention You Need in the Emergency Room

Your choice of words in the emergency room (ER) could affect the quality of your care—or even your odds of survival. And I don't mean being polite and saying please and thank you to everyone.

Busy ER doctors and nurses make rapid decisions about which patients are top priorities…and what tests and treatments patients require. How patients describe their conditions and concerns is crucial. A few well-chosen words could get one patient the prompt treatment he/she needs, while poorly chosen ones leave another suffering for hours—or facing a dangerous misdiagnosis. Frighteningly, the right or wrong language has been found to be a big factor particularly in women's survival after a heart attack. Women more often report breathing difficulty, fatigue or dizziness, rather than the classic chest pain, leading health-care providers off track. Of course, what you say and how you say it affects both sexes.

Here's the right language to use…

Speaking with the Triage Nurse

The single most important communication in the ER occurs almost as soon as you arrive, when a triage nurse (or other hospital employee) makes an initial evaluation of the severity of your condition, likely with the assistance of patient-evaluation software. This evaluation often takes just a minute or two, but if there are misunderstandings, it could lead to hours of delay if the nurse and the automated software decide that you're not in immediate danger.

Older patients are especially vulnerable during triage because they don't always experience the dramatic symptoms a younger person would in certain life-threatening situations.

Example: A young adult is likely to be in obvious agony when his appendix is about to burst, leading to quick attention in the ER…but older people often experience only discomfort and loss of appetite.

When the nurse asks what's wrong…

Joel Cohen, MD, former emergency room physician who now is medical director of DoctorCare, a geriatric house-call practice based in Scottsdale, Arizona. He is coauthor of *BoomER: Emergency Room Survival Guide for Baby Boomers and Older Folks.* EndlessKnotPress.com

137

• **Briefly describe your one or two most concerning symptoms.** Put these into context using phrases such as "the worst I've ever felt" or "I've never felt anything like this before," if appropriate.

Example: "I'm having upper-abdominal discomfort that's not like anything I've ever felt before." If it's bad, say it's bad.

If you're concerned that your symptoms could be related to a serious health condition that you have (or you had in the past...or your doctor has warned you that you are at risk of developing), mention this as well.

Examples: "I'm worried because the only time I felt something similar is right before my last heart attack" or "I'm worried because my doctor recently warned me that if I felt something like this, it could be a sign that I'm having a heart attack."

What not to say: Unimportant details about your health saga. A busy triage nurse might cut you off before you get to your most concerning symptoms...or get so buried in your details that he/she overlooks your key complaints.

Example: Some patients try to tell the story of how symptoms started small but grew over time—only to get cut off before they get to the part where the symptoms escalate. Get the important facts out fast.

When the triage nurse asks your pain level, likely on a one-to-10 scale...

• **Provide the honest number, then add a phrase that explains why this number should be taken especially seriously in your case, if appropriate.** Pain tolerances vary—one patient's seven might be worse than another's 10. If you have a high pain tolerance, that's something the triage nurse should know.

Examples: "My pain level is seven...but this is the worst pain I've ever experienced." Or, "I'll say seven, but I said three when I had a broken collarbone—this is bad."

What not to say: "10"—unless you truly are enduring what you believe to be the worst pain possible. When people say 10, tri-age nurses often are suspicious that they're exaggerators, complainers or pain-medication addicts in search of a fix.

Note: If you are instructed to use a one-to-10 scale, do not provide a number higher than 10 in an effort to express that you're in extreme pain. That just makes you seem like someone who can't answer questions accurately.

When the triage nurse tells you to take a seat and wait (or you're told to follow someone to a treatment room)...

• **Ask, "What's my triage level?"** ERs are not first-come, first-served. Most ERs assign each patient a number from one to five that represents the level of urgency. The higher your number, the longer you're likely to wait. One means that you require immediate care...two means you require care within the next 14 minutes...three means you need care within one hour...four means within two hours...and five means your case is considered "nonurgent" and you can safely be left waiting as long as 24 hours. (These time frames are guidelines, not guarantees—how long you actually wait depends on how busy the ER is.) If the ER waiting room is crowded and your number is five, it's probably smarter to head to a nearby urgent-care facility, where the wait might be shorter.

Warning: Do not leave the ER if there is any reason to suspect that your condition might be life-threatening despite the high triage level assigned to you. If the situation did become a life-threatening emergency, your odds of survival would be much greater in an ER waiting room than in your car on the way to urgent care. If you don't agree with your triage number, politely ask for the physician in charge to do a quick evaluation. You have the right to ask for reevaluation if you feel worse while in the waiting area.

What not to say: "How long will I have to wait?" ER staff have no way to answer this—a dozen urgent cases may be about to come through the door. Asking could get you labeled a pest.

Speaking with ER Doctors and Nurses

ERs can be hectic, and doctors and nurses rarely know their patients—a recipe for miscommunications, misdiagnoses and other mistakes. *Four things to ask or tell ER medical personnel…*

• **"Who are you, exactly?"** Each time someone new examines you and/or offers a medical opinion, ask who that person is and what his title is. If it turns out it's a student or resident—a doctor-in-training—ask, "Can I speak with the physician in charge after you are done with your evaluation?" You also have the right to ask for a consultation by a specialist such as a cardiologist for chest pain if your problem is possibly serious or you are not improving.

• **"What is this for? Who ordered it?"** Get these details whenever a hospital employee hands you a pill, starts to stick an IV into your arm or says he's going to take you for a test. ER staff sometimes get patients mixed up. If you're told it was ordered by a doctor whose name you don't know and/or it doesn't sound relevant for your health problem, ask, "Can you double-check that this is for me?" For medications, be sure you have alerted everyone to your medications. Confirm that there are no interactions.

• **"It's the worst I've ever felt."** Don't just say this (and/or "I've never felt anything like this") to the triage nurse, say it to doctors, too, assuming it's accurate. It sends the message that you're not a chronic complainer with an everyday issue—this is an extreme situation to be taken seriously.

• **"Could you run this by my primary care physician?"** If you're in the ER during your doctor's office hours, ask the ER staff to call your doctor to discuss their conclusions before sending you home. Most doctors' offices also can be reached after hours. Even an on-call provider should have access to your medical records and be able to offer the ER useful medical history. This is especially important if they're sending you home with prescription medications.

Three things you should not say…

• **Do not say: "I know which painkillers work best for me."** When patients request specific painkillers—especially opioids—it sends up red flags that these patients might be addicts fabricating medical problems to obtain drugs. (If you're allergic to specific painkillers, definitely do say that, even if the allergy is noted in your records.)

• **Do not say: "I need to see the doctor right now!" or "I'm going to sue!"** Being demanding or making threats in an ER will not get you what you want, but it might get you labeled a nutcase or a problem patient—which would make the ER staff even less eager to deal with you. If you must ask for rapid attention—maybe you've been waiting for a half-hour for a bedpan—a polite-but-urgent request to a nurse at the nurses' station is most likely to produce a rapid response.

Example: "I know you're busy, but I just can't bear it any longer, could you possibly…"

• **Do not say: "Aghhhh."** Don't scream or moan audibly if you can help it. ER staff sometimes take such vocalizations as signs that a patient is exaggerating or faking pain, perhaps to get quicker attention or because of a painkiller addiction. A silent-but-pained facial expression is a more effective way. It is best to seek ER care with a friend or relative to serve as your advocate.

Emergency Room Finder

The nationwide app, EMNet findERNow, quickly determines your location…finds the ERs that are closest in terms of distance and time…and provides directions and other information. Listings are researched by Boston's Massachusetts General Hospital.

EMNet findERnow.

Timing Your Doctor Visit

Patients who see their primary care physician later in the day are less likely to be sent for a cancer screening than those who go earlier. For example, colonoscopy and other colon cancer screenings were ordered more frequently when patients were seen at 8 am (37%) versus at 5 pm (23%).

Theory: Doctors—and patients—suffer from "decision fatigue," where they are less inclined to make new choices after a long day.

Mitesh S. Patel, MD, MBA, MS, director, Penn Medicine Nudge Unit, University of Pennsylvania, Philadelphia.

Is Ageism Making You Sick?

Sana Goldberg, RN, a registered nurse practicing in New Haven, Connecticut. A public health advocate and member of the International Honor Society of Nursing, Ms. Goldberg has published scientific papers in *Neuropharmacology* and *European Journal of Neuroscience*. She is author of *How to Be a Patient: The Essential Guide to Navigating the World of Modern Medicine.*

Older adults spend the majority of health dollars in the US. So you'd think that doctors and other health-care professionals would treat these individuals—their best customers—with lots of care and respect. But that's often not the case... and the consequences can be catastrophic.

Important new finding: When researchers from Yale School of Public Health and Yale School of Medicine looked at national data to assess the health effects of ageism (which their study defined as prejudice against people age 60 and older), the results were eye-opening.

Over one year, ageism played a role in more than 17 million cases of eight health conditions, including cardiovascular disease, diabetes, chronic respiratory disease and musculoskeletal disorders such as arthritis, according to their research, which was published in *The Gerontologist*. Ageism is estimated to drive up health-care costs by an astounding $63 billion a year.

The good news is, there's plenty you can do to protect yourself—or a loved one—from the perils of ageism.

A Dangerous Blind Spot

Most Americans have a blind spot when it comes to ageism. People usually don't recognize when they're being ageist...or when ageism is happening to them. *What to watch out for—in others and yourself...*

•**Second-rate treatment.** Age discrimination often shows up as inferior medical treatment.

Example: When you describe a new health problem, the physician says: "It's just your age" or "That's a normal sign of aging"—and doesn't adequately investigate or treat your problem.

A personal story: Not long ago, my mother—who is 65—was walking around for several months with severe pain in her upper thigh.

The doctor she talked to about the problem didn't believe she was in as much pain as she said she was. He chalked it up to arthritis and prescribed a course of steroids. Finally, she went to the emergency room—where X-rays showed that she had a broken femur (thighbone)!

•**Harmful stereotypes.** In the health-care setting, ageist stereotypes—that is, negative beliefs about an older person or older people in general—can be the driving force behind disrespectful treatment from doctors and other medical personnel.

Example: A doctor thinks all older people are somehow impaired in mind and body—and talks to you in a patronizing way, speaking in high-pitched, loud tones as if you were a child.

This type of treatment is more than a mere annoyance. In a study published in *Psychology and Aging*, people age 61 and older who were subjected to patronizing speech performed more poorly on a cognitive test and had higher levels of cortisol, a stress hormone that can trigger high blood pressure, headaches, weight gain and insomnia.

•**Negative self-perceptions.** Surprisingly, older adults often view old age and the aging process negatively themselves.

Example: You think aging—including your own old age—is inevitably associated with forgetfulness, incompetence, decline and disease. There's significant harm associated with that mind-set.

What the research shows: In a series of studies, people with self-directed ageism were found to be twice as likely to develop cardiovascular disease...have poorer day-to-day function...be less likely to follow health-promoting practices such as eating a balanced diet, exercising regularly and taking prescribed medications...be less likely to seek care for debilitating back pain...and be at greater risk for depression.

Put a Stop to Ageism

Even though health-care ageism is usually deeply ingrained, there are ways to counter it. Once you recognize that older adults are likely to encounter biases when interacting with health professionals, you've taken the first step to overcoming it. *Additional steps...*

•**Be honest about your own attitudes.** Are you guilty of self-directed ageism—for example, do you assume, on some level, that disease and decline are just a "normal" part of aging? If you do, you need to know that such assumptions may not be true, particularly with the advances of modern medicine. Even though health problems are more common in older adults, when you have a condition that interferes with a full, active, fulfilling life, it's important that you get the care you need and deserve.

•**Stand up for yourself.** Older adults should never be submissive at the doctor's office or the hospital. Don't seek conflict—but

don't avoid it either. Give yourself permission to challenge health-care providers who are not meeting your needs. And if a concern you've raised is dismissed, say something like: "This one thing is really important to me, so I want to make sure we discuss it."

•**Find the right advocate.** Whether you're going for an annual physical, major surgery or anything in between, get an advocate to go to the appointment with you. This will help ensure that you get top-notch treatment.

Helpful: Be choosy about your advocate. You want someone who is dependable, conscientious, loyal and sharp. Before an appointment, ask this person to help you practice the story you plan to tell the physician about your health problem and the questions you'll ask. And don't be shy about telling your doctor any details (even embarrassing ones) that might help you get the best care.

•**Don't wing it.** Many people don't take their doctor appointments seriously enough. You should always ask questions and, of course, write them down in advance.

Examples: What are my treatment options, and which one do you think is the most effective? What are the benefits, risks and side effects of the medicine you are prescribing? Are tests necessary? What will they show and how will they affect treatment? What costs can I expect, and does insurance cover them? If there is no one to take notes, you may want to record the conversation during a doctor appointment on your smartphone. If you do, just be sure to ask the doctor first.

•**Think ahead.** Before you leave any medical appointment, make sure you know the next steps for your care.

Ask questions such as: How long should it be before my next visit? Are there symptoms that mean I should return sooner than planned? How will I know whether this medication is working? What is the best way to reach you if needed?

•**Make sure you're seeing the right type of doctor.** After age 65, your primary care

141

provider should be a geriatrician—a specialist in aging. This doctor will coordinate your care with other specialists, such as a cardiologist or neurologist. The geriatrician also may oversee your care in a hospital setting if he/she has privileges at the hospital.

Ask for a reference from your primary care physician. Or consult the American Geriatrics Society's HealthinAging.org website to find a geriatrician in your area.

Why It's Smart to See a Geriatrician

Charles B. Inlander, a consumer advocate and health-care consultant based in Fogelsville, Pennsylvania. He was the founding president of the non-profit People's Medical Society, a consumer-advocacy organization credited with key improvements in the quality of US health care, and is author or coauthor of more than 20 consumer-health books.

Once we hit our 60s, 70s and beyond, our medical needs are often quite different from what they were when we were in middle age or early adulthood. Wouldn't it be smart to use medical professionals who specialize in care for older adults? The medical world appears to think so based on the increasing number of medical professionals who are getting trained in geriatric medicine. *What you need to know…*

• **The terminology is tricky.** There are essentially two types of health-care providers for older adults. Geriatricians are primary care doctors who hold MD or DO degrees and most often have become board-certified in internal medicine or family medicine before undergoing further training for a subspecialty in geriatrics. Geriatricians look at all the medical issues of an older person, including the appropriateness of a given procedure or a particular medication regimen. They are able to weigh the risk versus benefit for a particular course of treatment (such as chemotherapy for cancer or intensive an-

tibiotic therapy for an aggressive infection). Geriatricians most often work with other specialists, such as cardiologists and oncologists, to oversee an older adult's care.

Gerontologists aren't physicians but have special training in how to deal with a range of health-related issues in the elderly. Examples of these professionals include geriatric social workers (who work closely with patients and families to help them identify a nursing home or assisted-living facility, for example)…and personal care aides (who provide assistance in a person's home or facility, such as help with bathing).

Each of these professionals, depending on the state in which they work, must be licensed by the state or meet specific certification requirements.

Insider tip: Always ask what training the professional has undergone and if he/she is certified or licensed before choosing a geriatrician or gerontologist.

• **Find the right provider.** To find health-care professionals who specialize in geriatrics, check the website of the American Geriatrics Society, AmericanGeriatrics.org/public. Your state's department of health also can help you find licensed or certified providers and facilities. If the services are deemed medically necessary, insurance usually will pay all or part of the fees.

• **Your current doctor may be just fine.** If you're not yet 65 and are in relatively good health, you may not need a geriatrician. This is particularly true if your primary care doctor sees a lot of older patients and is affiliated with a hospital that has a geriatrics department. But if you, your spouse or an elderly parent has multiple medical needs (including a chronic health problem, such as heart disease, along with balance issues)…has trouble keeping on top of things physically or mentally…or simply wants someone who oversees an individual's entire health needs, switching to a geriatrician and using the services of gerontologists may be the best way to maintain independence and continue to enjoy life.

Is Your Doctor Overconfident?

David E. Newman-Toker, MD, PhD, professor of neurology and director of the division of neuro-visual and vestibular disorders at The Johns Hopkins University School of Medicine in Baltimore. He is also director of the Armstrong Institute Center for Diagnostic Excellence in Baltimore. His work has been widely published in professional journals including *JAMA, BMJ Quality & Safety, Stroke* and *Neurology*.

In the work world and in life, confidence is a highly appealing trait. But when it goes overboard, it can be dangerous—especially when it's a doctor who is wielding an infallible, all-knowing attitude.

A growing body of evidence suggests that diagnostic errors—diagnoses that are missed, wrong or delayed—may cause as much death and disability as all other types of medical errors combined. And a common cause of these errors, research shows, is an overconfident doctor.

Sobering study: To understand how doctors' confidence levels sync up with their accuracy in diagnosing medical conditions, 118 internal medicine doctors in the US were given diagnostic cases to solve online—two that were easy and two that were difficult. The doctors were given the patients' medical profiles (histories, physical exams and diagnostic tests) and could ask for additional resources if they needed help. The doctors got the right diagnosis in 55% of the easy cases, but in only 5.8% of the hard ones, according to the research, which was published in *JAMA Internal Medicine.*

The doctors then were asked to rate their confidence level for each diagnosis on a scale of zero to 10. For the easy cases, the average confidence level was just over seven. For the hard ones—the ones they got right only 5.8% of the time—the confidence level averaged 6.4, hardly dropping at all.

To learn how physician overconfidence can contribute to diagnostic errors, we spoke with David E. Newman-Toker, MD, PhD, a leading expert in patient safety.

How does doctor overconfidence contribute to diagnostic error?

There is a lot of research showing that people who have the highest confidence levels are less competent than their peers who are a little less confident. So having a little uncertainty is a good thing—you're less likely to assume that you're right, and it gives you some motivation to learn and improve. This is now being recognized in medical schools and residency programs. In the past, confidence and quick decisions were valued in medical training. Today, there is more of an emphasis on a willingness to express uncertainty. Doctors who get more help and more information become better doctors.

We can think of overconfidence as a special type of "cognitive bias" that makes us unaware of the risk we might be wrong. Bias happens to everyone—all people rely on past experience to make new decisions, and our brains often take "shortcuts" or go on "autopilot." But this can be a trap for doctors with years of medical experience. They may substitute past experience for critical thinking and that can be dangerous.

What other factors can lead to overconfidence?

The biggest issue in overconfidence is a lack of feedback. When a doctor makes the right diagnosis, the patient comes back and gives thanks and praise. When a doctor makes the wrong diagnosis, however, the patient often moves on to another doctor, and the first doctor never finds out.

For an emergency room (ER) doctor, overconfidence could be a factor when he/she, say, orders a CT scan for a patient with new dizziness to rule out a stroke. If the scan is normal, the ER doc may confidently dismiss it—and miss the diagnosis of stroke. A neurologist would know that an early CT scan (especially in the first 24 hours after symptoms begin) will miss at least 85% of the most common type of stroke, the type caused by a blood clot in the brain. An MRI would miss only about 15% to 20%. The ER doctor may have been overconfident because he did not know what he didn't know.

How can you spot an overconfident doctor and protect yourself from a medical mistake?

The three most important things patients can do is come prepared…ask the right questions…and stay vigilant. *When you have a new problem…*

•**Write down all of your symptoms on a sheet of paper in the order they happened—make a timeline if you can.** Take your time and include all the things that could be important. Giving your doctor a good starting point saves time and helps your doctor focus on your problem.

•**Write down key questions to ask.** If your doctor gives you a diagnosis, ask what else could be causing your symptoms. Ask what your doctor is most worried about. What is the worst thing that could be causing your symptoms? Why does your doctor think that condition is not the problem?

•**Stay vigilant.** If your doctor starts treatment and you are not getting better, don't assume it's just the wrong medication. It could be the right medication for the wrong diagnosis. Instead of accepting a change in medication or a higher dose, it's OK to question the diagnosis. Don't be afraid to ask for a consult with a specialist or a second opinion. If the doctor seems upset when you ask questions or the treatment being proposed is risky, consider getting that second opinion even before starting treatment.

Some situations are riskier and more error-prone than others. High-risk situations occur, for example, when your doctor is really busy and seems to be in a hurry…if you've been seen multiple times for the same symptoms without a clear diagnosis being made…and if your symptoms are new and serious enough that you've gone to the ER.

Finally, look out for overconfidence "red flags." If your doctor does not give you enough time, does not listen to your questions or gets in a huff when you ask for a consult or second opinion, get another doctor. If you do find out that your doctor made a mistake, let him/her know. That type of feedback may help your doctor avoid the overconfidence trap in the future.

4 More Health Numbers You Really Need to Know

Tom Rifai, MD, FACP, founder and CEO of Reality Meets Science, LLC, a health coaching and consulting company, and clinical assistant professor of medicine at Wayne State University, both in Detroit. Facebook.com/DrTomMD

You can probably recite most (if not all) of your personal health numbers—your body weight, cholesterol level, blood pressure and blood glucose—off the top of your head. You commit these metrics to memory because they provide at-a-glance insights into your cardiovascular and overall health.

Something else you need to know: There are other important numbers that tend to get overlooked. Staying on top of them will help you more accurately apprise your health status…and can motivate you to make personal changes that could very well save your life.

Also: Be sure to always ask your doctor for copies of your blood test results so that you can keep your own record of your numbers.

Four key health numbers to know—with appropriate coding, insurance should cover the cost of these tests, but check first if you have questions…*

1. Alanine transaminase (ALT). A routine physical exam usually includes a blood test to measure levels of a liver enzyme known as ALT. Keep tabs on this number because high (or rising) levels can indicate non-alcoholic fatty liver disease (NAFLD), a condition in which excess fat is stored in the liver.

This disease usually causes no symptoms in the early stages, so you won't know that you have it unless you get tested. NAFLD is serious business—it's a major cause of liver cirrhosis, liver cancer and liver transplants. And it affects 30% to 40% of US adults.

*Normal ranges may vary slightly depending on the lab. In addition, factors such as age, sex and race can influence what's normal. Ask your doctor to explain all of your tests.

What to do: This test is usually part of a routine physical, but the result may be passed over. Keep an eye on it!

Optimal ALT level: Approximately 7 U/L to 56 U/L (aim for the lower end of the reference range your lab uses).

Exception: People with risk factors for NAFLD, such as obesity, metabolic syndrome (a cluster of conditions including high blood pressure, elevated blood sugar and belly fat) or type 2 diabetes, may have the disease even when the test results are in the upper half of the normal range. Your doctor might recommend additional tests, such as an ultrasound of the liver, if he/she suspects NAFLD.

If you test high: If you're overweight and catch the disease early, losing just 10% of your waist circumference (or your total weight) will usually help the liver return to normal. If you're in the early stages of NAFLD, lowering cholesterol and triglyceride levels also helps.

2. Glomerular filtration rate (GFR). This is the most useful blood test for detecting kidney disease.

What to do: Get the GFR test every year. It measures the filtering capacity of the kidneys. Testing is critical because you can lose up to 75% of kidney function before you develop symptoms (such as frequent urination and/or swelling of the feet or ankles). Diabetes and high blood pressure are the main risk factors for kidney disease. Smoking, high cholesterol and obesity also increase your risk.

Optimal GFR level: Ideally, 90 or above. Below 60 for three consecutive months indicates chronic kidney disease, and 60 to 89 can be normal based on a person's age...or indicate stage 2 kidney disease. A higher number is better because it indicates how efficiently the kidneys filter toxins from the blood.

If you test low: Talk to your doctor about lifestyle changes that support kidney health—regular exercise, a healthy body weight, not smoking and a diet that includes potassium-rich foods such as fruits and vegetables (if you already have some loss of kidney function, you may need to restrict potassium). Your doctor also may recommend an ACE inhibi-

tor, such as *enalapril* (Vasotec), or a calcium channel blocker, such as *diltiazem* (Cardizem), to lower blood pressure. Because the kidneys are a complex vascular system, the odds of wear and tear increase significantly in the presence of elevated blood pressure.

3. LDL-P. A standard cholesterol test is fine for those with average cardiovascular risk, but you may need a more specialized test if you've been diagnosed with heart disease...have a family history of early heart attack or stroke (before age 55 for men and age 65 for women) in a first-degree relative (a parent or sibling)...or are at high risk due to metabolic syndrome.

The traditional test for LDL "bad" cholesterol measures the amount of cholesterol that's present in blood. LDL-P is an advanced lipid test that calculates the number of LDL particles themselves. The distinction is important because the particle number is directly linked to disease, even in patients with normal cholesterol readings.

What to do: If you have—or are at increased risk for—cardiovascular disease, ask about an NMR Lipoprofile, which includes an LDL-P test.

Optimal LDL-P level: Below 1,000 nmol/L.

If you test high: Genetics can contribute to high LDL-P, but people who exercise, eat well and manage their weight—and, in some cases, take a statin and/or aspirin—can lower their cardiovascular risks to close to normal.

4. Abdominal circumference. This isn't a blood test, but it's a crucial number because a person can have a normal body weight but a large midsection.

What to do: Use a tape measure to measure your midsection—without clothing, one inch above your navel. People with larger-than-expected bellies (as well as those who are both obese and "apple shaped") have a higher risk for heart disease than those with slimmer middles.

The internal fat that causes waistlines to expand, known as visceral fat, releases hormones, inflammatory chemicals and other compounds that increase risk for chronic disease. Excess belly fat in men is also linked to erectile dysfunction.

Optimal abdominal circumference: The US standard is less than 40 inches in men... and less than 35 inches in women. But I advise my patients to aim for the International Diabetes Foundation's target of less than 37 inches in men...and less than 32 inches in women.

If you measure high: Try to reduce your abdominal measurement by 10%. Regular exercise (including strength training) and healthful eating will help.

---

10 Ways Your Pharmacist Can Help You...

Heather Free, PharmD, practicing pharmacist in Washington, DC, and spokesperson for the American Pharmacists Association. Pharmacist.com

---

If you count on your pharmacist only to count your pills, you're missing out on an important medical ally. Pharmacists are highly educated about medications and the human body. And they tend to be a lot more accessible than doctors. You usually can consult with a pharmacist for free simply by showing up at a pharmacy—no need to be filling a prescription at the same time. These days, many pharmacists can provide a range of health-care services, thanks in part to changing state and federal laws.

Also: Technological advances are freeing up pharmacists to spend more time with their customers. *Ten things your pharmacist might be able to do for you...*

Prescription-Related Assistance

•**Find cheaper options on prescriptions.** Your doctor likely has no idea how much the pills that he/she is prescribing will cost you. Pharmacists not only see how much you must pay out of pocket—if appropriate, they can recommend low-cost generic drugs that may work just as well as the pricier name brands...advise you when paying out of pocket for a drug is cheaper than your insurance or Medicare co-pay...and/or offer money-saving pill-splitting strategies. Your pharmacist can call your doctor's office on your behalf to work with the doctor to find a more affordable but still effective medication, including to confirm whether it's OK to substitute a generic for a name-brand product.

Even if your pharmacist has not done this for you in the past, it's worth trying again. Legislation passed in late 2018 banned the "gag orders" included in many pharmacy/insurance company contracts—clauses that prohibited some pharmacists from sharing money-saving advice with their customers.

•**Prescribe certain medications.** Pharmacists in a few states are allowed to prescribe certain medications, saving patients the time and cost of seeing a doctor. This is most common with birth control pills (in California, Colorado, DC, Hawaii, Idaho, Maryland, New Mexico, Oregon, Tennessee, Utah, Washington and West Virginia, according to the National Alliance of State Pharmacy Associations)...tobacco-cessation products (in Arizona, California, Colorado, Idaho, Indiana, Iowa, Maine and New Mexico)...and the opioid overdose treatment *naloxone* (in most states).

In Idaho, pharmacists can prescribe drugs for a much wider range of common health issues, including strep throat and urinary tract infections...and Oregon has a formulary of drugs that pharmacists can prescribe, including diabetic testing supplies, inhalers and *epinephrine* injectors. Visit the National Alliance of State Pharmacy Associations (NASPA. us) for more information on resources available in your area.

•**Sort your pills into pill packs or other dose-by-dose dispensers.** Some pharmacies can, upon request, package pills in dose-by-dose blister packs or another system designed to make it easy to remember which pills you're supposed to take when. These packs also help you monitor whether you've already taken a day's dose. This service might be offered for free or for a fee.

•**Reduce pharmacy trips by coordinating prescriptions.** Many pharmacies offer "medicine synchronization"—they'll work with the insurance company to shift the refill dates of multiple ongoing prescriptions so that the customer has to stop by only once or twice each month to pick them up. That isn't just convenient…it reduces the odds that the patient will forget to refill a prescription and miss doses.

•**Review what you take to make sure they all work well together**—including prescription and over-the-counter (OTC) drugs and herbal and vitamin supplements. The typical person age 65 or older fills 20 or more prescriptions each year—and some of those drugs could impact the effectiveness of others. It isn't just prescription drugs that can be problematic—OTC drugs and herbal supplements can cause dangerous interactions as well.

Example: St. John's wort, a medicinal herb commonly taken for depression, can decrease the effectiveness of some blood pressure medications.

Your pharmacist likely can conduct a free "medical reconciliation" upon request, reviewing the drugs you're taking and confirming that they're compatible with one another and appropriate for your current medical conditions. It's worth having this done—the Institute of Medicine has estimated that at least 1.5 million preventable adverse-drug events occur each year due to a lack of review by medical professionals. You could ask your doctor to review your medicines, but a study published in *American Journal of Health-System Pharmacy* found that the reconciliation process is more accurate when a pharmacist conducts it. If you use OTC drugs or herbal supplements—and/or fill prescriptions at multiple pharmacies (which is not a good idea)—bring a list of these or the pill bottles themselves when you ask your pharmacist to conduct a reconciliation. Your records in the pharmacists' computer systems likely list only prescription drugs that you obtain at that pharmacy (or at other pharmacies in the same chain).

Beyond Prescriptions

•**Administer vaccinations.** Flu shots are not the only vaccination offered by many pharmacies. Details vary by state, but often vaccinations for diphtheria, hepatitis A and B, human papillomavirus, pneumonia, shingles and tetanus are available as well, plus vaccinations for international travel. While you may still pay a co-pay for the vaccine, you avoid the cost of an office visit.

•**Perform an annual wellness visit.** Some pharmacies now offer "wellness visits" that are just like the wellness visits provided at doctor's offices—only without the long delays often required to get on a doctor's schedule for a non-emergency appointment. During the visit, a pharmacist would take basic health measurements, such as blood pressure…ask a series of health-related questions…and do basic screening for signs of cognitive impairment. This wellness visit would be conducted by a pharmacist or potentially by another health professional employed by the pharmacy such as a nurse practitioner. Results are sent to the primary care physician for follow-up.

•**Conduct cholesterol, blood glucose, flu, HIV or hepatitis tests.** Some pharmacies now conduct tests such as these on a walk-in basis, no appointment or prescription necessary, often for just $10 to $30, which can be less than the co-pay that often must be paid to have these tests done at a doctor's office. Occasionally pharmacy tests are completely free. Pharmacies usually do not report these test results to doctors, but patients can use the results to determine whether they should see their doctors. If you are reactive to the flu test, the pharmacy can provide treatment.

•**Provide guidance with the selection and use of OTC drugs.** Pharmacists aren't just experts in prescription drugs—they're knowledgeable about OTC drugs. Unfortunately, few pharmacy customers bother to ask for their guidance before picking medicines off shelves.

Tip: Always ask a pharmacist's advice before choosing a cough-and-cold medication.

Many of these feature a cocktail of drugs, some of which you might not need…or might have side effects that you don't expect.

• **Provide specialized knowledge about specific health needs.** Like doctors, pharmacists can have board-certified specialties including cardiology, geriatrics, oncology, organ transplant, pediatrics and psychiatric drugs. If you have health needs related to one of these specialties, it could be worth seeking a pharmacist in your area who has that certification—he/she would be ideally suited to offer medicine-related guidance to patients in this area.

Example: A pharmacist certified in geriatrics will be well-versed in age-related decline in liver and kidney function and what that means for older patients' ability to process medicines.

Ask local pharmacies if they have a pharmacist who is board-certified in the specialty relevant to your health. You also can look for local pharmacists certified in this area on the Board of Pharmacy Specialties website (BPSweb.org). This site lists pharmacists by specialty, name and town but not by pharmacy. Enter the names of pharmacists you find listed here into a search engine along with your state and the word "pharmacy" to determine where these local specialists work.

The Truth About Generic Drugs

Joe Graedon, MS, a pharmacologist and cofounder with his wife, Terry Graedon, PhD, of The People's Pharmacy, PeoplesPharmacy.com, which educates consumers about the use of medications and natural remedies. He is an adjunct assistant professor at University of North Carolina Eshelman School of Pharmacy and coauthor of numerous books, including Top Screwups Doctors Make and How to Avoid Them.

From carcinogenic contaminants…to an increased incidence of side effects…and/or even poor efficacy, there can be problems with generic drugs, ranging from blood pressure and antiseizure drugs to heartburn medications and antidepressants.

What Can Go Wrong with Generics

There are three main reasons why generic drugs may not be as effective and safe as the FDA promises—possibly because generic drugs have thinner profit margins, with less money available for quality control. *The issues are…*

• **Instant release vs. timed-release.** Decades ago, most prescription drugs were instant release—the active ingredient was immediately released into the bloodstream. To maintain an effective level of medicine in the blood, you had to take pills two or three times a day. But in the 1980s and 90s, companies began to market timed-release or extended-release formulations, allowing for a once-daily dose. Today, most popular drugs are available in a timed-release form.

A hidden threat: The approval process the FDA uses for generic drugs is still based on the decades-old concept of instant release. If a generic drug reaches a "maximal concentration" in the bloodstream that is similar to its equivalent brand-name drug, the FDA approves it. But the hour-by-hour level of the drug in the blood may be quite different from the brand-name drug, possibly reducing effectiveness and increasing side effects.

• **Foreign manufacturing.** About 80% of drug ingredients—the active pharmaceutical ingredients (APIs)—are now made in foreign countries, including India, China, Thailand, Turkey, Brazil, Mexico, Bangladesh, Slovakia and others. Many pills are also manufactured abroad.

Unfortunately, FDA oversight of the foreign production of APIs and pills is inadequate. In the US, for example, the FDA makes unannounced inspections of drug manufacturers. Abroad, the FDA usually schedules its visits, allowing companies to prepare in advance. This contrasting oversight has led to products with inadequate levels of the active compound, contamination and falsification of testing data.

• **Transportation.** The FDA has stringent temperature and humidity guidelines for the transportation of drugs (generic and brand-name versions) to ensure that they stay intact. But the FDA exercises little oversight of those guidelines. For example, what happens if an API is manufactured in China…goes to India to be formulated into pills, which travel by container ship to Houston…then get shipped to a wholesaler or distributor in San Diego or Phoenix…and are finally distributed to pharmacies? No one knows the consequences of this odyssey.

How to Protect Yourself

It's difficult to figure out if a generic drug you're taking could harm your health. Complicating matters is the fact that there are no specific categories of generics that are worse than others. Problems have been found in many classes of generic drugs.

Case in point: Some of the worst offenders are foreign-manufactured angiotensin II receptor blockers (ARBs). There have been repeated reports of these popular medications, such as *losartan*, *irbesartan* and *valsartan*, typically used for high blood pressure and heart failure, being contaminated with carcinogens (nitrosamines). The FDA has now recalled untold numbers of these pills and has published a list of ARBs it considers safe. To see the list, go to FDA.gov and search "ARB Drug Products."

To minimize potential harm…

• **Assume nothing.** Don't assume that your generic drug is flawed—but don't assume that it's perfect either. Because of the failure of the FDA to protect us from harmful generic drugs, you need to personally evaluate the safety and effectiveness of your generic drug.

• **Ask for lab results.** You and your physician need to monitor your health with all of the data that is available. With that in mind, make sure your physician supplies you with all lab results so you can track any changes.

Example: HbA1c, a measure of long-term blood sugar levels—if it rises but you haven't made any changes in your diet or lifestyle, your generic diabetes drug may not be working.

• **Keep records.** Once you have your lab results, be sure to record them so you can closely track the effectiveness of the drug. If those numbers stay steady, it's likely the medicine is working. If they change significantly after you start a generic substitution or get a refill, tell your doctor immediately. You may need to revert to the brand-name drug or a different generic manufacturer.

Smart ideas: If you revert to the brand-name drug, consider buying from a Canadian online pharmacy, which will have lower prices. (You will most likely have to pay out of pocket, but the drug may be covered by a private insurer if you submit a receipt.)

Important: To make sure it's a reliable pharmacy, visit the website PharmacyChecker.com.

• **If you switch generics, ask your pharmacist for an "authorized generic drug"**—a type of generic that is identical to the original brand-name drug. (The authorized version is often made by the same manufacturer that makes the brand-name version.)

Example: Pfizer makes Viagra, and a Pfizer subsidiary makes its authorized generic, *sildenafil.*

• **Monitor symptoms.** Some conditions aren't measured in numbers.

Examples: You're taking a generic prostate drug for urinary symptoms, but you still have to get up several times a night to urinate—a sign the drug isn't working. Or you switch to a generic pain reliever, and your arthritis pain comes roaring back. In both cases, the generic drug is the likely culprit.

• **Challenge and rechallenge.** This is a time-honored way to assess your reaction to medication. If generic drug X causes a headache, going back on the brand name should solve the problem. To confirm that the problem lies with the generic, take the same one you used before to see if the symptom reappears. If it does, it's highly likely the generic is at fault.

●**Find out the manufacturer.** There may be dozens of different companies making your generic medicine. Ask the pharmacist to always put the name of the generic manufacturer on your prescription bottle. If a generic drug from a particular manufacturer works, stick with it…and ask your pharmacy to keep it on hand or order it just for you—not all drugstore chains, however, will be able to fulfill this request.

●**Seek allies.** If you decide not to use the generic, ask your doctor and/or pharmacist to go to bat for you if your insurance company balks at paying for the brand name. (If your doctor or pharmacist insists that all generic drugs are identical to their brand-name counterparts, ask him/her to read this article.)

Helpful: To find out the latest on recalled drugs, sign up for recall alerts at FDA.gov/safety/recalls-market-withdrawals-safety-alerts.

Antibiotics for a Toothache?

Antibiotics are often prescribed to relieve pain and prevent worsening of a toothache.

Now: A new review found that treatment by a dentist and, if needed, over-the-counter pain relievers, such as *acetaminophen* (Tylenol) or *ibuprofen* (Advil), are more effective at reducing pain and swelling and avoid the side effects and overuse of antibiotics.

Exception: Antibiotics may be needed if you are unable to see a dentist right away and/or have fever, swollen lymph nodes or extreme tiredness, symptoms that suggest the infection has spread beyond the tooth.

Peter Lockhart, DDS, chair, American Dental Association expert panel that developed the guideline, and research professor, Carolinas Medical Center–Atrium Health, Charlotte, North Carolina.

Beware These Rx Mistakes

In a review of 38,229 primary care patients age 65 and older, about half were prescribed potentially inappropriate medications, and the percentage was even higher among those who were hospitalized.

Examples of inappropriate prescribing practices: Receiving a higher dose of a current medication…and failure to stop or reduce a drug dosage after hospital discharge.

Self-defense: Carry a list of the medications you are currently taking (with dosages and reasons for use) whenever you see your primary care doctor or are admitted to the hospital—and review any changes with your doctor.

Frank Moriarty, PhD, senior research fellow, HRB Centre for Primary Care Research, Royal College of Surgeons in Ireland, Dublin.

Medicines That Cause Night Sweats

Pain relievers such as *acetaminophen*, aspirin and *ibuprofen*…tricyclic as well as SSRI antidepressants…migraine medications including *frovatriptan* (Frova) and *eletriptan* (Relpax)…and diabetes medications such as insulin, *glipizide* (Glucotrol) and *pioglitazone* (Actos) can cause overstimulation of sweat glands. (For more about night sweats, see page 12 in chapter 1, "Aging Well.")

Sharon Orrange, MD, associate professor of clinical medicine in the division of geriatric, hospitalist and general internal medicine, Keck School of Medicine, University of Southern California, Los Angeles.

Don't Die from Your Heartburn Medication

People who took a proton pump inhibitor (PPI), such as *omeprazole* (Prilosec) or *lansoprazole* (Prevacid), for more than 90 days were 17% more likely to die than those who took an H2 blocker, such as *cimetidine* (Tagamet) or *ranitidine* (Zantac), for the same amount of time, according to a 10-year study of nearly 160,000 participants.

Important: 80% of the PPI prescriptions were at the low-dose level found in over-the-counter formulations.

Ziyad Al-Aly, MD, director, Clinical Epidemiology Center, VA St. Louis Health Care System.

Safer GI Procedures

Ask for a disposable scope for GI procedures. Current reusable models of duodenoscopes—used for diagnosing and treating diseases of the pancreas and bile duct—cannot be sufficiently sterilized and have been known to spread infections from one patient to another. The Food and Drug Administration (FDA) recently approved two disposable duodenoscopes for gastrointestinal use. Tell your doctor that you are aware of the FDA recommendation, and request that a disposable scope be used.

Roundup of experts on medical devices reported in *The New York Times*.

Skip the Catheter for Faster Joint Replacement Recovery

People undergoing hip or knee replacement traditionally have received a Foley urinary catheter prior to surgery because it was thought to prevent postoperative complications.

Recent study: There was no difference in urinary complications, such as incontinence, in those who had a urinary catheter inserted prior to surgery and those who didn't, according to a study of 335 patients. Also, infection rate was higher in some patients who got the catheter.

Bonus: Catheter-free patients were able to get up and walk sooner.

Michael A. Charters, MD, orthopedic surgeon, Henry Ford Health System, Detroit.

Get Blood Cultures Before Beginning Sepsis Treatment

Recent finding: Among 325 patients admitted to the hospital with sepsis, those who had blood drawn before starting an antibiotic had more microbial pathogens needed to accurately identify the infection, compared with patients who had blood drawn within two hours of starting an antibiotic.

Takeaway: Treatment should begin as early as possible for potentially deadly infections, but determining the bacteria prior to treatment is also critical in identifying the most effective antibiotic.

Matthew Cheng, MD, clinical instructor in infectious diseases, Brigham and Women's Hospital, Boston.

Is That Newly Approved Treatment Really Safe?

Vinayak K. Prasad, MD, MPH, associate professor of medicine and public health at Oregon Health & Science University in Portland. Dr. Prasad is coauthor of *Ending Medical Reversal: Improving Outcomes, Saving Lives.* VinayakKPrasad.com

Every year, many new drugs and other medical treatments are approved after rigorous research studies and get adopted into practice. Some of the new treatments are then hyped by the companies that produce them and become very popular.

But here's the problem: Many of these treatments will be found to be ineffective or even harmful when further testing is done years later—this is known as medical reversal. Among established practices tested in studies that were published in top journals, up to 40% have been reversed.

Why medical reversals happen: Early research with a small number of participants may show that a new treatment or medication is better than existing treatment. The study seems sound, and the drug or therapy is widely adopted and heavily marketed to doctors and patients. But years later, when many patients are using the treatment, larger studies show that the therapy does not stand the test of time…and/or that the original results were misleading.

Case in point: In 2008, the FDA approved the drug *bevacizumab* (Avastin) as an add-on to standard chemotherapy for advanced breast cancer. Early studies found that it slowed the growth of breast cancer tumors by more than 20%, but follow-up studies found that the tumors eventually grew back and women did not live longer or better. After three years, bevacizumab was withdrawn by the FDA as a treatment for breast cancer.

Other reversals: Sometimes a therapy is taken off the market, but there are plenty of treatments that have been reversed in studies yet continue to be used in practice. *Examples…*

• **Heart stents are commonly placed into the narrowed coronary arteries of people experiencing chronic stable angina,** at a cost of at least $10,000, with the hope of preventing heart attacks, improving symptoms and lengthening life. However, since 2007, studies show that stents do not reduce the risk for heart attack or lengthen the lives of these individuals. These patients can avoid the risks of the procedure and do just as well with medications.

Note: Stents have been shown to help patients who are having a heart attack.

• **Arthroscopic knee surgery is one of the most common orthopedic procedures.** Millions of these surgeries have been performed costing billions of dollars. The procedure repairs the cartilage that cushions and stabilizes the knee with the hope of reducing pain. Tears in this cartilage due to aging are very common in people over age 50. However, since 2013, studies have found that when the tear was not caused by an injury, this surgery is no better than physical therapy.

To learn about many other medical reversals, go to MedicalReversal.com, a site run by a team of researchers.

To protect yourself: For any proposed new treatment, ask your doctor probing questions. *Examples…*

• **Is this treatment supported by a randomized clinical trial?** The most reliable studies are randomized clinical trials (RCTs). RCTs randomly assign patients to the new treatment or the standard treatment and compare results.

• **Was the study sponsored by a drug company or performed by independent researchers?** For more reliable results, look to studies done by reputable independent researchers such as the National Cancer Institute or the National Institutes of Health.

• **Will this treatment relieve my symptoms or help me live longer?**

• **How long have you been using this treatment?**

• **Are there follow-up studies that find that this treatment may not work?**

• **What did you recommend before this new treatment was available?**

• **Is there an older, less expensive treatment that is effective and has stood the test of time?**

• **Does the condition I have need to be treated now? Could a wait-and-see approach be an option?**

If your doctor dismisses your questions, find a new doctor or get a second opinion. Also, you can research clinical studies on a specific treatment on your own online. A summary of the study (called the abstract) will be more readable than the full description.

Helpful website: PubMed.gov.

Heal Faster from Surgery with This Plan

Michael Englesbe, MD, professor of surgery at University of Michigan, Ann Arbor, and founder of Michigan Surgical Home and Optimization Program.

When you're having surgery, you might think your only job is to show up at the right time. The rest is in the hands of the doctors and nurses, right? Wrong. You hold the key to having a successful surgery and faster recovery. The secret? You have to train for surgery—physically and mentally.

Surgery is tough on your body and spirit. I have found that physically, major surgery—one where you receive a general anesthetic—is as hard on your body as running a 5K race. You wouldn't run a race without taking steps to get in shape for it. Along the same lines, you need to prepare and get your body in shape for your operation. Most surgeries are elective, and you and your surgeon can pick a date a few weeks to a month out, giving you time to prepare.

Your whole body—not just the one spot where the surgeon cuts—is affected by the strain. A training plan that includes physical, spiritual and practical preparation has had great success at University of Michigan, where I started a program called Michigan Surgical Home and Optimization Program. We found that patients who got wellness coaching and followed the plan before surgery had shorter hospital stays and were more likely to go home and not to a nursing home. *Here's the plan…*

1. Get walking. Simply walking more before surgery can reduce your hospital stay by one day.

Don't worry if you're not currently fit or active. In my clinical experience, only about 5% to 10% of people having surgery are. What's important is improving your current level, not reaching a particular step goal. Walking is crucial because it strengthens muscles and bones and increases cardio fitness and en-

durance. The goal is simply to increase the number of steps you can currently walk. If you start with 1,000 a day, maybe you can soon do 1,200 or more.

If walking is hard for you, it's fine to do a half-hour a day of another activity, such as swimming. But the reason we stress walking is that walking is important in getting up and moving after surgery, so it's good to practice.

2. Don't try to lose weight—but do eat a protein-rich diet.

Good news: Unless your surgeon tells you otherwise, you don't need to go on a diet. In fact, it's not the best time to stress your body by cutting calories. Instead, focus on eating healthier before surgery. It's especially important to eat enough lean protein—especially skinless chicken breasts, turkey, fish and beans—because it helps build muscle mass, keeping you in optimal shape. It's not new information, but it bears repeating—eat at least five to seven ounces of protein a day.

Beyond that, opt for a whole-foods–based diet, with five to seven servings of fruits and vegetables a day and whole grains. Limit saturated fats like the kind you get in bacon and butter. Cut back on chips, cookies and other processed foods. The goal is to reduce the unnecessary work your body has to do before and after surgery.

3. Make sure your doctor knows as much as possible about you. Surgery is intimate. It's really important that your surgeon knows and understands you. If your doctors and nurses don't ask you questions, proactively tell them about yourself, including your profession, hobbies, travel plans. Doctors want to know ahead of surgery how we can help you fully enjoy your life.

Why that matters: Some big operations aren't for everyone, and the marginal benefits they'll give may not be worth the other issues surgery creates.

Example: My father is an 80-year-old guy with minimal health problems. One procedure a doctor suggested for melanoma would prevent him from ever playing golf again. He lives to play golf. Because my dad said, "One of my most important goals is continuing to play golf every day," the doctor knew that this procedure might not be right for him, especially because less invasive options for his care were available.

Sharing personal details and your hopes for how life will be after this procedure will remind everyone that there's a real person under the surgical robing. When I'm doing a liver transplant, it helps if I can say to the team, "That's Mr. Smith. He's a retired first-grade teacher. He really wants to get home in the next two weeks so that he can go to his daughter's wedding. That's his goal."

4. Come clean about your medications —all of them. Your surgical-care team will go through exactly which medications and supplements you should stop taking and when. For instance, you have to avoid fish oil supplements because they thin your blood and can increase bleeding. The problem is that patients don't always tell the whole truth about all that they take, either out of embarrassment or fear. You'd be shocked to know how many people lie about taking opioids for pain and benzodiazepines for anxiety.

Important: Be honest about your alcohol consumption, too. If you drink every day and find that you get tremors when you don't drink, then you can't just stop cold turkey— your doctor needs to know so that he/she can come up with a safe plan for you.

5. Line up your support team. The biggest thing people do wrong before surgery is trying to go it alone to spare their loved ones ("I don't want to bother anyone, so I'll just take a taxi to surgery"). That's a dangerous mistake that hurts everyone involved, but especially you. Having a support system actually helps you heal. Most of us get much of our energy and our fuel from our relationships.

You actually get better care when you have family members in the hospital. They can advocate for you and help you feel comfortable at a vulnerable time, including getting assistance for you if the nurses are busy. They can think to ask the questions that your postsurgery brain doesn't think of and they

may better remember the information and recommendations from the doctors. Happily, hospitals now make it easy for guests to visit and stay longer hours.

6. Optimize your attitude. I'm a conventional doctor, but I've come to realize that the secret sauce in having a great surgery is a combination of spiritual factors—including an all-around positive attitude and a feeling of empowerment. A study in *JAMA Network Open* looked at almost 7,000 people over age 50 and found that the ones who have a lot of goals and a strong life purpose live a lot longer than the ones who don't.

I see this every day as a transplant surgeon. We often can tell which patients are going to do better just by their attitude. One of the simplest things that you can do to improve your attitude before a health procedure is to focus on gratitude. Keep a journal, and ask yourself every day, *What went well today?* Write it down or keep a running list on your smartphone. Practicing mindfulness with techniques such as deep breathing and meditation also can help.

Sooner or later, we all may face a health challenge such as surgery, but training with these mind/body tools can help you feel stronger, calmer and more empowered—so that you can return faster to the life you love.

Opioids After Surgery? Not so Fast

Michael Kim, DO, clinical assistant professor of anesthesiology at Keck School of Medicine of University of Southern California in Los Angeles. Dr. Kim is the collaborative team leader for the Enhanced Recovery After Surgery program at Keck Medicine of USC.

Unless you live in a bubble, you know that the US is in the throes of an opioid crisis.

Even though doctors have begun to recognize that opioid use after surgery may play a part in the opioid crisis, more than two million Americans still begin to use and abuse opioids following surgery every year.

Now: Many medical centers have adopted a program known as Enhanced Recovery After Surgery (ERAS). ERAS involves a range of measures to provide a better surgery experience for the patient, resulting in shorter hospitals stays, a reduction in complications and readmissions and greater patient satisfaction. It also is curbing or eliminating opioid use for surgical procedures. Hospitals using an ERAS protocol are seeing opioid use drastically decline.

The Basics of ERAS

Although the specific ERAS plan differs depending on the type of surgical procedure and the individual patient's needs, there are some basic principles. *Five key steps of ERAS…*

•**Preadmission.** If your surgery is not an emergency, your pain-management plan should start before your procedure. For example, before surgery, you will talk to your surgeon and also get a pre-op anesthesia consultation with the anesthesiologist. At this time, your medication needs will be assessed. Knowing what to expect—and working with your team on a pain-management plan—reduces a lot of the anxiety and fear that contribute to pain after surgery.

Before surgery, you'll likely be asked to stop smoking and drinking alcohol. Tobacco and alcohol use generally does not affect the type of drugs that are administered during surgery, but eliminating both may reduce complications from anesthesia. A few weeks before, you also may be started on an exercise plan (such as daily walking) and/or a healthful diet to prepare your body for the stress of surgery.

Several days before surgery, you may be started on a nonopioid pain medication, such as over-the-counter *acetaminophen* (Tylenol), a nonsteroidal anti-inflammatory such as *celecoxib* (Celebrex) or the nerve-pain drug *gabapentin* (Gralise). This allows the medication to saturate your tissues before surgery and reduces the pain and inflammation reaction during surgery.

•**Preoperation.** Previously, it was common to have nothing to eat or drink after midnight the day before surgery. This was done to prevent any potential risk for aspiration (unintended inhalation of liquid or solid material into the trachea and lungs). An ERAS protocol recognizes that this level of fasting is not necessary. It can cause your body to use up valuable proteins, fats and nutrients that it needs to undergo surgery.

You may be able to have a light diet of a few crackers up to six hours before surgery and drink clear liquids, such as water or apple juice, up to two hours prior to surgery. In addition, you may be instructed to drink a high-carbohydrate drink the day before surgery and another three to four hours before surgery.

•**During surgery.** A lot can be done during surgery to reduce your pain afterward. Your anesthesiologist may use nonopioid pain medication, such as acetaminophen, celecoxib or gabapentin, just prior to surgery and give you medications to prevent nausea and vomiting when you wake up.

You also may get a nerve block just before the procedure begins to reduce pain when you wake up. The anesthesiologist or surgeon will give the nerve block at the beginning or after the surgery, and its effects can last from hours to a few days. Your anesthesiologist will constantly check your fluid levels, blood glucose and body temperature. Preventing cold stress during surgery reduces the surgical stress.

•**After surgery.** An ERAS plan kicks into high gear following surgery. *It typically includes the following promptly after surgery…*

•Mobilization. This can mean sitting in a chair instead of lying in bed and getting up to walk as soon as you can, even if you use a walker. If you can walk, you will be encouraged to go as far as comfortably possible at least twice on the first day after surgery.

•Nutrition. Depending on your surgery, you may be given clear fluids to drink within two hours after surgery. If you can't drink, you may get fluids through an IV.

Many patients can have a full diet the day after surgery.

•Removal of tubes and drains. If you have IV tubes, a Foley catheter, a surgical drain or a nasogastric tube, your surgical care team will try to get these out as soon as possible (usually 24 to 48 hours after surgery) to reduce the risk for infection. Some may go home with a drain, based on their procedure.

•Pain management. For medication, opioids are no longer the first choice. Other options include acetaminophen, an over-the-counter or prescription-strength nonsteroidal anti-inflammatory drug or gabapentin.

In many cases, these non-narcotic options may be as effective as an opioid. Opioids, if needed, may be used for "breakthrough" pain (a pain flare-up that occurs despite the regular use of pain medication). You may also be given a local anesthesia patch to wear.

•**Recovery at home.** Your discharge instructions will depend on the type of surgery you have, but opioids will not be an automatic part of the plan. A non-narcotic pain reliever will be the first choice.

If you need an opioid for breakthrough pain, you will be prescribed the lowest effective dose for a shorter amount of time.

If you are scheduled for surgery: Ask your surgeon if your hospital has an ERAS program. To learn more about ERAS, go to the website of the ERAS Society USA, ERAS USA.org.

How to Overcome Needle Phobia

James Hamilton, MD, a retired family physician who lives in Durham, North Carolina. His seminal academic paper, "Needle Phobia: A Neglected Diagnosis," published in *The Journal of Family Practice* in 1995, established needle phobia as a formal medical condition and has been cited in hundreds of academic journals.

Dread getting injections or blood tests? You're not alone. A 2012 survey found that around one in four adults experiences "needle phobia," and some research points to rates as high as one in three. This aversion can turn deadly when it makes people avoid immunizations and dental or medical care.

For many needle-phobic patients, injections cause a vasovagal reflex (also called vasovagal syncope)—their blood pressure plummets, their pulse weakens, they feel light-headed and they even might faint.

What to do: Try the following options until you find the solution or combination of solutions that work for you.

•**Numb your arm.** Hold an ice pack against the skin that's about to receive an injection for two minutes before the shot.

•**Confuse your nerves and brain with vibration.** Buzzy, a small battery-powered vibrating device, works when held against the arm receiving the injection or giving blood. The vibrations can block nerves from sending pain signals…and prevent the brain from focusing as intensely on any pain signals that are received. The device works best chilled to also get the benefits of icing, and it may be worth the investment for those who need frequent blood tests or injections. ($44.95 for consumer versions, BuzzyHelps.com.)

•**Pinch yourself.** I find that for some patients, pinching themselves immediately prior to the injection on a different part of the body helps. The brain can't focus on two strong stimuli at once, so there's a good chance that it will ignore the injection.

•**Desensitize yourself to needles.** Desensitization is a well-established technique for phobias.

How it works: Slowly increasing your exposure to needles in a relaxed setting can reduce your reaction to them. Start by just thinking about needles/syringes for a few minutes as you sit in a peaceful spot breathing deeply. Repeat this several times a day until you can do it with no light-headedness or fear, then move on to looking at pictures of needles…followed by looking at pictures of people receiving injections… then videos of people getting injections.

• **Distract yourself.** Any mental distraction can reduce your reaction to an injection—an unrelated conversation with a friend...a video on your phone...looking in a direction other than the needle.

Intriguing: Thinking about something that makes you angry is a good distraction when you're about to get a shot. Anger can trigger the fight-or-flight response, which boosts heart rate and blood pressure—potentially overcoming the vasovagal reflex's falling blood pressure and heart rate.

• **Take it lying down.** If shots make you light-headed, get injections while lying down with your legs elevated and shirt collar and belt loosened. This position can offset the falling blood pressure of the vasovagal reflex.

Take Photos for Better Care

Patients' medical photos empower and reassure them and can improve the patient-doctor relationship, leading to better care.

Examples: Parents took pictures of their children's surgical wounds after laparoscopic appendectomies so surgeons could review healing. Parents felt more confident with the medical service, and taking photos also was a good reminder to check how the surgical site was healing. A woman who felt doctors were not listening to her complaints about her six-week-old baby took a video of the child's constant vomiting, and the doctor who saw it recognized that the infant needed surgery. Both clinicians and patients benefit when patients provide visual material to doctors and the doctors take the time to review it and incorporate it into medical records.

Study by researchers at Queensland University of Technology, Brisbane, Australia, published in *Journal of Medical Internet Research.*

Don't Ignore Pins and Needles

Janice F. Wiesman, MD, FAAN, clinical associate professor of neurology at NYU Grossman School of Medicine in New York City and author of *Peripheral Neuropathy: What It Is and What You Can Do to Feel Better.*

Do you feel "pins and needles" on the soles of your feet? Don't ignore it!

There are two main culprits...Peripheral neuropathy (PN), a nerve disorder, often causes numbness, weakness, pain and tingling in the extremities. Common causes of PN are nerve damage caused by diabetes...heavy alcohol use...and medications, including certain chemotherapy drugs, cholesterol-lowering statins and fluoroquinolone antibiotics. Vitamin B-12 deficiency or excess levels of vitamin B-6 also can lead to PN. Some supplements and energy drinks have very large amounts of B-6. Impaired kidney function and bone marrow cancer are less common causes of PN.

With spinal stenosis, another possible culprit, arthritis causes overgrowth of the bone that surrounds the nerves, compressing them as they exit the spinal cord and run into the legs, then feet.

See your primary care doctor. If PN is suspected, blood work will help identify the underlying cause. Your doctor also may order an electrical test of your nerves and muscles. If more testing is indicated, you'll likely be sent to a neurologist. Spinal stenosis is typically diagnosed with a spine MRI and treated by a neurologist.

Depending on the cause, treatment may include an anti-inflammatory, such as *ibuprofen* (Motrin)...*gabapentin* (Neurontin), an anticonvulsant also used to treat pain...and/or *duloxetine* (Cymbalta), an antidepressant that can be used for pain. Controlling an underlying cause of neuropathy, such as diabetes, or changing a drug identified as a possible cause will also give relief.

Eating a well-balanced diet and getting regular exercise will help deliver nutrients and oxygen to nerve endings in your feet, easing symptoms.

Also helpful: A vibrating foot bath. Some people find that acupuncture helps, too.

Get Prompt Help for DVT

Patients with deep vein thrombosis (DVT)—blood clotting that often occurs in the legs—had a 20% lower risk for continued clotting when compression therapy was started, along with medication, within 24 hours of diagnosis, according to a new study of 600 DVT patients.

How it works: Compression therapy, which involves bandaging the legs or wearing compression stockings, reduces swelling and pain and prevents residual clots by improving blood flow in the legs.

Arina ten Cate-Hoek, MD, clinical epidemiologist, Maastricht University, Maastricht, the Netherlands.

The Truth About Cementing Spinal Fractures

Alan Hilibrand, MD, orthopedic surgeon specializing in surgical and nonsurgical care of the spine based in Philadelphia, and spokesperson for the American Academy of Orthopaedic Surgeons.

Study titled "The Efficacy and Safety of Vertebral Augmentation: A Second ASBMR Task Force Report," by researchers at Monash University, Australia, published in *Journal of Bone and Mineral Research*.

People with osteoporosis are prone to painful spinal compression fractures. Standard routine care is frequently surgery—either vertebroplasty or kyphoplasty, procedures that literally glue the bones back together. However, which is better…and whether either is any better than more conservative therapies…has not been clear. An international task force of orthopedic specialists now has answers.

Roughly 750,000 US adults suffer from vertebral compression fractures most of which are caused by osteoporosis. In fact, these kinds of fractures are the most common complication of osteoporosis and can result from such simple activities as a minor fall, carrying something heavy or even bending the wrong way. Kyphosis (curving of the spine) and/or loss of height are often used to detect that such a fracture may have occurred. One-third of compression fractures cause acute and chronic back pain.

Unfortunately, there aren't many treatment options for spinal fractures. Among them are two surgical procedures, where bone cement is injected into the broken vertebrae to stiffen up the bone in the hope that stopping it from moving will reduce or eliminate the pain. Percutaneous vertebroplasty involves injecting bone cement directly into the injured vertebra. Balloon kyphoplasty, a newer procedure, involves inserting a balloon into the crushed vertebra and inflating it to expand the bone to its original shape before injecting the cement.

Because there is no consensus among surgeons as to which procedure is better—nor any agreement as to whether either is better than less invasive approaches—The American Society for Bone and Mineral Research recently created a task force to look into the effectiveness of vertebroplasty and kyphoplasty, as well as other treatments for spinal compression fractures. An international team of researchers looked at 28 studies that addressed the effectiveness of either procedure, as well as other treatments for spinal compression fracture, based on improvement in pain, mobility and/or quality of life.

Results: Compared with placebo (sham surgery without the injecting of the cement) vertebroplasty was no better at improving pain, mobility and quality of life. Kyphoplasty may be marginally better, but the procedure is newer and there were no placebo-controlled trials.

The researchers do not suggest completely ditching vertebroplasty and kyphoplasty for spinal compression fractures. These procedures may still help some people when nothing else does. What the task force recommends is trying more conservative approaches—such as bracing, rehab exercises to strengthen the trunk and offload pressure on the spine, anti-inflammatory drugs and/or painkillers—before going for surgery. In fact, time itself will help your body heal.

Faster, Better Recovery from Hip and Knee Replacement

Daniel Wiznia, MD, orthopedic surgeon who specializes in reconstructive surgery of the hip and knee and associate professor of orthopedics and rehabilitation at Yale School of Medicine, New Haven, Connecticut.

Since most knee and hip replacements are elective surgeries, you have the luxury of taking your time to choose the right doctor and hospital, as well as the time to optimize your presurgical health, all of which can make a big difference in your recovery. *My inside secrets on how to do both...*

Choose the Right Team

It may be convenient to have your joint replacement done at the local community hospital, but a large orthopedic hospital or university teaching hospital is a better option. These doctors perform many more surgeries, plus these centers are where the thought leaders are, so you can benefit from the latest advances, state-of-the-art equipment and a team of specialized professionals.

Presurgery Preparation

Patients who are the healthiest going into surgery have the best outcomes, so you want to do everything possible beforehand to make yourself a safe candidate. While that can take several months for some, it's worth it to re-

duce the risks. *At Yale Medicine, we have a checklist of modifiable risk factors that we use to help patients overcome, including...*

Excess weight: Being overweight or obese increases your risk for complications, such as infection and delayed wound healing during surgery and postsurgery, and simply makes recovery more difficult. We like patients to have a body mass index less than 38. For patients at an unsafe weight, we provide nutrition counseling to teach them to eat healthier and drop pounds gradually for sustainable weight loss. For patients unable to exercise due to severe arthritis pain or who struggle to lose weight through diet alone, we might recommend bariatric surgery.

Poor diet: Even if you're at a healthy weight, we want to optimize your diet. Adequate nutrition and vitamin reserves sourced from protein, fruits and vegetables help you recover faster and heal your incisions. I have my patients eat an egg every day for two weeks prior to surgery to ensure that they have enough protein stores. If you suffer from anemia, low blood counts or low iron, we may also suggest that you take some vitamins to improve that, such as iron, folate, B-12, calcium, vitamin D and vitamin C, and perhaps a protein supplement. Any supplements should be coordinated with your primary care doctor.

Exercise: Conditioning with a physical therapist before surgery helps strengthen muscles and improve balance so that you recover faster. This is especially important if you are using a cane, walker or wheelchair before surgery. Increasing your mobility presurgery helps reduce your risk of falling and improves postoperative pain control.

Substance use: Patients need to wean off narcotic pain medications, alcohol dependency, tobacco and other recreational drugs prior to surgery, and we provide counseling for that. Tobacco use increases your chances of postsurgical lung complications and infection and delays wound healing. Patients must stop smoking for at least eight weeks before surgery.

Even if you drink alcohol only in moderation, you should avoid it altogether two weeks prior to surgery. Alcohol increases your risk for complications.

Dental care: Have a checkup, cleaning and any necessary dental work done prior to your surgery. Bacteria in your mouth can travel through the bloodstream and would be attracted to your joint implant, increasing your risk for infection. Patients should wait around six months after their joint replacement to have any other dental work.

Be Proactive Postsurgery

Many knee- and hip-replacement patients go directly home the day after the surgery—and some even go home the same day. We have found that patients recover faster, have fewer complications and are happier if they are discharged to home rather than a rehabilitation facility. A strong support system also promotes healing.

Physical therapy: Getting moving again is the most important thing you can do to reduce inflammation, swelling and pain. You'll start with a walker and progress to a cane. Usually patients do away with these devices by about four weeks. The physical therapist at the hospital will teach you specific exercises. Depending on your insurance, you will continue with physical therapy either at home or at an outpatient rehab facility. For the fastest and best recovery, perform your routine for 20 to 30 minutes two to three times daily. You'll also need to walk (with your walker or cane as needed) another 60 to 90 minutes daily. Don't worry about distance—the number of times you walk is more important than how far.

Pain relief: Less pain helps you heal faster, but at Yale and other leading surgical centers, we champion a narcotic-sparing approach due to the dangers of opioid pain relievers. We use peripheral nerve blocks during surgery to help reduce pain afterward and give *acetaminophen* (Tylenol) intravenously, which provides better pain relief than taking it orally. Once home, patients may be prescribed acetaminophen, a nonsteroidal anti-inflammatory (such as *ibuprofen*) and *gabapentin* (Neurontin), a non-narcotic neurological medicine that can help reduce pain for two to three weeks. Your goal should be to taper off narcotic medication by the end of the second week after surgery and take acetaminophen or an NSAID only as needed.

Diet: Follow the same high-protein, fruit- and vegetable-loaded eating plan as you did before surgery. It can be hard to eat while you're in pain, but your body requires adequate calories to help it heal after surgery. Avoid sugar and refined carbs, both of which can increase inflammation and slow healing.

Chapter 8

HEART HEALTH FOR WOMEN

Women: Don't Let Your Doctor Miss Your Heart Disease

"Time is muscle." That was the mantra I learned in my fellowship training.

What it means is: The longer a heart attack victim has to wait before being treated, the greater the potential damage to the heart muscle. To me, as a young doctor on call in the hospital overnight, it meant that the longer it took me to get out of the on-call room bed, get to the patient in the ER, evaluate and treat, the greater the chance that the patient's heart could be scarred for life. Talk about pressure! I used to sit up all night and wait even if things got quiet, just in case someone came in with a heart attack. Some doctors nap when they are on call, but I would sit with a huge cup filled with ice, then ½ water and ½ apple juice that I would find unused on patient food carts. I would alternate drinking that apple juice with cups of coffee all night long. I had jelly beans in my lab coat pocket for quick energy, and I would chew packs and packs of gum throughout my shift until morning came and the new

team arrived. To me, this was my only option. Time is muscle, and I wasn't going to have anyone's heart muscle destroyed unnecessarily on my watch!

This vigilance, no matter how crazy it might have looked to my colleagues, paid off on multiple occasions. Women often came into the ER with shortness of breath, nausea, vomiting, sweating and chest discomfort, and I needed to make sure I evaluated them in time. Although their symptoms were often atypical (although not, as it turns out, atypical for women), many of these women were indeed having heart attacks. We were learning then, and women's symptoms were often misdiagnosed as being something other than heart disease. Statistics show that within the first month after suffering a heart attack, women are twice as likely to die. Within the first year after a heart attack, they are 50% more likely to die. The more I learned, the more shocked I became. I felt that I needed to do everything I could to help change these stats. It was devastating—and it became my life's work.

Suzanne Steinbaum, DO, cardiologist in private practice in New York City and a national spokesperson for the Go Red for Women campaign. She is author of *Dr. Suzanne Steinbaum's Heart Book*. DrSuzanneSteinbaum.com

But that was a long time ago—about 20 years ago, in fact. Surely things have changed. It's a whole new century with 20 more years of research and technological progress. Surely by now, we have moved beyond these statistics—doctors must easily recognize a heart attack in a woman. Patients who suffer heart attacks must have a much better chance of post-event survival. Right?

Studies show otherwise. On those front lines, where EMTs in the field and doctors in the ER see heart attack victims all the time, it is still all too common that cardiac care for women gets unnecessarily delayed due to misdiagnosis or ignorance of the esoteric nature of symptoms in women. And that means more heart muscle damage. More subsequent risk of death. Time is muscle.

In her *Wall Street Journal* essay, *I Had No Idea I Was Having a Heart Attack*, Robin Oliveira, a retired nurse, describes the challenging and often typical scenario of a woman suffering a heart attack: the symptoms that don't seem obviously heart-related (nausea, vomiting, extreme fatigue, shoulder and back pain)…the lack of urgency and immediate diagnosis on the part of EMTs and ER doctors…and the reality of the neglect that women suffer all too often when they have a heart attack or heart disease. The author relates her own worrisome family history of heart attacks—her mother died of a heart attack at 53, and her father died of a heart attack at 62. Even though she took cholesterol-lowering medication and was a medical professional, she did develop heart disease and she did have a heart attack.

Yet even women with a family history of heart disease are still, frustratingly, misdiagnosed, resulting in treatment delays. What are we to do about this problem? Do we have options? Do we have any power?

Fortunately, we do. The reality is that for Ms. Oliveira and other women like her (and for all women), heart disease doesn't just appear out of nowhere. There are signs and there are warnings. The scary part is that we don't always see them and can't always feel them. The only way to catch them is to be proactive and brave in assessing your own personal heart truth. If a doctor or an EMT may not recognize your heart issues, then the simple fact is that it may be up to you.

I had a patient tell me the other day that she thought I had a scary job. Recalling those fellowship days in my early career, I used to think so too! But now I know that there is a predictable process by which heart disease develops, and understanding it can help to prevent those scary moments from happening. Today, instead of staying up all night popping jelly beans and chewing gum to stay awake, I spend my energy getting out this one message: *There are ways to protect yourself!* Heart disease almost always develops not just due to a possible genetic susceptibility but because of lifestyle factors. *It all goes back to basics…*

1. Get tests to understand your cholesterol level, blood pressure, blood sugar and a coronary artery calcium score (a screening test for plaque in the arteries). Tell your doctor you want to establish a baseline so you can best monitor your own health.

2. Stop smoking. (That goes without saying…)

3. Exercise regularly—at least three to five days a week—and get your heart rate up!

4. Get to a healthy weight.

5. Manage your stress.

6. Eat a heart-healthy diet full of vegetables, fruits, whole grains and healthy fats.

7. If you need medication to lower your risk factors, don't dismiss this option! It could save your life.

8. If you think something is wrong, seek medical attention immediately. Don't make excuses.

9. Take your health seriously. Be proactive. Let your voice be heard and advocate for yourself.

10. Don't put yourself on the bottom of the list. Make your health a priority.

Although it would be nice if doctors caught every heart attack within seconds, the truth is that you, who might actually need care and help someday, may have to demand it. Although Ms. Oliveira needed help and care and didn't get it as quickly as she should have, she was lucky enough to receive medical attention within the time frame necessary, without dying and without having muscle damage. Not every woman is so lucky.

Bottom line: For now, at least, this one is on us, ladies. It's in our laps, in our hands and, yes, in our hearts. We need to be the force that drives this story. We need to be more in charge of our health. We need to demand care and attention, and we need to take advantage of the many known preventive strategies available to us. We need to ask for tests that can detect disease before it gets too advanced. We need to take medication if we need it, eat a diet that works for us and is nutritionally complete, exercise to keep our hearts strong, get to a healthy weight where we feel good and our heart isn't unnecessarily burdened—in other words, know and manage our risk factors and get regular and routine follow-up.

Today, my job isn't nearly as scary as it used to be, but the landscape for women is just as scary as it was 20 year ago. I know that with aggressive prevention, we could get this disease under control. I can't speak for the many clinical care teams taking care of women's hearts across the country and the world. Each team and each scenario has its challenges. But the simple fact is that time is muscle, and that is something every woman should understand. Let's stop depending on a system that is not yet quite adequate and tackle this disease on our own time. Let's take charge of our own health. Let's demand early prevention and early detection. Let's prevent this story from happening to any woman ever again. When that happens, my job won't be scary at all.

10 Small Changes for a Healthier Heart

Joel K. Kahn, MD, holistic cardiologist and clinical professor of medicine at Wayne State University School of Medicine in Detroit. Dr. Kahn lectures throughout the country on the body's ability to heal itself through proper nutrition. His latest book is *The Plant-Based Solution*. DrJoelKahn.com

Every year, roughly 610,000 Americans die of heart disease. It is the leading cause of death in the US for both sexes. But there is good news. Research shows that even little shifts in diet and lifestyle can significantly boost your heart health.

Big bonus: Several require little or no effort. *Prominent cardiologist Dr. Joel Kahn suggests 10 surprising lifestyle tweaks that can make a big difference...*

1. Start fidgeting. Yes, you may have been told to sit still as a child, but that was then. Heart disease studies in the UK compared women who habitually sat still with women who regularly fidgeted (e.g., swinging legs, tapping toes, shifting weight) while seated. Over 12 years of follow-up, fidgeters developed heart disease significantly less frequently than women who sat still. Why? Fidgeting is a physical activity, and every bit of movement helps keep blood and oxygen circulating, even if you're glued to a computer all day.

Extra benefit: Little movements burn calories. Fidgeters generally burn around 300 extra calories per day. It's all about movement.

2. See a dentist. You probably already know that periodontal (gum) disease—which half of American adults have—means that you have two to three times greater risk for heart disease than people with healthy gums. But what you may not know is that patients with periodontitis who received treatment—such as special cleanings or, in more advanced cases, surgery—showed an improved cardiovascular risk profile. That's good news! What's the connection? Periodontal disease is a hidden source of inflammation and infection that can age the body, the brain and the heart. There is a growing connection between regular oral health checks and avoiding arterial and heart disease. Simply brushing twice a day and flossing daily, along with limiting sugary beverages and snacks, will reduce your risk significantly. Your dentist can tell you how often you need cleanings, based on your assessed risks for periodontal disease. Insurance usually covers two a year, but if you need more, it's an inexpensive investment in your health.

3. Add ground flaxseed to your food. Just two tablespoons of ground flaxseed a day sprinkled on your cereal, salad, yogurt, smoothie or other foods can make a healthy difference. Ground flaxseed, with its nutty taste, is packed with heart-healthy nutrients, including protein, fiber and omega-3 fatty acids. A meta-analysis of 15 trials published in *Clinical Nutrition* found significant reductions in both systolic blood pressure and diastolic blood pressure after regular supplementation with flaxseed powder or flaxseed oil. Drink lots of water to avoid possible digestive problems.

4. Drink two cups of hibiscus tea daily. The hibiscus plant is a significant source of antioxidants. Hibiscus tea tops the rankings for antioxidant power, even beating matcha (a drink made from powdered green tea leaves), according to NutritionFacts.org. Hibiscus tea also lowers cholesterol and blood pressure, according to a randomized controlled trial reported in *Journal of Human Hypertension.* At the end of the trial, 21% of participants had normalized their blood pressure. This brightly colored tea has a pleasantly tart, fruity taste, hot or cold.

5. Sit in a sauna. Scandinavians and others have sweated it out in the moist heat of saunas for centuries to soothe muscles and relax. But saunas offer other significant benefits as well. Studies from Japan (using dry sauna) and Finland (using wet sauna) demonstrate stronger hearts and longer lives. Why is the sauna experience so powerful? Research published in *Alternative Medicine Review* found that sauna users (with radiant

heat or far-infrared units) received multiple health benefits including relief from COPD, chronic fatigue and chronic pain. Try sitting in a sauna at least once a week for 15 to 20 minutes per session.

6. Eat garlic daily. Garlic is a well-known immune system booster and antioxidant. It even can lower blood pressure and cholesterol. In studies at UCLA, aged black garlic extract helped maintain clean arteries in patients with metabolic syndrome by lowering the accumulation of plaque that can cause heart disease. Aged black garlic is available online, but you also can use regular garlic for heart-healthy benefits.

7. Walk barefoot in the grass. Believe it or don't, but growing evidence reveals that direct contact of your body with the earth (called grounding or earthing) helps your heart, eases inflammation and can create a healthier circulatory system. The connection helps reduce blood viscosity—elevated viscosity hinders delivery of oxygen to blood cells. Going barefoot 30 or 40 minutes a day may reduce cardiac events, according to *The Journal of Alternative and Complementary Medicine.* So shake your shoes off, and get your toes on the ground.

8. Give your digestive system a rest. Periodic and intermittent fasting has many benefits, including disease prevention. Studies show that practicing time-restricted eating for at least 12 hours a day (for example, fasting from 8 pm to 8 am) promotes healing and repair of the body. It's an obvious statement, but fasting for certain hours each day means that most people eat less. Fasting and its associated weight loss have been shown to lower blood pressure and reduce the risk for heart disease, diabetes and other diseases.

9. Stand for five minutes every half hour while awake. By now, most people have heard that being sedentary is an independent risk factor for heart disease and stroke. But did you know that this is true even if you exercise regularly? Moderate-to-vigorous physical activity in the morning or evening does not compensate for prolonged sitting, according to an American Heart Disease Scientific Statement. And yet Americans are sedentary for about six to eight hours a day—it's 8.5 to 9.6 hours for those age 60 and over. Move every half hour to help maintain healthy blood sugar and weight. Simply walk away from your desk or stand and stretch for a few minutes.

10. Get busy in bed. A study published in *The BMJ* from Caerphilly, Wales, followed the sex lives of 918 men ages 45 to 59 for 10 years. The results indicate that frequent (twice a week or more) orgasmic activity can reduce the risk for heart attack by 50%. Research hasn't confirmed whether women would reap the same benefits, but it can't hurt to try.

Late Dinners Linked to Increased Heart Risk

The study "Evening Caloric Intake Is Associated with Cardiovascular Health in Women: Results from the American Heart Association Go Red for Women Strategically Focused Research Network" was presented at the American Heart Association's annual meeting in Philadelphia, November 2019.

All jokes aside about "early-bird specials," early-evening eaters may be on to something! At least when it comes to heart problems in women.

That's the finding from researchers who recently studied the link between evening mealtimes and women's risk for heart disease.

Study details: The heart health of 112 women (average age 33) was evaluated by researchers at the beginning of the 12-month study and again at the end. The women kept food diaries recording everything they ate—and the time of day—for a week around the time of the two cardiac assessments.

Through the assessments, a heart health score was created for each woman based on her body mass index (BMI), cholesterol, blood pressure and blood sugar levels as well as lifestyle factors such as not smoking, being physically active and eating a healthy diet. At the end of the study, the research-

ers calculated the percentage of calories the women consumed after 6 pm and 8 pm…and compared that data with the women's follow-up heart health scores.

The findings: The women who consumed a higher proportion of their daily calories after 6 pm were more likely to have a higher BMI…higher blood pressure…worse long-term control of blood sugar…and poorer overall heart health, according to the study, which was presented at the American Heart Association's annual meeting. The results were similar when women consumed more calories after 8 pm than earlier in the day.

Also: The link between late-day calories and adverse cardiac health markers was even stronger for the Hispanic women in the study.

"So far, lifestyle approaches to prevent heart disease have focused on what we eat and how much we eat," said Nour Makarem, PhD, lead author and associate research scientist at Columbia University's Vagelos College of Physicians and Surgeons in New York City. "These preliminary results indicate that intentional eating that is mindful of the timing and proportion of calories in evening meals may represent a simple, modifiable behavior that can help lower heart disease risk."

Preeclampsia Linked to Cardiovascular Disease

Women who had preeclampsia during pregnancy were significantly more likely to eventually develop hardened arteries, aortic stenosis, mitral regurgitation and heart failure. Women should tell their doctors about this history…obtain blood pressure screening at least once a year…and ask about lifestyle strategies to reduce risk.

Pradeep Natarajan, MD, director of Preventive Cardiology at Massachusetts General Hospital, Boston, and author of a study of more than 220,000 women published in *Journal of the American College of Cardiology*. MassGeneral.org

Little-Known Heart Attack and Stroke Triggers

Barry A. Franklin, PhD, director of Preventive Cardiology/Cardiac Rehabilitation at Beaumont Health in Royal Oak, Michigan.

Cardiovascular disease causes one out of every three deaths in the US—and it has three main henchmen…

Heart attack, when a blocked cardiac artery cuts off blood flow to the heart muscle, affecting about 735,000 people each year.

Sudden cardiac death (SCD), commonly known as cardiac arrest, when chaotic activity in the heart's electrical system causes it to stop functioning—a condition that strikes 325,000 people yearly.

Ischemic stroke, when blood flow is blocked to the brain, occurring in nearly 800,000 people every year.

If you ask most cardiologists what leads to these "acute cardiovascular events," they'll talk about conventional risk factors, such as elevated cholesterol, high blood pressure, a sedentary lifestyle, diabetes and smoking.

There's more to the story: Roughly half of all acute cardiovascular events are precipitated by little-known physical, emotional and chemical stressors, according to research. Exposure to these stressors can trigger a sudden, potentially harmful increase in the activity of the sympathetic nervous system, the "fight-or-flight" mechanism that prepares the body to respond to stress by temporarily accelerating heart rate, raising blood pressure and increasing blood clotting.

Because an estimated 85% of adults over age 50 have some degree of atherosclerotic cardiovascular disease, largely due to the risk factors listed above, the already-compromised arteries of the heart muscle or brain may not be able to handle these abrupt physiological changes…and you can end up suffering a heart attack, SCD or stroke. *What you need to know…*

Physical Triggers

Major surgery is the leading little-known physical trigger. Surprisingly, it's not just heart surgery, but any invasive surgery that requires general anesthesia.

Important finding: Among more than 10 million adults (age 45 and older) who underwent a major noncardiac operation (such as orthopedic, gynecologic, vascular and neurosurgery), 3% of patients (or one in 33), on average, had either a heart attack or stroke while hospitalized, according to a nine-year study published in *JAMA Cardiology*.

The risks were especially high for certain types of operations—nearly 8% of patients undergoing vascular surgery suffered a heart attack or stroke while hospitalized… and more than 6% undergoing chest (thoracic) surgery. Patients who were at greatest risk were older, obese, smoked and/or had chronic conditions such as diabetes, kidney disease or high blood pressure.

What can happen: The surgery may cause arterial plaque to rupture and form a blood clot, triggering a heart attack or stroke.

And the risk for an acute cardiovascular event remains elevated for some time. One in 20 patients (5%) who had major noncardiac surgery had a heart attack within 30 days of the surgery, according to a study published in *Annals of Internal Medicine*.

Self-defense: To protect yourself against an acute cardiovascular event during or after major surgery, improve your aerobic fitness—which is associated with lower resting heart rates—before surgery. For example, in the study mentioned above, every 10 beat-per-minute increase in resting heart rate before surgery (for example, 80 versus 70 beats per minute) was linked to about a 30% relative increase in the odds of a heart attack during hospitalization after surgery.

You can achieve a good level of fitness simply by walking briskly (where you can have a conversation, but you'll be breathing harder than usual) for at least 30 minutes, five or more times a week.

Emotional Triggers

Intense negative emotions—such as grief and anger—also stimulate the sympathetic nervous system, raising the risk for an acute cardiovascular event.

Compelling study: When researchers at Harvard Medical School tracked nearly 2,000 people (mean age of 62) over a five-year period, the risk for heart attack increased by 21-fold the day after the death of a "significant person," such as a spouse, and declined on each subsequent day, according to research published in *Circulation*. The risk was greatest among those who already had heart disease.

When researchers reviewed nine studies on anger and acute cardiovascular events, they found that rates of heart attack, stroke and arrhythmia (a risk factor for SCD) all increased—some by nearly eight-fold—in the two hours after outbursts of anger compared with other times, according to research published in *European Heart Journal*.

Women with diagnosed heart disease are particularly vulnerable to negative emotions. Those who had the highest levels of "psychological distress"—depression, post-traumatic stress, anxiety, anger, hostility and perceived stress—were 44% more likely to have a heart attack or stroke than those not experiencing those negative emotions, noted a study published in *Journal of the American Heart Association*.

How to protect yourself: If you have cardiovascular disease, stay fit (as described earlier) and take your prescribed medications, whether it's a beta-blocker, statin or low-dose aspirin. These drugs may reduce one's vulnerability to an acute cardiovascular event when an emotional trigger occurs.

To reduce, or even prevent, the adverse consequences of negative emotions, complementary approaches include meditation, deep breathing, yoga, tai chi, mental stress-reducing exercises and anger-management interventions.

Chemical Triggers

Air pollution and secondhand smoke are the two main chemical triggers of acute cardiovascular events.

Startling new findings: When levels of air pollution—from traffic and non-traffic emissions—in urban areas in New York state were tested and correlated with levels of hospitalization for acute cardiovascular events the next day, the higher pollution levels were linked to a more than doubled rate of hospitalization for arrhythmia and a nearly quadrupled rate of hospitalization for stroke, according to research published in *Environment International*.

Two years after smoke-free legislation was implemented in Uruguay—prohibiting people from smoking indoors in the workplace or in public places—hospitalizations for heart attack decreased by 22%, according to research published in *Tobacco Control*.

How to protect yourself: Limit your outdoor activities when pollution is high…and steer clear of people who are smoking. To monitor air quality in your local area, check the website AirNow.gov. As mentioned earlier, it's also crucial to get (and stay) fit and take your cardioprotective medications, as prescribed.

Other strategies to protect yourself against triggered cardiovascular events include avoiding unaccustomed heavy physical exertion (such as snow removal) and prolonged periods of sleep deprivation. It also helps to strive for strict enforcement of environmental regulations regarding air pollution.

The Right Eating Habits Help Your Heart

Skipping breakfast and eating a late dinner hinders heart attack recovery.

New study: Heart attack sufferers with these eating habits were four to five times more likely to die, have another heart attack or suffer from angina within 30 days of hospital discharge. Each habit alone was also linked to these outcomes.

Marcos Minicucci, MD, professor of medicine, São Paulo State University, Brazil.

Early Monday OK for Your Heart

Peak time for cardiac arrest is no longer early Monday. In a study of more than 2,600 cases of cardiac arrest (when the heart stops beating), the events were evenly spread across the hours of the day, as well as days of the week.

Possible reasons: Access to technology and a 24/7 culture of being "on" have altered our body's natural rhythms.

Sumeet Chugh, MD, cardiologist and associate director, Cedars-Sinai Smidt Heart Institute, Los Angeles.

Heart Disease Starts Long Before the Diagnosis…So Stop Waiting

Suzanne Steinbaum, DO, cardiologist in private practice in New York City and a national spokesperson for the Go Red for Women campaign. She is author of *Dr. Suzanne Steinbaum's Heart Book.* DrSuzanneSteinbaum.com

I will never forget the time when my son Spencer was five years old and I told him that I was going to work to take care of people's hearts. His response—only a five-year-old could have put it so simply—was, "Why can't the people take care of their own hearts?" As much as it made me laugh then, in the seven years since that time, I have not stopped thinking about it.

Why can't people take care of their own hearts? I think the answer is complicated, but rooted in one simple problem: They don't really know how.

People have become much more proactive about prevention in the world of cancer, diligently planning their mammograms, colonoscopies and skin screenings. Yet people are far less proactive about heart health. Since heart disease kills more people than cancer—and is, in fact, the number one killer of women as well as men—perhaps our health diligence needs to be spread around a bit more. For example, we've all heard about the latest diets, but that hasn't helped most people become any more aware of how the food they eat impacts the health of their arteries.

For many years, I have suggested that we change the paradigm for how we define heart disease. What if heart disease was not just something of concern after a diagnosis, whether a heart attack, a valve issue, heart failure or another form of illness, in which heart functioning has become dangerously dysfunctional? What if, instead, we could diagnose someone who doesn't exercise— or who has high cholesterol or high blood pressure or any other risk factors for heart disease—with actual heart disease, long before they fell sick? The traditional paradigm is that we wait until disease strikes to do something about it. But from my vantage point as a preventive cardiologist, that is simply too late.

If heart disease were diagnosed according to how you live your life, would that change how you approached your days and made your decisions? Would you still choose the doughnut over the fruit…the French fries over the salad…the Netflix binge over the evening walk or the after-work gym session…if those choices would mean you have heart disease right now?

Consider the American Heart Association's "Life's Simple 7," which are seven factors that, when optimized, are generally considered to prevent 80% of heart disease cases. *These seven factors are…*

- **Cholesterol level**
- **Blood pressure**
- **Blood sugar level**
- **Body mass index (your weight)**

- **Whether you exercise**
- **What you eat**
- **Whether you smoke.**

What if, when your numbers were optimal and you exercised for 150 minutes a week, ate a healthy diet and didn't smoke, you would be considered heart-healthy? And what if, when you have abnormally high cholesterol, blood pressure, blood sugar or body mass index, or if you don't exercise, if you eat junk food, or smoke cigarettes, your doctor could write "diagnosis: heart disease" in your chart?

Of course, this scenario I propose probably won't happen, but if you think about it, you will see the logic of it. If you have high cholesterol, high blood pressure or high blood sugar, it's likely due to your lifestyle choices. If you are overweight or obese, it's likely due to your lifestyle choices. If you don't exercise, that's almost always a decision under your control. The same goes for what you choose to eat and whether you choose to smoke. We know all of these things are risk factors for heart disease, so if you are making decisions that put you at risk, you are essentially inviting heart disease.

So I say, consider yourself already there.

Let's circle back to the question, How should people take care of their own hearts? The answer is simple. Exercise...eat healthy food...don't smoke...and monitor your cholesterol, blood pressure and blood sugar. Work to get to a healthy weight and, if you have questions, ask your doctor for answers.

As doctors, we need to get better at providing information and resources, such as how to get access to the healthy food we suggest, when to get basic tests done, how often to exercise and how to lose weight in a healthy way. First and foremost, we need behavioral changes to go beyond being just a concept, to something we actually do every day as a treatment paradigm for a disease state. We need to see these behavioral changes as urgent. As life-saving. Because that's exactly what they are.

Re-defining heart disease as something that exists before a heart attack happens can be incredibly empowering. Let's consider heart disease as inevitable in the presence of risk factors. If we do this on a grand scale—even lobbying for insurance companies to pay for the testing and diagnostic studies needed for screening for eventual heart disease before the actual diagnosis is made—maybe we could actually demote heart disease from its current title as the number one killer of "the people." What a victory that would be!

In the meantime, take a good hard look at yourself. How are you doing with Life's Simple 7? Where do you fit in? If you have any of these risk factors—if you aren't optimizing your numbers and behaviors—know that every day you procrastinate managing your diet ("I'll start tomorrow"), or starting an exercise program ("when I get motivated"), or trying to lose weight ("when the weather gets nice"), or managing your stress ("when I can learn how to meditate"), you are one day closer to heart disease.

Look at it differently. If you say to yourself that this is heart disease—that you have heart disease right now, and that you are sick when these numbers are elevated—maybe your motivation will be different. Maybe you will shift your priorities.

If we want the people to take care of their own hearts, then I say let them—but let them do so with full awareness of the need, the urgency and the power they have to make the lifestyle changes that will translate into success. Give the people the ability to make it happen and the knowledge that if they don't make it happen, then they do have heart disease...because eventually they will.

I want to be able to say to my son, "Spencer, finally the people are taking care of their own hearts. I don't think I need to go to work today. Let's go for a walk in the park!" Maybe I'll see you there, too.

Heart Attacks That Start Slowly Could Be More Deadly

Study titled "The Association Between Symptom Onset Characteristics and Prehospital Delay in Women and Men with Acute Coronary Syndrome" led by researchers at University of Illinois at Chicago, published in *European Journal of Cardiovascular Nursing.*

Sudden chest pain or discomfort is a classic red flag for heart attack, but sometimes the symptoms start out mild and develop gradually. How do slower symptoms affect treatment and survival?

To find out, researchers recently looked at the time that elapsed between the first symptoms that occurred in 474 heart attack patients (average age 62) and their arrival at emergency departments (EDs) at various locations across the US.

The study, which was published in *European Journal of Cardiovascular Nursing,* found that people who experienced gradual symptoms, which tend to start with mild discomfort that slowly worsens, took eight hours, on average, to get to an ED versus 2.6 hours for those with abrupt symptoms that were characterized by sudden and severe pain from the beginning.

"Both are a medical emergency and require urgent help," explained Sahereh Mirzaei, PhD, RN, study author and a clinical practitioner in the open-heart intensive care unit at the University of Illinois at Chicago. "But our study shows that gradual symptoms are not taken seriously."

Other study findings…

• **Slow-to-develop symptoms are common.** Even though 56% of the study participants experienced abrupt symptoms, including sudden chest pain, 44% suffered gradual symptoms, such as mild and slowly progressive chest discomfort or pain.

• **Abrupt symptoms are linked to physical activity.** Sudden heart attack symptoms were more likely to occur after some type of exertion such as shoveling snow, climb-

Give Your Heart a Fiber Boost

Better Gut Health Helps Your Heart

Heart failure patients often have less diversity in their gut microbiota.

New finding: Reduced gut bacteria was linked to lower dietary fiber intake, according to stool samples taken from more than 300 participants with and without heart failure.

Self-defense: Choose fruits, vegetables, cereals and other high-fiber foods to stimulate healthy gut flora.

Cristiane Mayerhofer, MD, cardiologist, Oslo University Hospital, Rikshospitalet, Norway.

Fiber May Help Lower Heart Disease Risk

The popular fiber supplement psyllium has been shown to help reduce LDL ("bad") cholesterol and two other lipids that are associated with heart disease. Those benefits are in addition to psyllium's treatment of constipation, the purpose for which it usually is used.

Analysis of the findings of 28 studies of people with normal and high cholesterol, led by researchers at St. Michael's Hospital, Toronto, Canada, published in *American Journal of Clinical Nutrition.*

ing stairs, heavy gardening or jogging. This can signal a serious type of heart attack that requires prompt restoration of blood flow to blocked arteries.

• **Driving to the ED is a mistake.** A major cause of delay for all patients was driving to the ED instead of calling for an ambulance. Only 45% of the study participants called for emergency medical services. Differences in delay time between men and women were not significant.

• **The uninsured are at greater risk.** Being uninsured was linked with a longer delay.

Key takeaways…

• **Don't delay.** When medical care for heart attack symptoms is not sought promptly, there can be dire consequences. For example, the American Heart Association has set a goal of two hours for getting a patient with heart attack symptoms to the ED. Research has shown that every 30-minute delay reduces life expectancy by one year. After six hours, standard treatment with angioplasty, in which a catheter is inserted and the blocked artery is opened by inflating a tiny balloon, does little to reduce the rate of heart attack deaths.

•**Call 911.** Driving to the hospital was linked to slower arrival times at the ED. Despite repeated warnings that driving is not safe and delays treatment, studies consistently show that most people with heart attacks arrive at the ED by car. Calling 911 has several advantages, according to the National Heart, Lung, and Blood Institute. For one, it allows the 911 operator to give you advice (such as taking an aspirin if you're not allergic). Once emergency medical services (EMS) personnel arrive, they can assess your condition and start lifesaving medicines and other treatments right away. In addition, people who arrive by ambulance often receive faster treatment at the hospital.

Heart attack symptoms—either sudden or slow—are a medical emergency. *They include...*

•**Chest pain, discomfort or pressure**

•**Pain or pressure in the throat, neck, shoulder, arms or back**

•**Shortness of breath**

•**Pain may include nausea, vomiting or cold sweats.**

Chili Peppers May Prevent Fatal Heart Attacks

People who ate them at least four times a week were 44% less likely to die from a heart attack over an eight-year period, compared with people who did not eat the hot peppers. Chili peppers also were associated

with a big reduction in the risk for death from cerebrovascular disease—61%—in people who ate them at least four times every week. It is possible that the ingredient that gives the peppers their heat—capsaicin—may have protective effects. Animal studies have found it is associated with lower cholesterol and with blocking expression of a gene that causes blood vessels to tighten.

Marialaura Bonaccio, PhD, epidemiologist, IRCCS Neuromed Mediterranean Neurological Institute, Pozzilli, Italy, and leader of a study of 22,811 people, published in *Journal of the American College of Cardiology.*

Reduce Blood Pressure, Preserve Mental Ability

People who have hypertension at midlife appear increasingly likely to suffer cognitive decline decades later. Two recent studies linked higher blood pressure at ages 36 or 44 with an increased risk for cognitive impairment at around age 70. A third study found that people treated intensively to reduce their systolic pressure (the upper number) to 120 mm Hg or lower developed fewer lesions associated with cognitive decline than those

Blueberries for Heart Health

Overweight adults with high blood pressure, elevated blood sugar and/or other cardiovascular risk factors ate a cup or a half-cup of blueberries, or a placebo, daily for six months.

Result: The one-cup group reduced their risk for cardiovascular disease by nearly 15%, while the half-cup and placebo groups showed no improvement.

Theory: One cup of blueberries daily provided adequate levels of heart-healthy anthocyanins.

Aedín Cassidy, PhD, professor of nutrition, Norwich Medical School, University of East Anglia, Norwich, England.

treated to keep systolic pressure at or below 140 mm Hg.

Roundup of several recent studies, reported in *University of California, Berkeley Wellness Letter.*

Breathing Technique Can Lower Blood Pressure

Inspiratory Muscle Strength Training (IMST) involves breathing in vigorously through a special handheld device originally developed to help critically ill people breathe without ventilators. This technique also has been shown effective in helping develop the weak breathing muscles of people with obstructive sleep apnea. Now early results of a new study show that regular use of IMST can lower systolic blood pressure (the top number) nearly twice as much as aerobic exercise does. IMST users also had better large-artery function and lower heart rate and oxygen consumption during exercise than study subjects not using the technique. Inspiratory muscle train-

Timing Your Blood Pressure Medication

Compared with people who took their blood pressure medication in the morning, those who took one or more blood pressure–lowering drugs at bedtime had 34% lower risk for heart attack...and 49% lower risk for stroke, according to a six-year study of nearly 20,000 men and women with hypertension.

Reason: Sleep-time blood pressure is the most significant marker for cardiovascular risk.

Important: Talk to your doctor before changing the time of day you take your medication.

Ramón C. Hermida, PhD, director, Bioengineering and Chronobiology Labs, University of Vigo, Spain.

ers already are commercially available—ask your doctor if you should consider IMST.

Daniel Craighead, PhD, postdoctoral researcher, integrative physiology department, University of Colorado at Boulder and leader of a study of 50 people, presented at the recent Experimental Biology conference in Orlando, Florida.

Mouthwash/Blood Pressure Alert

Recent finding: After one week of using an oral rinse containing the antiseptic *chlorhexidine*, which is used to fight plaque and gingivitis, participants' tongues had a decrease in "friendly" bacteria that produce nitric oxide (NO), a substance that helps maintain normal blood pressure. In addition, their systolic (top number) blood pressure increased significantly—by 5 mm Hg to 26 mm Hg. Once the mouthwash was stopped, NO-producing bacteria in the mouth were replenished and blood pressure returned to normal after seven days.

Nathan Bryan, PhD, adjunct professor of molecular and human genetics, Baylor College of Medicine, Houston.

Yogurt for Heart Health

Eating yogurt may reduce heart disease risk in people with high blood pressure. Men with high blood pressure who ate at least two servings of yogurt each week had 21% lower risk for heart attack or stroke. Risk was cut by 17% for women. The reason is unknown, but probiotics from fermentation in yogurt production may play a role.

Lynn L. Moore, DSc, MPH, director of nutrition and metabolism at Boston University School of Medicine and coauthor of a study published in *American Journal of Hypertension.*

Cutting Back on Salt May Harm You

Michael Alderman, MD, emeritus professor at Albert Einstein College of Medicine, New York City, and former president of the American Society of Hypertension. He has studied extensively the effects of sodium on hypertension.

Salt has a reputation for being bad for your health. The main cause for alarm is sodium, which at very high levels can throw the body's fluid balance out of whack, causing high blood pressure, heart disease and even death. Government organizations say that we consume too much salt and recommend cutbacks. But in fact, sodium is a nutrient that's essential for myriad physiological processes in our bodies, and getting too little salt is also harmful to our health. The truth is, most of us are fairly conservative with the salt shaker.

Although it's true that cutting back on sodium can lower blood pressure in people who have hypertension, no studies have shown that doing so will help reduce heart attacks or death. What's more, cutting back too much also is likely to have some unexpected side effects—higher cholesterol, triglyceride and blood sugar levels.

Recent research summarizing six decades of studies that included more than one million people worldwide suggests an optimal range for sodium intake that's associated with the lowest risk for disease and death from all causes. That sodium "sweet spot" is roughly 3,500 mg to 4,500 mg a day. (Most people consume 3,600 mg to 3,700 mg daily.) That's a lot higher than the 1,500 mg to 2,300 mg a day recommended by the American Heart Association (AHA), the World Health Organization and numerous other health bodies.

Instead of trying to lower your sodium, it may make more sense to increase your intake of potassium, which helps control blood pressure by upping your ability to process sodium out of your body and by relaxing blood vessel walls. (Fruits and vegetables such as bananas, oranges, spinach and cucumbers are good sources.) Research has shown that higher levels of potassium are linked to fewer cardiovascular events and deaths across the globe.

Red...White...or No Meat?

According to a recent study, healthy adults, ages 21 to 65, ate a diet rich in red-meat protein (such as beef)...a white-meat diet (chicken)...and then a no-meat diet, for four weeks each, with a "washout" period of two to seven weeks in between.

Result: LDL cholesterol levels were similarly higher (6% to 7%) after eating the red or white meat, versus the nonmeat diet.

For cholesterol control: Aim for a diet limited in meats and rich in plant-based proteins, such as nuts, beans, lentils, quinoa and tofu.

Ronald M. Krauss, MD, director of atherosclerosis research, Children's Hospital Oakland Research Institute, California.

No Fasting Needed Before Cholesterol Test

Prior to a cholesterol blood test, fasting has traditionally been advised for nine to 12 hours beforehand.

Recent finding: Nonfasting cholesterol levels were similar to fasting levels measured four weeks apart in the same participants, according to a study of more than 8,000 people with cardiovascular risk factors. This research supports the recent guideline change from the American College of Cardiology/American Heart Association that no longer requires fasting before a cholesterol test.

Samia Mora, MD, director, Center for Lipid Metabolomics, Brigham and Women's Hospital, Boston.

Triglycerides: The Heart Threat You Should Not Ignore

Michael Ozner, MD, a board-certified cardiologist, Fellow of the American College of Cardiology and of the American Heart Association, medical director of the Center for Prevention and Wellness at Baptist Health South Florida in Miami and voluntary clinical assistant professor of medicine/cardiology at University of Miami Miller School of Medicine. Dr. Ozner is also author of *The Great American Heart Hoax, Heart Attack Proof* and *The Complete Mediterranean Diet.* DrOzner.com

When it comes to heart disease risk, most people are aware of the threat high cholesterol poses—in fact, nearly one in three American adults over age 40 takes medication to help control his/her cholesterol…and new guidelines were recently announced to provide better cholesterol management.

What you may not know: According to the latest research, high triglycerides are just as threatening to your heart. But unfortunately, they're frequently downplayed by doctors and their patients.

Background: In prehistoric times, triglycerides (fats, also called lipids, in the blood) were a way for our hunter-gatherer ancestors to store fat—a must when food was sparse and famine common. But the stored fat that saved our ancestors from starvation is killing us now.

Fatty, sugary food is superabundant, and we eat too much of it. As a result, more than 70% of adults in the US are overweight or obese—which means they're storing harmful amounts of triglycerides that increase risk for cardiovascular disease.

Up until now, scientists had not proven that lowering triglycerides also lowers the risk for cardiovascular disease…

Important new finding: In a study published in *The New England Journal of Medicine,* researchers looked at more than 8,000 patients with heart disease, diabetes and other risk factors for heart attack and stroke. All participants were taking a statin, and their low-density lipoprotein (LDL) "bad" cholesterol was at a healthy level (below 100 mg/dL). However, they still had high triglyceride levels.

Adding a triglyceride-lowering drug to their regimen—4 g of *icosapent ethyl* (Vascepa), a highly purified fish oil that delivers the healthful omega-3 fatty acid EPA—lowered triglycerides by 20% compared with a placebo. Over the six-year study, first-time heart attacks were reduced by 31% and strokes by 28%, and there were 20% fewer deaths from cardiovascular disease in patients taking the triglyceride-lowering drug. Additionally, the level of C-reactive protein, a biomarker for artery-damaging inflammation, was reduced by an average of 20%.*

In follow-up research, the results were even better—there was a 30% reduction in the combined rate of first as well as second and subsequent cardiovascular deaths, nonfatal heart attacks or strokes, procedures such as stenting and hospitalization for unstable angina.

Bottom line: The higher your level of triglycerides, the higher your risk for cardiovascular disease. Based on this new research, lowering high triglycerides will likely become standard practice to curb risk for and treat cardiovascular disease.

Get Your Levels Tested

A normal triglyceride level is generally below 150 mg/dL. But research shows that about one-third of Americans have triglycerides in the danger zone—150 mg/dL and above.

To get your levels tested: Your doctor should order a blood test to measure all blood fats that impact the heart, including total cholesterol, LDL cholesterol, HDL cholesterol and triglycerides. Apolipoprotein B levels, which measure the number of potentially harmful particles that carry cholesterol and triglycerides, are often measured as well.

*The research was sponsored by Amarin, the manufacturer of Vascepa.

The frequency of testing depends on the age and cardiovascular risk of the patient.

While triglyceride levels have previously been measured in standard blood tests, doctors didn't realize their importance in the treatment of cardiovascular disease.

If your triglycerides are high…

Note that several classes of medications can raise triglyceride levels.

For example: Beta-blockers and diuretics (used for high blood pressure)…estrogen (for menopause)…retinoic acid and retinoids (for psoriasis and other skin problems)…and bile acid sequestrants (used mainly for lowering cholesterol). If you're taking any of these drugs and your triglycerides are high, your doctor may change the dose or prescribe an alternative drug.

Other risk factors for high triglycerides that your doctor should check for include prediabetes and diabetes, kidney disease, thyroid disorder and a family history of very high triglycerides. If an underlying condition is treated, high triglycerides can be resolved.

If the above causes have been ruled out, under the guidance of your doctor and for the amount of time he/she suggests, try the triglyceride-lowering lifestyle plan below. *This healthy plan is also a good way to help protect against developing high triglycerides…*

•**Eat a Mediterranean diet.** The main reason for high triglycerides is a poor diet—namely one that emphasizes processed foods, trans fats (found in baked goods and fried foods), saturated fat (found in meat and dairy products) and sugar and refined starches. Your best strategy is to eliminate or minimize your intake of all these types of foods.

To keep triglycerides under control, I favor the Mediterranean diet, which is rich in vegetables, fruits, whole grains, beans, nuts and seeds, fish and olive oil. In a study published in *Journal of Nutrition,* people who followed a Mediterranean diet for six months had a significant reduction in triglycerides compared with people who ate their usual diet.

•**Exercise regularly.** Regular exercise lowers triglycerides…LDL cholesterol…inflammation…and stress hormones. It also helps control weight, a risk factor for high triglycerides. To start, aim for 20 minutes of moderate exercise (like brisk walking), three to five times a week. Over time, increase to at least 30 minutes, five times weekly. In a recent study published in *Journal of Clinical Lipidology,* daily 30-minute walks lowered triglycerides.

•**Get seven to eight hours of sleep every night.** A new animal study from Japan and published in *American Journal of Physiology—Endocrinology and Metabolism* shows that sleep deprivation increases triglycerides. In a similar study, people with sleep apnea—a disorder in which breathing repeatedly stops during sleep—had higher triglycerides than those without this sleep condition. Sleep apnea is linked to increased cardiovascular disease and is best treated with a continuous positive airway pressure (CPAP) device. See a sleep specialist for advice.

•**Discuss medication.** If the lifestyle measures above don't adequately lower your triglyceride levels, talk to your physician about medication, such as a statin, fibrate and/or the prescription omega-3 fatty acid Vascepa. It is FDA-approved for patients with triglycerides of 500 mg/dL and above (this level can cause pancreatitis, a potentially life-threatening disease that must be treated) as well as for people at high risk for cardiovascular disease who have well-controlled LDL cholesterol on statin therapy but continue to have triglyceride levels of 150 mg/dL and above.

Note: Vascepa is pharmaceutical grade and is not the same as the omega-3 fish oil supplements that you can buy in the store.

Get Up and Move for Your Heart's Sake

Risks from prolonged sitting can be offset by about 20 to 40 minutes of exercise a day. If you regularly sit for six hours or more per day, you need 150 to 300 minutes of moderate-intensity exercise per week to offset the negative effects on your cardiovascular system.

Study of 150,000 people in Australia by researchers at University of Sydney, Australia, published in *Journal of the American College of Cardiology*.

E-Cigarettes May Harm the Heart More Than Regular Cigarettes

Study titled "Chronic E-Cigarette Users Demonstrate More Consistent Coronary Endothelial Dysfunction Than Chronic Combustible Cigarettes," by researchers at Smidt Heart Institute at Cedars-Sinai Medical Center in Los Angeles and presented at the 2019 American Heart Association Scientific Sessions in Philadelphia.

If you're a cigarette smoker looking to quit, e-cigarettes, also known as vape pens, may seem like a good alternative.

Battery-operated or rechargeable e-cigarettes do not contain any tobacco. Instead, a cartridge of liquid nicotine, flavorings and other chemicals is heated to make a vapor, which is then inhaled by the user. The ease of use, lack of ash and smoky odor and variety of flavors make these electronic nicotine delivery systems appealing to many people, including teenagers.

But a study presented at the 2019 American Heart Association Scientific Sessions concludes that using e-cigarettes may carry as much risk for heart disease—and maybe even more—as traditional tobacco cigarettes.

This finding comes at a time when, despite increased reports of lung-related e-cigarette injuries, manufacturers continue to claim that these electronic systems are safe and can help cigarette smokers to quit.

Recent study: Researchers at the Smidt Heart Institute at Cedars-Sinai Medical Center in Los Angeles measured blood flow to the heart—a marker of how well the heart is functioning—of regular smokers ages 18 to 38 before and after smoking either e-cigarettes or traditional cigarettes. The measurements were taken while the participants were at rest and after they performed a handgrip exercise. The tobacco cigarettes caused blood flow to decrease after physical stress, but not while at rest. The e-cigarettes, however, caused impaired blood flow both after physical stress and while at rest. Decreased coronary blood flow increases the risk for heart disease.

"It's not just the nicotine that makes e-cigarettes harmful to the heart and lungs. It's the completely unknown bucket of manufactured products used to form vapors that is likely causing the most harm," said senior study author Florian Rader, MD, MSc, medical director of the Human Physiology Laboratory at the Smidt Heart Institute.

Note: The Centers for Disease Control and Prevention recently identified vitamin E acetate as a "very strong culprit" in lung injuries related to vaping.

And because e-cigarettes are associated with blood flow dysfunction not just during physical stress but at rest as well, they may be even more harmful than traditional cigarettes, despite what their distributors would like you to believe, the study reports.

The researchers add that because the practice of vaping is still relatively new, scientists may not yet know all of the ways it can damage hearts and lungs. Dr. Rader advises, "The use of any electronic nicotine delivery system should be considered with a high degree of caution until more data can be gathered."

Bottom line: At this point, we need to assume that cigarettes of any kind may hurt your health. If you don't smoke or vape, don't start. If you need help quitting, you can find useful tools and tips at SmokeFree.gov.

Your Heart Needs Sleep

Getting less than six hours of sleep in 24 hours can up your heart attack risk by 20%. Ten or 11 hours can also increase heart attack risk by 34%, although we don't know the reasons for this yet. Staying in the healthy zone and sleeping six to nine hours per night can offset other risks for heart disease—even if those risks are genetic.

Céline Vetter, PhD, assistant professor of integrative physiology and director of the Circadian and Sleep Epidemiology Lab at University of Colorado, Boulder, and senior author of a study published in *Journal of the American College of Cardiology.*

Glucosamine May Reduce Heart-Disease Risk

Glucosamine is a dietary supplement known to lessen joint pain, but a large study found that regular users were 15% less likely to experience cardiovascular events. Earlier research suggests that these benefits might be related to glucosamine's ability to reduce inflammation or its ability to mimic a low-carbohydrate diet that is related to lower risk for heart disease.

Lu Qi, MD, PhD, professor of epidemiology at Tulane University, New Orleans, and coauthor of a study published in *The BMJ.* SPH.Tulane.edu

"I've Done Everything Right...Why Am I Having Heart Problems?"

Suzanne Steinbaum, DO, cardiologist in private practice in New York City and a national spokesperson for the Go Red for Women campaign. She is author of *Dr. Suzanne Steinbaum's Heart Book.* DrSuzanneSteinbaum.com

Every so often, despite everything we advise, despite every preventive measure taken, despite the best of intentions, the unpredictable happens. We can tell patients what to eat and how to exercise, and they follow our advice to the letter, yet they get sick anyway, even diagnosed with the exact disease they're fighting so hard to prevent. It's frustrating, to say the least. This doesn't happen often, but it sometimes does, and if it has happened to you, I want you to know you are not alone.

You may have heard that 80% of the time, heart disease is preventable. This is true, but some people are led to believe that this number is actually 100%. Unfortunately, 20% of the time, people will have a very difficult, if not impossible, time making an impact with lifestyle choices alone. Eighty percent chance of success—those are good odds, but they are no guarantee. As I write this, I can see the faces of my patients who fit into this category. Even after trying so hard, they are left with a diagnosis of hypertension, atrial fibrillation, high cholesterol or even heart disease.

Disease processes are driven by two things: Genetic propensity and lifestyle. Yet, these two factors do not occur completely separately. Epigenetics is the study of the influence of lifestyle on gene expression, meaning how you choose to live can "turn on" genes that make certain conditions more likely, or can leave those genes "dormant" and unexpressed. But a perfect lifestyle cannot always keep those genes from expressing themselves, resulting in the occurrence of these risk factors and diseases. In most cases, you can prevent heart disease, but in some cases, even for those who try their hardest, the internal genetic makeup wins out.

Giving up on lifestyle improvements is certainly not the answer. For one thing, 80% is a promising statistic that makes a strong case for lifestyle intervention. This is true for everyone but especially for the genetically susceptible. For another, even when risk factors appear or disease surfaces, lifestyle changes can make a profound difference in how well someone weathers a health crisis. Getting high blood pressure, high cholesterol or heart disease is certainly no reason to give up on a healthy lifestyle—in fact, it is the best reason to ramp up your efforts because we know it improves outcomes.

One of my patients, who is in her early 50s, has spent years fighting her genetic code. Both hypertension and heart disease run in her family. She exercises five days a week and eats a mostly vegetarian, low-salt diet. She came to my office with a blood pressure cuff, a journal recording her blood pressure readings four times per day, and her diet plan. She explained to me that she had been making deliberate attempts to prevent hypertension because both her mother and father had high blood pressure and her mother had died of a heart attack. She was now postmenopausal, and showed me in her book the progressively increasing blood pressure readings she experienced over the past year.

What began in the 120s (120 is the highest "normal" systolic blood pressure reading) was creeping up into the 140s (140 or higher is considered significant high blood pressure) despite maintaining the same healthy diet and exercise routine. She was understandably frustrated and angry. She thought that doing everything she could would be enough and yet, in her case, she was going to need medication to intervene. But did I advise her to give up on her excellent lifestyle habits? Of course not! If she had not been doing those things, her numbers could have been even worse. And, although I can't prove it, she could have prevented herself from getting a heart attack already.

Even when medication is required, lifestyle choices could minimize your dosage requirements or the need for multiple drugs. Lifestyle can optimize your situation, even when your genetic susceptibilities aren't ideal.

Another patient with a history of atrial fibrillation was a runner and healthy eater. She came to my office due to her symptoms, except rather than being frustrated by her diagnosis, she just assumed that she would end up with the "family arrhythmia." Yet, this expectation did not make her give up on her efforts. After watching her father suffer a stroke, all she wanted was to live a healthy and stroke-free life. For her, that was reason enough to stay completely focused on being as healthy as she could be for the rest of her life. Her lifestyle very well may prevent a stroke like her father had, even if it has not prevented her atrial fibrillation.

In other words, lifestyle changes matter, whether you prevent disease or risk factors completely or you don't. Continue (or start!) your exercise program, keep choosing healthy foods in moderate portions and maintain or even increase your stress management efforts. Stay hydrated and get adequate sleep. Don't take supplements, herbal preparations or vitamins without reviewing the potential side effects with your doctor. Do all these things and I assure you that 80% of the time, you will be able to keep the cardiac risk factors and medical diagnoses in check. And if you can't, you will certainly minimize the risks you have and give yourself the best possible chance at success. You are in the driver's seat as you navigate your future. Just know that sometimes, in spite of all that you do, you might need treatment. You might need medication. And that is okay.

The last point I want to make is an important one: People sometimes believe that "succumbing" to medication means they have somehow failed. This is absolutely untrue, so don't let yourself be coerced into believing this potentially dangerous point of view. Medication does not mean that you have failed or have not tried hard enough! It simply means that you have to add one more useful intervention to your efforts to keep yourself on track. Trust your doctor if you are told that medication is important for you.

Meanwhile, continue to do everything you can to stay as healthy as you can and stay in touch with your doctor about your dosage requirements. Don't give up, get depressed or feel defeated.

Always remember: Genes are not destiny, and if you didn't do everything you were doing, things could be much worse! Stay the course and take care of yourself. You are worth every effort.

New AFib Guidelines: *Warfarin* Not the Best Drug?

Ijeoma A. Ekeruo, MD, assistant professor, department of internal medicine, division of cardiology, McGovern Medical School at UTHealth, Houston.

For more than 50 years, the gold standard drug to prevent stroke for patients with atrial fibrillation (AFib) has been *warfarin* (Coumadin). Now new guidelines for treating AFib bump that drug out of first place in favor of newer anticoagulants. If your doctor prescribed warfarin for your AFib, should you change medications? *Facts to consider...*

Warfarin works by blocking the effect of vitamin K, which is involved in the cascade of proteins called "clotting factors" that help blood to clot. Vitamin K levels fluctuate naturally, and consuming dietary sources—including leafy greens—also influences levels of the vitamin in the body. Since the effectiveness of warfarin depends on how much vitamin K is in the body, dosage of the drug has to be carefully monitored—too much can lead to bleeding, while too little doesn't protect against stroke. So patients need to have their blood levels of warfarin checked often and, if necessary, the dosage adjusted. And they need to keep dietary sources of vitamin K at a steady level.

Nonvitamin K Anticoagulants

Alternative anticoagulants known as direct oral anticoagulants (DOACs) block clotting factors without depending on vitamin K. There's no need for blood tests or dietary restrictions.

It would seem like a no-brainer to just switch patients over to these new medications. But without years of clinical trials attesting that they are safer and more effective than warfarin, doctors have been holding off. Now the American Heart Association has published updated guidelines for treating AFib that strongly recommend DOACs over warfarin, with some important qualifications. *According to the available research, all four DOACs are about equally effective for AFib, but with some differences to consider...*

- *Dabigatran* (**Pradaxa**). FDA-approved in 2010, the drug showed lower rates of stroke and systemic embolism compared with warfarin but had similar risks of bleeding. It can cause nausea or heartburn and is not recommended for patients with kidney problems. It is taken twice a day.

- *Rivaroxaban* (**Xarelto**). Approved in 2011, it's taken only once a day. Another plus is that there are established dosing recommendations for patients with compromised kidney function, although it's not advised for patients on dialysis or with severe renal dysfunction.

- *Apixaban* (**Eliquis**). Approved in 2012, it was shown to be superior to warfarin with regard to stroke and systemic embolism... and also caused less bleeding and resulted in lower mortality. While it, too, is not recommended for patients with severe kidney dysfunction, apixaban is the only DOAC recommended for patients with AFib on dialysis. It is taken twice a day.

- *Edoxaban* (**Savaysa**). Approved in 2015, edoxaban is unique among DOACs in that it can be used by patients who have some kidney damage and at a reduced dose by patients with more severe decreased kidney function. It is taken once daily and not recommended for patients on dialysis.

Important: The guidelines advise that patients with a heart valve problem stick with warfarin. There's not enough evidence to say that DOACs are safer or more effective for this condition.

Side Effects

When first introduced, there was concern about life-threatening bleeding from DOACs because there was no reversal drug as there is for warfarin. However, research finds the risk of bleeding from DOACs to be lower than with warfarin. Also, *idarucizumab*

(Praxbind) is now an approved antidote for dabigatran...Andexxa is approved for rivaroxaban and apixaban...and other reversal drugs are being developed. Still, bleeding is a serious concern when taking any anticoagulant. *Signs to watch for include...*

• **Unexpected bleeding,** such as from the gums, bladder/urine...or sudden swelling of the joints,

• **Unexplained bruising,**

• **Bloody or black and tarry stool.**

DOACs are very expensive, so check with your insurer regarding coverage before talking to your doctor about changing your prescription.

Aspirin for Heart Health

Christina C. Wee, MD, MPH, associate professor of medicine at Harvard Medical School and director of the Obesity Research Program in the Division of General Medicine at Beth Israel Deaconess Medical Center (BIDMC), both in Boston. She is also associate program director for the Internal Medicine Program at BIDMC and deputy editor of *Annals of Internal Medicine.*

Taking a daily low-dose (81-mg) aspirin has long been considered a bedrock therapy for people striving to prevent cardiovascular disease (including heart attack and stroke). The reasoning was simple. Aspirin interferes with the formation of blood clots that develop inside blood vessels and can lead to a heart attack or stroke.

Here's the rub: Interfering with blood clotting also can lead to harmful bleeding—especially from the stomach. So it's been a balancing act to identify the people who are most likely to get more help than harm from aspirin therapy.

Until recently, most studies found that the benefit of low-dose aspirin therapy outweighed the risk of bleeding for people with a history of cardiovascular disease (a past heart attack or stroke) and for those with risk factors such as elevated cholesterol, diabetes, high blood pressure or a strong family history of heart attack or stroke.

New thinking: As researchers have continued to investigate this widely used therapy, a more nuanced view of the individuals who can benefit from daily aspirin—and who is at risk of experiencing more harm than good—has emerged.

What you need to know about a more customized use of aspirin therapy...

How We Got Here

While aspirin therapy has been recommended for decades, the backdrop for its use in preventing cardiovascular disease has changed during that time. The risk of bleeding from aspirin has stayed about the same, but the risk for cardiovascular disease has been going down due to better treatment of key risk factors. Statin drugs have lowered cholesterol, and doctors have been doing a better job of treating diabetes and high blood pressure. Many people have stopped smoking, eliminating another major risk factor.

This means that the risk-benefit balance has shifted for people taking a daily low-dose aspirin to prevent a first heart attack or stroke (primary prevention). However, the therapy should still be used by those who have already had a heart attack or stroke.

This more customized view resulted from three landmark studies that came out in 2018, looking at primary prevention in adults with diabetes...adults at average risk for cardiovascular disease...and older adults. Taken together, these studies found few benefits compared with a consistent risk of bleeding.

Note: These studies do not apply to those with preexisting heart disease or stroke. The new studies prompted the American Heart Association (AHA) and the American College of Cardiology (ACC) to update their 2019 guidelines for aspirin therapy in primary prevention.

Why Is the Bleeding Risk So Concerning?

With daily aspirin therapy, the main risk for internal bleeding is from a peptic ulcer. These ulcers, which are more common as people age, occur in about one out of 10 people. Bleeding can lead to anemia and the need for hospitalization and blood transfusion if it's acute.

Back in 2015, AHA guidelines said it was reasonable to use aspirin for primary prevention in anyone with an increased risk for cardiovascular disease and without an increased risk of bleeding. The AHA and ACC now say that people ages 40 to 70 should take it only if they are at significant risk for a first heart attack or stroke, and they are not at increased risk of bleeding, due to such factors as use of blood-thinning medication and a history of peptic ulcer or kidney disease, which also increase bleeding risk. And people over age 70 are strongly discouraged against routine aspirin use for primary prevention.

The big takeaway is that you should not start daily aspirin therapy to prevent heart disease on your own. Unless your primary care doctor has ruled out bleeding after taking your medical history and has calculated that you are at high enough risk for cardiovascular disease, the risk of using aspirin therapy is greater than the reward.

What About People Already Taking Aspirin?

As the landscape for recommended aspirin use has changed, it's worth noting that a lot of Americans are now taking it outside the guidelines. A recent study by researchers at Beth Israel Deaconess Medical Center and Harvard Medical School analyzed health data from 2017 for more than 14,000 adults over age 40 to determine how many people in the US were taking a daily aspirin for primary prevention—and estimated the total number of aspirin users from this representative survey.

Based on the study's findings, published in *Annals of Internal Medicine*, an estimated 30 million Americans over age 40 with no history of heart disease or stroke were taking a daily aspirin. This included close to 10 million people over age 70. More than six million Americans were taking aspirin without a doctor's approval. Researchers also found that Americans with a history of peptic ulcer—putting them at increased risk of bleeding—were not significantly more likely to report reduced use of aspirin.

This research, along with the new guidelines, is a warning that millions of Americans are probably using daily aspirin contrary to the new guidelines and are subjecting themselves to more risk than benefit by doing so. The researchers urge doctors to ask their patients about aspirin use and counsel them about the risks and benefits.

What Should You Do?

If your doctor has told you to take a daily aspirin because you have cardiovascular disease (that is, you've had a heart attack or stroke or undergone bypass surgery or received a heart stent), the warning above does not apply to you. To be safe, have another discussion with your doctor to make sure his/her recommendation has not changed based on the new guidelines.

If you do not have cardiovascular disease and you have been taking a daily aspirin, here's what you need to do…

• **If you are over age 70,** talk to your doctor. You probably do not need to be on aspirin if you don't have preexisting heart disease or stroke.

• **If you are any age and you are taking aspirin for heart health without your doctor's approval,** talk to your doctor to find out if your risk outweighs your benefit.

• **If you are age 40 to 70 and have any bleeding risk,** but no cardiovascular disease, talk to your doctor. You probably need to stop aspirin.

Doctors are doing a better job of reducing heart attack and stroke risk factors. To help reduce your own risk factors, don't smoke… eat a heart-healthy diet…and get regular exercise. If you are at low-to-moderate risk for cardiovascular disease, adding a daily aspirin may no longer be worth the risk. Risk assessment is complex but typically includes your doctor's clinical evaluation based on a risk calculator such as the tool provided on the ACC's website. Go to ACC.org and search "risk estimator."

Note: These guidelines do not include recommendations for aspirin use to treat other conditions such as headache and fever and to help reduce risk for colon cancer in people who are at increased risk. Consult your doctor for advice on these uses.

Dog Owners Live Longer After a Heart Attack Than People Without Dogs

Compared with people who did not own a dog, dog owners had a 21% lower risk of dying after a heart attack and an 18% lower risk of dying after a stroke in an 11-year study.

Bonus: Dog owners living alone fared even better. They were about 30% less likely to die after a heart attack or stroke than non–dog owners living alone.

Tove Fall, VMD, PhD, professor of epidemiology, Uppsala University, Sweden.

Heart Patients: Block Out the Nighttime Light

Exposure to hospital light at night could harm recovering cardiac patients. Mice subjected to seven nights of even dim light after cardiac arrest had increases in mortality, compared with those that had no light disruption.

Theory: Nighttime light disruption upends our circadian rhythms, which in turn negatively impacts our immune systems and can lead to inflammation.

Self-defense: Since patients can't control hospital lighting, they should wear a sleep mask while there to block nighttime light.

Laura K. Fonken, PhD, assistant professor in the division of pharmacology and toxicology at University of Texas at Austin and lead author of the study published in *Experimental Neurology*.

Chapter 9

INFECTIOUS DISEASES

Strengthening the Gut Microbiome in the Era of COVID-19

At the time of writing this, COVID-19 has swept the globe, infecting millions of people worldwide and killing hundreds of thousands. While we've done plenty to mitigate our risk of infection—from practicing social distancing to perfecting personal hygiene to focusing on immune health—one factor may be overlooked by many: Bolstering the health of our gut microbiome to avoid an inflammatory storm.

Consider this: Some people infected with COVID-19 show no signs and some have only minor flu-like symptoms. Others who contract the novel coronavirus—people with conditions such as diabetes, hypertension, kidney disease or those at an advanced age—can have an acute systemic inflammatory response that may result in death. And others still, including people between the ages of 20 and 60 who become infected but have no known underlying medical conditions, "develop serious illness requiring intensive care treatment," the Lippincott

Nursing Center reports. What dictates the severity of responses?

One theory that's currently being investigated is the concept of an inflammatory or cytokine storm—in short, an excessive immune response to potential danger. As medical experts at NPR report, "Now doctors and researchers are increasingly convinced that, in some cases at least, the cause is the body's own immune system overreacting to the virus. The problem, known broadly as a 'cytokine storm,' can happen when the immune system triggers a runaway response that causes more damage to its own cells than to the invader it's trying to fight." And this surge in an immune response can lead to the fatal shutdown of multiple organs.

As you may know, your immune system is your body's natural defense system against infection and illness, and includes two main parts that work in concert with each other—your innate immune system (which you are born with) and your adaptive immune system (which, as John Hopkins Medicine

Laurie Steelsmith, ND, LAc, licensed naturopathic physician and acupuncturist in private practice in Honolulu. She writes Bottom Line's "Natural Healing Secrets for Women" blog and is coauthor of three books—*Natural Choices for Women's Health, Great Sex, Naturally* and her latest, *Growing Younger Every Day*. DrSteelsmith.com

puts it, "you develop when your body is exposed to microbes or chemicals released by microbes"). Other than your nervous system, your immune system is the most intricate network in your body, working tirelessly at patrolling for invaders. But when it goes into overdrive in an attempt to keep you healthy, it can get stuck doing so—failing to shut off and sending off the alarm long after it's needed.

This occurs in your innate immune system, which holds a multi-protein complex, known as the NLRP3 inflammasome, that instigates an inflammatory form of cell death and triggers the release of proinflammatory cytokines. While researchers are still learning more about this phenomenon, it's believed that this happens when the immune system encounters a new pathogenic trespasser, which then causes cytokines to surge—and we all know now that COVID-19 is heretofore unknown. (Indeed, cytokine storms are thought to explain the devastating effects of the 1918 Spanish flu pandemic.)

So how can you do all that you can to help your body have a proper immune response to infections, rather than an extreme, possibly deleterious reaction? Part of this may rest in the health of your gut microbiome.

Your gut microbiome—the community of bacteria that lives in your gut—plays a vital role in a number of functions, including your mood, the amount of energy you derive from your diet and, yes, your immune system. At the same time, your immune system and the gut work in a symbiotic relationship, moderating one another and working to support each other—an interaction that's underscored by the fact that, according to *Cellular and Molecular Immunology*, 70% to 80% of the body's immune cells are contained in the gut.

To build and maintain this healthy crosstalk, it's important to first think of your GI tract as a system as intricate as a rainforest, with a multifaceted system of life. It's been adapted to accommodate a wide range of microbes, and to upset its delicate balance may lead to a host of health problems, including an exaggerated response to an invader.

This internal ecological system is influenced by the way you live your life and the decisions you make on a daily basis. What you eat, how often you move, the quality of your sleep, your external environment, your emotions and moods, the medications you take, your social life—all can contribute to your gut health. While several factors can impact your gut health and influence a decreased or dysregulated immune system—including nutrient deficiency (such as a zinc deficiency, as seen in those with pyrrole disorder, as well as those who eat diets low in antioxidant-rich fruits and vegetables), stress, insulin resistance, food allergies and intolerances (which can create systemic inflammatory effects, impact the intestines and contribute to irritable bowel syndrome), over-the-counter medications such as antacids and NSAIDs, toxin exposure (to, say, heavy metals, pesticides and prescription medication) and genetics—you can take your gut health into your own hands.

Given that it's your gut we're talking about, it makes sense that its health is to a large part dependent on your diet. In fact, the single most important factor for a strong microbiome is what you eat. A microbiome in equilibrium is full of bacteria that produce specific short-chain fatty acids that positively affect wellness. These include acetate, propionate and, especially, butyrate—highly biologically active compounds that promote gut health, blood sugar regulation, optimal blood fat levels, appetite control and immunity. This friendly flora needs nourishment, which can then have a huge impact in shifting the inflammatory cascade. *In addition to a healthy diet, rich in organic food, here are a few foods to nurture it right…*

Green Tea

EGCG—the chief catechin in green tea—has been linked to a variety of health benefits. Functioning as a powerful antioxidant, it not only protects cells from oxidative damage but also encourages gut health. A 2019 review of studies and trials published by *Nutrients* found that green tea consumption resulted in the reduction of Firmicutes (an unfriendly bacteria) and improved levels of Bacteroidetes (a friendly bacteria)—changes, the authors say, that could help prevent gut dysbiosis (microbial imbalance). Green tea can also inhibit NLRP3 inflammasome activity and increase Nrf2 (which decreases inflammation). What's more, a randomized control study out of Japan on 200 healthcare workers showed the incidence of influenza was lower in the group that took 378 mg of green tea catechins and 210 mg of the amino acid L-theanine per day. The amount of EGCG in each cup of tea depends on the quality of the tea. Some resources suggest 50 mg to 100 mg, and others as high as 180 mg.

Pomegranate

Also rich in antioxidants, pomegranate can have a positive impact on gut flora by acting as a prebiotic—compounds that help "good" bacteria flourish in the intestines. A 2015 study published in *Anaerobe* reveals that pomegranate extract and pomegranate juice increased the mean counts of Bifidobacterium and Lactobacillus (friendly bacteria) and inhibited unfriendly bacteria such as the B. fragilis group. Another study in *Anaerobe* found that pomegranate stimulates the growth of a bacteria known as Akkermansia Muciniphila—an intestinal bacteria superstar that supports microbiome health and offers protection from disease.

To boost your own intestinal health, you can drink eight ounces of pomegranate juice daily or take it as a supplement, 400 mg to 800 mg a day.

Note: Check with your doctor before making pomegranate a regular part of your diet. Pomegranate can lower blood pressure so if you are on a bp-lowering medication, your blood pressure could become too low if you drink a lot of pomegranate juice. Pomegranate may also interfere with some medications.

Broccoli Sprouts

Broccoli sprouts—small, immature seedlings of the broccoli you typically eat—contain sulforaphane, a sulfur-rich compound, found in cruciferous vegetables, that has been shown to have immune-enhancing benefits, and inhibit multiple inflammasomes that cause cytokine storms (one of which is the aforementioned multi-protein complex known as the NLRP3 inflammasome). Use them in lieu of lettuce or bean sprouts in a sandwich, on top of your avocado toast, in a salad or as a soup topper. They have a spicy, almost radish-like, flavor so don't put them in your smoothie. And they are very easy to grow on a counter at home.

Turmeric

One of the boons of turmeric—or, more specifically, the phytochemical curcumin that's found in it—is that it operates as an anti-inflammatory. Used in Ayurvedic medicine as a digestive healing agent, it began being recommended as treatment for acid reflux, flatulence and functional dyspepsia by the World Health Organization in 1999. What's more, it works synergistically with EGCG, vitamin C and quercetin to stimulate the production of immune-boosting enzymes. To have more turmeric in your diet, enjoy eating curries, add it to smoothies or make "golden milk."

Walnuts

Eating a handful of walnuts per day—roughly 16 walnut halves—boosts the bacteria species that generates butyrate, thus changing the microbiome for the better. Other nuts that encourage a healthy microbiome include pecans, almonds, cashews, pistachios and hazelnuts.

Foods Rich in Quercetin

Quercetin is one of the most abundant antioxidants in many grains, fruits and vegetables (it also gives some of these their pigment) and naturally supports your ability to ward off free radical damage. It also increases gut microbial diversity, which protects your gut and immune health. While quercetin supplements are available, you can up your intake of it through the consumption of foods with a high quercetin content, such as apples, onions, grapes, broccoli, berries, cherries, citrus fruits and capers. Other options include tea (black and green), red wine, spinach, kale, buckwheat and olive oil.

Prebiotic and Probiotic Foods

Prebiotics—a type of fiber the human body cannot digest—work as food for probiotics, microorganisms that help the body cultivate and maintain a healthy colony of bacteria. Prebiotics are present in many high-fiber foods, including Jerusalem artichokes, garlic, onions, leeks, barley, banana and flaxseeds. Foods rich in probiotics, meanwhile, include yogurt, kefir, miso, tempeh, Kombucha and fermented foods such as sauerkraut and kimchee.

Eat your way towards an effectual immune response? Absolutely.

For updates on COVID-19, check the CDC site (CDC.gov/coronavirus).

How to Kill the New Coronavirus: When You're Home…When You're Out

Charles Gerba, PhD, a professor of microbiology and immunology and environmental science at University of Arizona College of Agriculture and Life Sciences, Tucson, Arizona. He is coauthor of *The Germ Freak's Guide to Outwitting Colds and Flu.*

It's hard not to get hysterical about the spread of the coronavirus. It's a novel virus—which means it's never been seen before—and the illness it causes, COVID-19, can be serious for people over 60 as well as those with underlying health conditions, especially diabetes, heart disease and respiratory illnesses like asthma, bronchitis and emphysema.

Because this coronavirus is so new, we don't have much data on it. We do know about other coronaviruses—including the one that causes SARS and the ones that cause many colds in the US every year—so we're presuming this coronavirus acts in similar ways. Based on these assumptions, there are things you can do to protect yourself from getting sick, both at home and when you're out and about.

At Home

Like the common cold and influenza virus, COVID-19 can survive very well in cool, dry temperatures—anywhere from a few hours to nine days, depending on the temperature and location.

COVID-19 enters your body when you touch a surface where the germ is living and then touch your nose, eyes or mouth. That's why not touching your face and washing your hands often is crucial. So is killing the virus to stop its spread. *Here's how…*

• **Clean high-traffic surfaces at least daily.** These include counters, desks, tabletops, phones, computer keyboards and mouse, tablets, television remote controls and your bedside table. You should also swab down the bathroom and kitchen sink, bathroom fixtures and the toilet. If someone in your house is sick with COVID-19, clean these areas two or three times a day.

• **Use a disinfectant wipe when you clean.** You want to concentrate on smooth, nonporous surfaces. The easiest way to clean these surfaces is to use a wipe that contains quaternary ammonium compounds (quat), which is found in most disinfecting wipes, such as from Clorox and Lysol. Why wipes? Because you are more likely to let the disinfectant dry naturally after you use one, which gives it time to kill the virus. Sure, you can use a quat-based spray on surfaces, but you have to wait about 10 minutes before you wipe it dry. Avoid white vinegar sprays for now because we don't know if it's effective against this virus.

• **Don't worry too much about soft surfaces.** Blankets, sheets, carpets, someone's jacket—it's harder for a virus to transfer to your fingers from these types of surfaces. Pillowcases could be a concern, although there is no data on this. You could change them nightly to be safe. Also, don't worry about mail and packages being contaminated even if the mail carrier is sick and doesn't know it yet.There is low transfer of virus from paper to the hands because paper is porous and absorbs a lot of the fluid the virus may be suspended in.

• **Use liquid soaps.** That way, when you and your family members wash hands, you're not contaminating each other.

• **Put a bottle of hand sanitizer next to entrances.** We have done studies on virus contamination of surfaces in homes, and once-a-day use of hand sanitizer seems to be enough to break the movement of viruses around the household. Place hand sanitizer near the front door, and ask everyone to use it when they come inside so no one brings viruses into the household. Even better, have everyone wash their hands thoroughly as soon as they come into the home. Don't rely on an air purifier to kill the virus. It won't unless it has a HEPA filter.

• **It is not necessary to shower as soon as you get home since it is largely your hands that spread the virus.** But if you are taking care of an ill person with coronavirus, change and wash your clothes every day.

When You're Out

It takes, on average, five days for people infected with COVID-19 to show symptoms, according to researchers from Johns Hopkins. So even if people aren't coughing and sneezing, they still could be passing on the virus. *Besides staying away from crowds and washing your hands as soon as you get home, here's how best to stay healthy…*

• **Always have a bottle of hand sanitizer in your purse or pocket.** Use one that contains 60% to 70% alcohol, and squirt it on your hands often—when you get off the bus, when you leave the grocery store, when you walk out of a public restroom. Keep one in your car, too.

• **Take extra care at the store.** Some areas that might contain more COVID-19, at least based on studies done on viruses that cause colds—self-checkout counters and serving spoons at the prepared food stations. Apply hand sanitizer after using those. Consider going to the supermarket at off hours to minimize exposure to other people.

• **Swab down your car—especially if you've driven a sick person to the doctor or your children/grandchildren anywhere.** A car isn't a particularly germy place if you're the only person in it. But it can become a virus magnet once children or sick people go for a ride. Use disinfecting wipes to clean the often-touched areas—steering wheel, controls, armrests, door handles and the child/baby seat if there's one.

• **Don't go too crazy.** You don't have to wipe down the seat at the theater or on the train or in an Uber or taxicab—this virus isn't butt-borne. And you don't have to wear gloves so you don't touch the gas pump, door handles or elevator buttons with your bare hands. You could carry along tissues and use those, but honestly, if you squirt some hand sanitizer afterward and try not to touch your face you should be OK.

Incubation Period for New Coronavirus Determined

Once a person is exposed to the virus, symptoms of COVID-19 begin after a median of 5.1 days, according to an analysis of 181 cases. The study found that 97.5% of people who develop symptoms of COVID-19 do so within 11.5 days, which supports the 14-day quarantine or active-monitoring period being used for people at high risk. Strains of coronaviruses that cause the common cold have a mean incubation period of about three days…while the median incubation period for influenza A is 1.4 days, and 0.6 days for influenza B.

Justin Lessler, PhD, associate professor of epidemiology, The Johns Hopkins Bloomberg School of Public Health, Baltimore.

For the Cleanest Hands—Sing This!

Nisha Thampi, MD, assistant professor of pediatrics and pediatric infectious diseases consultant, University of Ottawa, medical director of the infection prevention and control program, division of infectious diseases, department of pediatrics, CHEO (formerly Children's Hospital of Eastern Ontario).

With new infectious diseases threatening our health daily—such as SARS, MERS, the new coronavirus—frequent handwashing is more important than ever. Unfortunately, not everyone has this healthy hygiene habit…and few wash their hands as thoroughly as needed. Here's an easy, fun, musical way to make sure you're getting rid of all the germs, literally "out of the mouth of babes!"

Hands are arguably the most common way to transmit germs, according to the World Health Organization (WHO). Children are especially significant spreaders of germs. For one thing, they have not learned hygiene habits that adults (hopefully) practice, such as coughing into the elbow.

About 10 years ago, the WHO came up with a six-step hand-washing procedure that is practical and effectively reduces germs that cause infectious diseases. Studies find that when children practice handwashing correctly, it reduces upper-respiratory and gastrointestinal infections and also cuts down on number of days lost from school.

Bonus: Learning the WHO method as a child will hopefully become ingrained and practiced automatically in adulthood for even longer-term germ reduction benefits!

However, it's hard to get kids to remember all the steps…and to do them for the 30 seconds necessary to effectively get rid of the germs. Nisha Thampi, MD, at CHEO, a pediatric academic health center in Ottawa, Canada, and her "research assistant" eight-year old daughter came up with a brilliant—and fun!—solution. Their research was published in *BMJ*.

Solution: Since learning through memorization of songs and lyrics is a proven way to teach children, the research team created lyrics to a familiar children's folk tune as a mnemonic that would be easy for children to learn. They used the French children's folk tune, "Frère Jacques" ("Brother John" in English). To test the effectiveness of their method, the researchers applied fluorescent markings to their hands before washing.

Results: After washing while singing the song and performing the steps, the markings were notably decreased on the palms, back of the hands and fingertips compared with washing hands without following the six steps. To further explore how easy the song is to teach to young children, Dr. Thampi's daughter taught the song to her four-year-old brother.

Dr. Thampi is working on a larger study to examine the impact of the song on handwashing behaviors among preschool-aged children in Ottawa, Canada, with the hope of having it incorporated into future public health campaigns in schools. She also has received requests to translate the song into other languages.

Ready to learn—and teach—the handwashing song? You probably already know the tune, but here are instructional lyrics:

Lyrics—and instructions:

Scrub your palms

between the fingers.

Wash the back! (wash back of one hand)

Wash the back! (wash back of other hand)

Twirl the tips around, (scrub fingertips of one hand into palm of other hand)

Scrub then upside down. (scrub fingertips of other hand into opposite palm)

Thumb attack! (scrub one thumb)

Thumb attack! (scrub other thumb)

Note: If soap and water aren't handy, Dr. Thampi recommends using an alcohol-based hand sanitizer and doing the six steps until hands are completely dry.

Stay Healthy When You Fly

Philip M. Tierno, Jr., PhD, clinical professor of microbiology and pathology at New York University Langone Medical Center. He is author of *The Secret Life of Germs: Observations* and *Lessons from a Microbe Hunter.* Med.NYU.edu

As the country opens up to travel, more people are flying. Airline passengers spend hours stuck in a small space with fellow travelers, breathing the same air and touching the same surfaces—surfaces that might not get cleaned well or often. And their body's natural defenses against germs are compromised by the environmental conditions on planes. Beyond a pandemic and other germs, the shrinking airline seats, when combined with lack of movement, can lead to other serious health issues as well.

Luckily, there are ways to protect yourself, particularly on longer flights…

•**Stay hydrated.** You need moist mucous membranes to create a line of defense against germs that are inhaled. The air in airplane cabins is very dry—often only about 20% humidity or less. Healthful levels should be closer to 40%. Low humidity dries out the mucous membranes in passengers' noses and throats, limiting their ability to shield them from germs in the air they breathe. Drink four to eight ounces of fluid—preferably water—per hour. Avoid alcoholic beverages that can dehydrate the body.

Warning: Water is, of course, an excellent beverage for hydration—but consume bottled water, not water from the plane's bathroom tap, which can be contaminated with germs.

•**Turn your air vent on, but don't point it at your face.** In past decades, the standard advice was to leave the air vent above airline seats turned off—it blew air that could contain germs from passengers seated throughout the plane. That risk has been greatly reduced because commercial aircraft now have very effective air-filtration systems. In fact, breathing filtered air blowing from the vent above your seat could reduce your exposure to germs from a sick passenger seated near you. Still, filtration systems are not perfect, and this blowing air could further dry out your mucous membranes, so a prudent compromise is to turn your vent on but not aim its stream of air directly into your face.

•**Find the healthiest seat.** What's the healthiest seat on the plane? People often ask whether aisle seats or window seats are the better choice from a health perspective. The answer is, it's a trade-off—aisle seats make it easier to get up and move around, avoiding blood clot risk…but window seats mean that you have fewer passengers seated near you, decreasing the odds that you'll be near someone who is contagious.

Also: Politely ask a flight attendant if you can switch seats if someone near you on the plane is repeatedly sneezing or coughing. Passengers within three seats to the front or sides of someone who is contagious—or within one to two seats behind such a person—face much higher infection risks than passengers seated elsewhere on the plane.

•**Don't forget your mask.** Be sure to wear your mask, especially if you are seated near someone who is coughing or sneezing and you cannot switch seats, perhaps because the flight is full. At-risk or elderly passengers should wear a mask even if no one around them appears to be sick. Not all contagious people show obvious signs of an illness.

•**Get up and move every hour or two.** Stroll up the aisle and back or at least stand and stretch. Spending long hours stuck in a cramped airline seat isn't just uncomfortable…it can lead to a potentially fatal blood-clot condition called deep vein thrombosis—even in travelers who have no history of circulatory problems. If it isn't possible to move around because the "fasten seat belts" sign remains on, at least flex and stretch the muscles of your legs, feet and toes and do some shoulder rolls.

Note: Qantas, which plans to start running the world's longest flight—from Sydney to London in 23 hours, 40 minutes—has created a video to help passengers benefit from easy-to-do inflight exercises. Go to YouTube/Gv7enzI7Yq8.

•**Wear eyeglasses rather than contact lenses.** The low humidity on airplanes can dry out your eyes, creating discomfort for contact lens wearers. If you must wear contacts on a flight, apply eyedrops periodically to keep your eyes moist.

•**Hand sanitizer and/or sanitizing wipes reminders.** Everyone should know by now to carry and use hand sanitizer during flights immediately before eating, drinking, removing contact lenses or doing anything else that involves touching your eyes or face on flights. At this writing, the TSA allows passengers to bring up to 12 ounces of hand sanitizer aboard (check with the airline beforehand). Or bring a three-ounce bottle of 60% or higher rubbing alcohol and paper towels. Use a quarter-size drop for each hand cleaning—most people don't use enough. Also wipe down the seat-back tray table before using it—these are rarely cleaned by airlines and could be contaminated with germs from passengers on prior flights.

•**Washing your hands thoroughly with soap and water ordinarily is as effective as using hand sanitizers or sanitizing wipes, but hand washing can be problematic on commercial aircraft.** It sometimes isn't possible to get to the bathroom to wash your hands immediately before eating or drinking—the food cart might block your path… the handles of airplane bathroom doors and soap dispensers are themselves often contaminated with germs…and sometimes there are germs in planes' tap-water reservoirs. Always wash your hands thoroughly as soon as you deplane.

Don't Touch That Pen!

At the hospital or a doctor's office, use your own pen—not theirs—to fill in forms. Writing implements in medical settings harbor vast amounts of germs.

Miryam Z. Wahrman, PhD, professor of biology at William Paterson University, Wayne, New Jersey, and author of The Hand Book: Surviving in a Germ-Filled World.

Lower Risk for COVID-19 Naturally

Zinc and glycyrrhizin (from licorice root) may reduce risk for coronavirus. In studies on 2003 SARS coronavirus, zinc killed the virus on contact. Sucking a zinc lozenge when in crowds may offer some protection. Drinking licorice tea each morning and taking vitamins A, C, D, E, zinc and elderberry (available in a combination called ViraPro) makes your body less hospitable to viruses—another line of defense.

Jacob Teitelbaum, MD, Hawaii-based holistic physician and author of numerous books including the newly updated Real Cause, Real Cure *(BottomLineStore.com). Vitality101.com*

Flu Mystery Solved

Why is the flu so easily transmitted during winter? There have been many theories, but research now says that low humidity plays a key role because of its effects on immunity. In lab studies performed on mice, low humidity impaired the animals' ability to repair viral damage.

Proceedings of the National Academy of Sciences

5 Smart Ways to Avoid Germs at the Gym

Bryan Combs, PhD, CRNP, a nurse practitioner and assistant professor of nursing at the University of Alabama at Birmingham School of Nursing. His research has been published in *Orthopedic Nursing, Workplace Health and Safety* and other leading professional journals.

Hopefully as you read this, after massive closures due to the coronavirus, gyms and fitness centers are open and in full swing to meet your workout needs. A trip to the gym is supposed to improve your health. So why do so many people get sick after hitting the treadmill, pumping some iron or sweating their way through spin class?

No matter how clean your gym looks, there's a good chance that it is crawling with microbes ranging from garden-variety cold and flu viruses to the infamous fungi that lead to athlete's foot and a host of bacteria such as staphylococcus (more commonly known as "staph") and *Escherichia coli* (E. Coli).

Interestingly, many people assume that winter is the worst time of year for germy gyms—and certain pathogens, such as the infamous coronavirus, are more likely to be hanging around during that time. But the truth is, gyms are a hotbed of icky microbes year-round.

That doesn't mean you should sacrifice the health benefits of regularly working out at your local gym or fitness center. Just be sure to follow these five steps to avoid picking up a nasty bug from the germiest places at the gym.

***STEP #1:* Wipe down gym equipment before using it.** Whether it's an elliptical machine, stationary bicycle, weight machine or free weights, never assume that it was cleaned by the previous user. Any piece of gym equipment that a person can touch could be teeming with germs. Don't believe it?

Consider this: When researchers took 288 samples at 16 fitness facilities in Ohio, S. aureus bacteria, which causes everything from skin infections to pneumonia, were found in the greatest concentrations on the following equipment—half of treadmill handles ...56% of weight plates...and 63% of medicine balls, according to a 2019 study published in *BMC Infectious Diseases*.

What to do: To protect yourself, always use a disinfectant spray or towelette to clean any piece of exercise equipment before you touch it. And, of course, be a sport and do that for the next person.

Helpful: If the gym doesn't keep a disinfectant spray or wipes on hand, bring along a travel-sized antibacterial hand sanitizer to apply to your hands between machines and/or a time or two during your workout.

***STEP #2:* Beware of gym towels.** When your face is dripping with sweat, it's handy to grab one of those towels that your gym may have on hand for a quick dry-off. Think twice before doing this. You probably assume that those towels are germ-free because they are freshly laundered, but that may not be the case.

"While the towels have been washed, a lot of gyms use the same container to carry dirty towels to the washing area and to bring clean towels back, so they can become contaminated again," explains Bryan Combs, PhD, CRNP, a nurse practitioner and nursing instructor at the University of Alabama at Birmingham School of Nursing.

What to do: To be safe, bring your own clean towel...and make sure you wash it after each workout.

***STEP #3:* Don't go barefoot.** By now, everyone knows that you need to wear flip-flops or some other waterproof shoes in the shower. But don't get careless and walk barefoot in the locker rooms either. Both are ideal places to pick up athlete's foot or even a methicillin-resistant *Staphylococcus aureus* (MRSA) infection, which can spread by skin contact.

What to do: Wear shoes in the shower—and the locker room. You can buy a pair of shower shoes for less than $20 online and in stores.

STEP #4: Watch that water bottle. Staying hydrated is good for you, but an unwashed water bottle can make you sick. That's because it's common for people to use the same water bottle each time they go to the gym. But how often do they wash the outside, which may be covered with bacteria or viruses? Most likely, not very often.

What to do: Wash the outside of your water bottle with dish soap and hot water after every workout. It's also a good idea to rinse the inside with hot water—just as you would any drinking glass.

STEP #5: Don't forget about your gym bag. Surprisingly, your own gym bag may carry the most bacteria.

Here's why: Your gym bag does double duty, carrying your clean clothes to the gym and your dirty, smelly ones back home. It probably also holds your sweaty shoes. But do you ever clean your gym bag? Probably not.

What to do: To prevent the spread of germs, opt for a plastic or vinyl gym bag and clean the inside and outside with a disinfectant spray after each use, if possible, or at least a few times a week if you're a frequent gymgoer. As an alternative, choose a cloth bag that you can wash in hot water and bleach at least once a week and then dry in a hot drier.

Pneumonia Rx Danger

Two-thirds of pneumonia patients receive antibiotics for longer than necessary when discharged from hospitals. The median prescription was two days longer than needed. Excessive antibiotic use increases the risk for antibiotic resistance, infections and—in the case of fluoroquinolones—torn tendons, ruptured arteries and suicidal thoughts. If an antibiotic prescription following hospitalization for pneumonia extends more than five days total (seven days for those with severe issues beyond pneumonia), ask why.

Valerie Vaughn, MD, MSc, an assistant professor at VA Ann Arbor Healthcare System and University of Michigan Medical School. UofMHealth.org

Healthier Behind the Wheel

The luxury carmaker Jaguar announced that new models might incorporate a type of ultraviolet light that sterilizes air and surfaces and could reduce dangerous "superbugs." The car company is considering this among other "well-being" features.

USA Today

Tiny But Deadly

Mosquitoes are humans' deadliest enemies. The diseases they carry may have killed almost half the 108 billion human beings who have ever lived.

Roundup of experts on mosquito-borne disease, reported in *Nature*.

The Natural Way to Boost Your Immune System When the Grandkids Come to Visit

Jamison Starbuck, ND, a naturopathic physician in family practice in Missoula, Montana, and producer of *Dr. Starbuck's Health Tips for Kids*, a weekly program on Montana Public Radio, MTPR.org. She is a past president of the American Association of Naturopathic Physicians and a contributing editor to *The Alternative Advisor: The Complete Guide to Natural Therapies and Alternative Treatments*. DrJamison Starbuck.com

Not long ago, my patient Kathy guiltily admitted that she sometimes dreads visits from her grandchildren—when the kids leave, her husband is exhausted and she ends up in bed, sick with a cold or bad sore throat. Kathy's situation is not unusual. Parents, grandparents and all adults who

Keeping Your Hands Clean in the Hospital

Ask for Hand Sanitizer in the Hospital

Hospital hand sanitizers are used less often than they should be because they cannot be placed close to patients. Fire marshals require sanitizer dispensers to be removed altogether or located far from patients' bedsides because hand sanitizers contain at least 60% alcohol and are flammable. Fire regulations also limit how much hand sanitizer can be kept on site.

Result: Sanitizer dispensers usually are in hallways—but greater use of sanitizers closer to patients could be more effective at germ control. In one study, 50% more hand sanitizer was used when the product was hung over patients' beds on a trapeze-bar construct.

The New York Times

Hospital Patient Handwashing Alert

Early in their hospital stay, 14% of patients had so-called "superbug" antibiotic-resistant bacteria on their hands, according to a study of nearly 400 hospital patients. Nearly one-third of commonly touched objects in their rooms, such as the nurse call button, were also positive for methicillin-resistant Staphylococcus aureus (MRSA) or other types of bacteria that can lead to deadly infection.

If you are in the hospital: Wash your hands frequently with soap and water (the preferred method) or waterless hand sanitizer.

Lona Mody, MD, associate division chief, Geriatric & Palliative Care Medicine, University of Michigan Medical School, Ann Arbor.

share close quarters, hugs and kisses and frequent meals with little ones often find that their immune systems are unable to defend against the onslaught of contagious ailments that kids carry around.

Here's what I suggest to help my patients strengthen their immune systems...*

• **Don't forget the basics of healthy eating and hydration.** When you're busy with childcare, it's easy to fill up on quick "kid" snacks and forgo healthy meals...and many grandparents and parents forget to hydrate sufficiently. Make sure to nourish yourself (and your little ones) with healthy food, such as plenty of fruits and vegetables, lean meat, beans and whole grains, and to hydrate well—water is always best. Aim to drink half your body weight in ounces daily.

• **Take antioxidants daily.** *A common regimen:* 1,000 mg of vitamin C...400 international units (IU) of vitamin E...and 10,000 IU of vitamin A.

Note: It's beneficial to take these antioxidants all the time, not just when around young kids.

Additional help: The week before your grandkids come to visit, or at the first sign of a child getting ill, start taking an immune-boosting herbal tincture. I particularly like a combined formula of astragalus, ligusticum, lomatium and elder. However, if you can't find a combo formula, taking just two or three of the four herbs is beneficial. Take 60 drops of a combined tincture in two ounces of water, twice daily, in between meals. Continue to take the tincture throughout the child's visit, or his/her illness, and for three days afterward.

• **Get good sleep!** This can be hard to do with the excitement of visitors or when the kids are sick. A safe, non–habit-forming natural sleep aid is the amino acid L-tryptophan. You may already know that tryptophan is abundant in turkey and thought to be responsible for that sleepy feeling after the Thanksgiving meal. Tryptophan promotes

*Before taking any supplement or herbal remedy, check with your doctor.

the production of serotonin, a neurotransmitter that facilitates relaxation. Take 500 mg of L-tryptophan at bedtime, with water, away from food.

• **Manage your stress.** Caring for kids can be fulfilling and lots of fun, but it can also cause impatience, confusion, irritability and self-criticism. This emotional stress takes a toll on the immune system. Another amino acid, gamma-aminobutyric acid (GABA), can help manage these strong emotions. Take 200 mg of GABA up to four times a day, as needed, for emotional stress.

Kathy followed my plan and six months later happily reported back that she was no longer getting sick after her grandkids came to stay. She had convinced her husband to do the protocol as well, and except for the very messy house after the kids depart, they both now thoroughly look forward to visits with the grandchildren!

Common Flu-Shot Side Effects

Soreness or aching in your arm usually lasts a day and indicates that your immune system is responding properly to the shot. Redness, pain or swelling at the injection site may last a few days—this too shows that your immune system has been activated. Low-grade fever is possible but uncommon—if the fever is above 101°F, you are probably sick with a virus different from the flu virus. Nausea, headaches or fatigue occasionally occur.

Caution: Severe allergic reactions to flu shots or their components are rare but do occur. Anyone who develops breathing trouble, wheezing, hives, high fever, swelling around the eyes or lips, or a fast heartbeat should get to a doctor or emergency room quickly.

Centers for Disease Control and Prevention, Atlanta.

Legionnaires' Disease Is on the Rise

Theresa Rowe, DO, assistant professor of geriatrics at Northwestern University Feinberg School of Medicine, Chicago.

During the summer, risk of the respiratory infection Legionnaires' disease rises, thanks to high temperatures and moisture. Cases of this virulent and sometimes deadly bacterial infection are growing—the rate of reported cases has grown by almost nine times since 2000. Why? For one thing, an aging population is more susceptible due to weakened immune systems. The bacteria usually are transmitted by breathing in water droplets from a water source that isn't properly maintained—such as the plumbing and HVAC systems in a hotel, cruise ship, hospital or nursing home.

Protect Yourself at Home...

• **Keep the hot-water-temperature dial set no lower than 120°F**—high enough to prevent bacterial growth and low enough to prevent scalding.

• **Don't shut off water heaters when you go for extended trips.** The water can stagnate and grow bacteria.

• **Change the water in your hot tub every three months or more often if heavily used.** Follow the manufacturer's instructions regarding filter changes and use of chemical treatments.

Protect Yourself on the Road...

Responsibility for a facility's plumbing and HVAC system is out of your hands, but there are ways to protect yourself...

• **Contact *Passport Health* for news of outbreaks in the region you're thinking of visiting.** Consider an itinerary change if necessary.

• **Check for signs of rust, dirt or slime in public showers.** If noted, tell management and do not use them.

• **If you plan to swim,** pack pool test strips to make sure that the levels of chlorine, bromine and pH are in the safe range before you take a dip.

• **Symptoms of Legionnaires' disease mimic flu—fever, cough, muscle pain, shortness of breath, confusion and nausea.** Don't ignore symptoms, especially if you've spent time in a large public facility within the 10 days prior to becoming ill. It requires treatment with specific antibiotics.

Power Soup That Helps Boost Immunity

Jackie Newgent, RDN, CDN, a registered dietitian, classically trained chef and author of several cookbooks, including *The Clean & Simple Diabetes Cookbook.* Check out her plant-based recipes on her blog at JackieNewgent.com.

If there's ever been a time when you need a well-functioning immune system, it's now. And the first place to start strengthening your immune system is with the foods you eat. Immune-boosting foods protect us in several ways—they provide antioxidants and reduce inflammation in the body…they stimulate the immune system to do its job…and they help to fight infection. We asked Jackie Newgent, RDN, CDN, a nutritionist and classically trained chef known for creating delicious healthy dishes, to come up with a list of 10 of her favorite foods that help boost immunity. Her list includes a bit of everything—from spices and protein-packed picks to vegetables and even tea.

Best of all: These foods can be eaten separately…or together in a delicious soup that helps boost immunity. The recipe is below!

10 Immune-Boosting Foods

Find out how these 10 super-germ-fighting foods do their job…

• **Lentils provide a significant amount of iron.** Getting iron from the food you eat can help your body fight fatigue.

• **Garlic and onion both contain compounds called allyl sulfides,** which work to protect immune function.

• **Mushrooms contain a naturally occurring compound called lentinan,** which stimulates immune function. They also contain a significant amount of zinc, a nutrient that also can help the immune system. Studies suggest that the white button mushroom, in particular, can help the body fight viruses.

• **Spinach is an amazing source of folate.** This nutrient can help increase the body's ability to fight infection.

• **Sweet potatoes are rich in beta-carotene,** a carotenoid that has a positive effect on immune cell function.

• **Tomatoes get their red pigment from the phytonutrient lycopene.** Regular consumption of tomatoes has been associated with enhanced immunity due to lycopene's role in immune cell function.

• **Yogurt that contains probiotics from live friendly bacteria helps to improve your body's immune response**—and protect you from infection. When choosing yogurt, read the label carefully. Look for brands that ideally contain at least two probiotic types and no added sugars, including high-fructose corn syrup.

• **Green tea is loaded with flavonoids that have powerful antioxidant and antiviral properties.** When regularly consumed, green tea may help protect against the flu.

• **Cinnamon is a warming spice,** so called because it seems to warm our bodies by playing a role in promoting circulation. Cinnamon's antioxidant and anti-inflammatory properties help stimulate the immune system.

Amazing Immunity-Boosting Soup

1 Tablespoon olive oil or avocado oil
1 large onion, chopped
2 large garlic cloves, finely chopped

½ teaspoon ground cumin

½ teaspoon ground cinnamon

4 cups reduced-sodium vegetable broth

¾ cup dry brown or green lentils

4 ounces cremini, shiitake or white button mushrooms, stemmed and sliced

1 (15-ounce) can diced tomatoes

1 medium garnet yam or sweet potato, scrubbed, unpeeled and diced

1 cup freshly brewed green tea, unsweetened

1 (5-ounce) package fresh baby spinach

Sea salt and freshly ground black pepper to taste

⅓ cup reduced-fat plain Greek yogurt and/or 6 lemon wedges (optional)

In a large saucepan, heat the oil over medium-high heat. Add the chopped onion, and cook until lightly browned, about eight minutes, stirring occasionally. Add the garlic, cumin and cinnamon, and cook one minute longer, stirring constantly. Add the broth and lentils. When the liquid boils, reduce the heat, cover and simmer for 25 minutes.

Add the mushrooms, tomatoes, diced yam and tea. Cook until the lentils are soft and the yam just holds its shape, about 12 minutes.

Stir the baby spinach into the soup by the handful. Cover and heat for five minutes. Add seasoning as desired.

To serve, divide the soup among six wide, shallow bowls. Add a dollop of Greek yogurt to each bowl and/or serve with lemon wedges, if desired. Makes six servings.

HPV Vaccine Is Important for Boys as Well as Girls

Cancer caused by the human papillomavirus is wrongly thought of as only a female issue. But of the 34,800 HPV-caused cancer cases in the US every year, 40% are in men. HPV is sexually transmitted, usually through oral sex. In men, the cancer that HPV most commonly causes is of the mouth and throat. But the vaccine against HPV, Gardasil, is not approved to prevent mouth or throat cancer—only cervical cancer—so it is generally only given to girls. Also, insurance may not cover an unapproved use. It takes decades between an HPV infection and the time cancer develops, so early vaccination is a good idea.

Maura Gillison, MD, PhD, professor of medicine, department of cancer medicine, The University of Texas MD Anderson Cancer Center, Houston, and leader of a study published in *JAMA*.

The Search for Flu Strains Continues

Scientists travel to county fairs each year, where they swab the snouts of pigs and look for new—and dangerous—strains of flu. The 2009 flu pandemic began in pigs and eventually caused 12,000 human deaths.

The Ohio State University College of Veterinary Medicine

Why You Need a Tetanus Shot

Mark K. Slifka, PhD, professor of microbiology and immunology, Oregon Health & Science University, Beaverton.

Tetanus is a serious bacterial infection that can be life-threatening if not treated promptly. The bacteria that cause tetanus are typically transmitted via soil, dust or manure. Rusty nails are widely thought to cause tetanus, but rust itself does not necessarily carry the bacteria—any sharp object that's rusty could have been exposed to dirt, dust or manure that contains the bacteria that cause tetanus.

In the US, the current recommendation by the Advisory Committee on Immunization Practices is for adults to be revaccinated for tetanus every 10 years throughout adulthood. In other countries, such as the UK, there is no recommendation for adult booster vaccination against tetanus once a person has completed his/her childhood vaccination series.

If you don't remember when you got your last tetanus shot (or if you don't know whether you got the full childhood series), you should get a booster. A booster dose may be given when someone is exposed to the bacteria to help prevent severe disease, but the vaccine works best when given before exposure to allow time for protective levels of antibodies to build up.

Even though tetanus is rare in the US, the majority of reported illnesses occur in people who didn't receive the full childhood vaccination regimen or didn't complete their booster shots in adulthood. Side effects from the shot are rare but may include fever and/or swelling at the injection site. If you have questions about your vaccination history, consult your doctor.

Hepatitis C Treatment Keeps Getting Better

Eric Lawitz, MD, a professor of medicine at University of Texas Health San Antonio and vice president of scientific and research development for the Texas Liver Institute, also in San Antonio. He has more than 300 publications in leading scientific journals and serves as a reviewer for many journals, including *The New England Journal of Medicine*, *The Lancet* and *Journal of Hepatology*. TXLiver.com

Sometimes progress seems to happen very slowly...and then all at once. Such is the case with treatments for the potentially lethal hepatitis C virus.

For years, Americans with hepatitis C suffered through grueling therapies requiring as many as 18 pills a day, as well as injections of the medication *interferon*, known for dreadful side effects such as extreme fatigue, rashes, muscle aches, anemia, anxiety and depression. During this time, hepatitis C killed more Americans than any other infectious disease.

A new era: The dismal track record for hepatitis C therapies began reversing five or so years ago with a variety of much more effective antiviral medications...but with a catch. The first-generation antivirals were genotype specific, which means different treatment regimens were required depending on the specific genotype of the patient's infection. Hepatitis C genotypes are strains that represent the genetic variation of the virus. People can be infected with one of six major genotypes of hepatitis C, which include multiple subtypes of each genotype.

Now: Second-generation antivirals have come on the scene, curing the vast majority of patients with all genotypes of the disease... and regardless of their previous interferon therapy and despite the presence or absence of severe scarring of the liver (cirrhosis), a serious complication that can develop within 20 years of contracting the infection.*

The Game Changers

The first round of game-changing drugs treated genotypes 1 to 6. The first pill to treat all six genotypes of hepatitis C was FDA-approved in 2016. *Sofosbuvir/velpatasvir* (Epclusa) is a 12-week regimen for patients with or without cirrhosis.

The latest breakthrough drug is *glecaprevir/pibrentasvir* (Mavyret), which was approved by the FDA in 2017 as an eight-week regimen effective for all hepatitis C genotypes in people without cirrhosis. (Patients with cirrhosis require 12 weeks of treatment with the drug...those with genotype 3 who have been treated with interferon take the drug for 16 weeks regardless of the presence or absence of cirrhosis.)

The cure rate for the latest two drugs is about 98% in many populations. For the 2% who fail the first round of therapy, there is a three-medication antiviral combination of *sofosbuvir/velpatasvir/voxilaprevir* (Vosevi), and this cures 96% of the remaining 2% who failed the first-line therapy. All told, this

*Impressive cure rates can be achieved only if the treatment course is completed.

leaves only one in 1,000 hepatitis C patients uncured.

New Thinking on Testing

Along with the new medications, there's no longer a need for needle biopsy. Doctors have traditionally relied on a liver biopsy, which involves extracting a small piece of tissue with a needle, to determine the extent of a hepatitis C patient's liver damage. Now the FibroScan, a painless, noninvasive test that measures the amount of liver scarring, is the preferred way to determine the presence or absence of cirrhosis. If your doctor does not advise FibroScan testing, ask for it! Insurance typically covers the cost.

The Follow-up

Hepatitis C patients who have liver cirrhosis before successful treatment are at higher risk of developing liver cancer, as cirrhosis is a risk factor for cancer. If you have cirrhosis, you should receive twice-yearly screening via a blood test and ultrasound. The extra caution is well worth it, since small liver tumors can be removed surgically, treated locally or with a liver transplant, while large cancers tend to be life-threatening.

Important Note About Testing

Hepatitis C is often present for decades before symptoms (such as fatigue, nausea and/or jaundice) or complications occur, suggesting a weakening liver or development of liver cancer. Speak to your doctor about testing for hepatitis C.

Syphilis and Gonorrhea Are at Epidemic Levels

Until recently, these sexually transmitted diseases were declining in the US, with syphilis nearly eliminated. But both are increasing significantly. Gonorrhea cases rose 5% in 2018 over the previous year (latest data available) to more than 580,000...and syphilis increased 13.3%, to 115,000 cases. Combined cases of gonorrhea, syphilis and chlamydia—the most common STD, with 1.7 million cases reported—reached an all-time US high in 2018.

Sexually Transmitted Disease Surveillance Report by the US Centers for Disease Control and Prevention, Atlanta.

Protect Yourself from Germs in Public Bathrooms

Philip M. Tierno, Jr., PhD, clinical professor of microbiology and pathology at NYU Langone Health in New York City. He is author of *The Secret Life of Germs*. Med.NYU.edu

Public bathrooms can be a hotbed of viruses and bacteria. *My advice...*

• **Don't fret so much about the toilet seat.** Unless there's noticeable liquid or a smear of something gross on the seat, it is less contaminated than most people fear. That's because there's usually a low germ count on smooth-surfaced toilet seats and you have a protective skin barrier.

• **Flush with your shoe.** The flush handle is often contaminated, so flush with your shoe instead of your hand. If balance is a problem for you, at least use toilet paper to press the handle, then drop it quickly into the bowl.

• **Use paper towels.** The soap dispenser, faucet handle and door handle are often contaminated. Use a paper towel instead of your bare hand.

• **Avoid electric hand dryers.** Research shows that these machines can actually spread bacteria into the air and onto your hands.

• **Count to 30.** Even if your hands get contaminated, it's not a problem as long as you wash them with soap and water before touching your eyes, nose or mouth or a break in the skin (the conduits of entry into your body). Use the same paper towel you dry your hands with to open the door.

Good idea: Consider carrying your own paper towel in a pocket or bag in case the bathroom doesn't have any.

Where Germs Hide in Your Home

Sheets are a breeding ground for microscopic dust mites—wash sheets in hot water weekly, and keep humidity below 50%. Showerheads may contain bacteria that can cause lung infections—clean heads by submerging them overnight in vinegar if the manufacturer says that will not harm the finish. Refrigerators can have mold and bacteria growing in them—wipe up spills immediately, clean regularly with hot soapy water and throw out spoiled food at least weekly. Hand towels may hold germs for hours after use—avoid sharing them, and change and wash them regularly. Remote controls are covered with germs—disinfect them weekly with antibacterial wipes. Vacuum cleaners may contain bacteria, molds and allergens—clean them regularly and consider wearing a mask while vacuuming.

FamilyHandyman.com

Do Adults Need a Measles Shot?

William Schaffner, MD, professor of preventive medicine and infectious diseases, Vanderbilt University Medical Center, Nashville.

The recent spate of measles cases—the worst outbreak in 25 years—has generated a great deal of concern.

The good news is that most adults are at low risk for measles, and few cases have spread into the general population. The majority of recent cases have occurred in unvaccinated children in certain close-knit communities with some adults in those communities getting the illness.

Most unvaccinated people will become ill if they come in contact with someone who is infected. But for people born in 1957 or earlier, it's highly likely that they had measles as a child, and once you've had the disease, you're immune to getting it again.

That said, some adults are at higher risk for measles—namely those living in a community with a measles outbreak, health-care workers, college students living in close quarters and those planning international travel. If you're in any of these categories—and don't remember whether you had measles as a child—check your records to be sure that you got two doses of the measles, mumps, rubella (MMR) vaccine.

If you're not sure if you got two doses of the MMR vaccine or had measles as a child, there's no harm in getting vaccinated.

Exceptions: The vaccine is not recommended for pregnant women and adults who have a weakened immune system, a bleeding disorder or recently received a blood transfusion. A blood test also can confirm whether you have immunity to measles.

Measles Does Long-Term Damage to Immune System

The measles infection eliminates up to 73% of children's protective antibodies, deleting the immune system's "memory" of other diseases. Children who have measles are more vulnerable to other infections long after measles is gone.

Stephen Elledge, PhD, geneticist, Harvard Medical School, Boston, and coauthor of a study published in *Science*.

The Truth About Fecal Transplants

Henning Gerke, MD, gastroenterologist, University of Iowa Health Care, and clinical professor of internal medicine, gastroenterology and hepatology, University of Iowa, Carver College of Medicine, Iowa City.

Admittedly, a fecal transplant—putting someone else's poop into your body—sounds unpleasant. However, it may be the only way to cure some very serious gastrointestinal conditions that resist conventional treatment. And the procedure is not really as gross as what you're probably imagining.

The medical name for the procedure is fecal microbiota transplantation (or FMT)—and the serious condition it most commonly treats is C. difficile (C. diff), a bacterial infection that sickens half a million Americans and kills up to 30,000 each year. In fact, both the Infectious Diseases Society of America and The Society for Healthcare Epidemiology of America have recently added FMT to their official guidelines for treating C. diff.

An Ancient Therapy Made Modern

The concept of curing illness with donor fecal matter dates back to 4th-century China, when a cruder version of the procedure (which truly was gross—it involved making a soup!) was used to treat severe food poisoning and diarrhea. Today's procedure administers FMT via colonoscopy, enema or a tube run through the nose and into the stomach. (An oral capsule is being tested in clinical trials.) The procedure is simple and usually performed outpatient. In most cases, the patient leaves the hospital the same day and C. diff symptoms ease within days.

The fecal matter used in FMT comes from either a local donor (someone you know or the hospital's donor program) or from a national nonprofit stool bank called OpenBiome. In all cases, donors are screened first for illnesses, the same as for blood donors.

With a local donor, medical staff mixes the stool with saline (often in a basic kitchen blender) to prepare for a transplant. OpenBiome stool donations are filtered and homogenized, then sealed and kept frozen.

The risk for side effects is low—for instance, abdominal discomfort or a mild fever. FMT has become so accepted as a treatment for C. diff that 97% of Americans live within two hours of a facility that performs the procedure, according to OpenBiome.

How FMT Works

The main culprit behind C. diff and many other gastrointestinal upsets is a disruption of the gut microbiome. This can be caused by medical conditions, such as a compromised immune system, diabetes or obesity... or from taking certain drugs, such as antibiotics. FMT transplants gut organisms from a healthy donor into a sick patient's gut, repopulating the disrupted gut and helping to restore the natural balance. Numerous studies show FMT to be about 70% to 90%—or more—effective for treating recurrent C. diff infections. (If you're wondering why probiotics don't help, they contain only a few strains of microorganisms, not the wide, diverse spectrum contained in the stool of a healthy donor.)

C. diff bacteria actually are present in a normal, healthy gut in small numbers. But when antibiotics—even a single course—kill off healthy gut bacteria while they're killing the pathogens that made you sick, C. diff can take over, triggering severe diarrhea. Ironically, the standard first line of treatment for C. diff is more antibiotics, which explains why recurrent C. diff is a common problem. Especially vulnerable are children, people over age 65 and those who have a compromised immune system.

The FMT Frontier

While the effectiveness of FMT has only been established for treating C. diff—which is the only FDA-approved use outside of research—the procedure shows promise for other conditions. Because your gut microbiome is critical to your whole immune system and your general health, scientists are studying how FMT might also treat irritable bowel syndrome (IBS), Crohn's disease, diabetes, obesity, peanut allergies and melanoma.

The National Institutes of Health is currently funding a large study that is being conducted by the Fecal Microbiota Transplantation National Registry under the guidance of the American Gastroenterological Association's Center for Gut Microbiome Research & Education.

The study plans to track about 4,000 FMT patients for a decade after their transplants. The researchers will be gathering data on FMT's effectiveness for C. diff and other illnesses, including information on the short- and long-term effects. Currently, more than 20 hospitals, medical centers and medical schools across the country are participating—a number that's expected to grow to 75.

Meanwhile, you can search for a doctor who performs FMT by going to OpenBiome. org.

Statins Increase Risk for Skin Infections

Statins increase the relative risk for staphylococcal skin infections by 40%, reports Humphrey Ko, BSc (Pharm) (Hons). The risk was statistically significant and similar over three, six and 12 months of taking these drugs, which previously had been linked to diabetes risk. This study shows increased risk for skin infections, whether or not patients had diabetes.

Humphrey Ko, BSc (Pharm) (Hons), a doctoral candidate at School of Pharmacy and Biomedical Sciences at Curtin University in Perth, Australia, and lead author of the study published in *British Journal of Clinical Pharmacology.*

Avoid Athlete's Foot

Forgot your flip-flops and worried about the fungus you might pick up walking barefoot on the locker room floor? Use hand sanitizer to clean your feet before putting your shoes back on.

Jeffrey Benabio, MD, FAAD, dermatologist and physician director of Health Care Transformation at Kaiser Permanente, San Diego.

Say Goodbye to Toenail Fungus

Douglas F. Tumen, DPM, a board-certified foot surgeon and fellow of the American College of Foot and Ankle Surgeons. He is a founding partner at Hudson Valley Foot Associates in upstate New York and author of *Ask the Foot Doctor: Real-Life Answers to Enjoy Happy, Healthy, Pain-Free Feet.* AskTheFootDoctor.com

Most people know the telltale signs of toenail fungus, but few are aware of the best ways to get rid of this wily infection.

The condition is more common as we age, with about half of adults over age 70 dealing with this unsightly problem.

Onychomycosis (the medical term for nail fungus) is notoriously difficult to treat—some people spend years, or even decades, trying to eradicate their thick, brittle and crumbly toenails that may have turned yellow or brown.

But some therapies are more effective than others. In fact, new research shows that even particularly stubborn toenail fungus can now be eliminated with few risks for side effects.

How the Battle Begins

The environment inside your shoes is ideal for fungus—warm, humid and dark. What's more, the hard nail structure makes it difficult for topical drugs to penetrate effectively.

Your feet encounter fungus every day—in the shower (be it public or in your home)…

in your gym locker room…at nail salons…or when going through airport security if you're barefoot when you pull off your shoes. These are common ways to contract athlete's foot.

Toenail fungus, however, more often results from repeated nail injuries, such as your toes hitting the inside of your shoes when walking or running…or banging your toe into a chair or other furniture. Such injuries weaken the nail bed, allowing fungus to invade the toenail. Long toenails and snug shoes make the toenails vulnerable to these injuries, so proper nail care, including keeping your toenails trimmed, and proper shoe fit are crucial.

Important: A fungal infection can spread from one toenail to another, and early treatment helps minimize this. People with diabetes, poor circulation or compromised immunity should seek medical advice for toenail fungus.

To give yourself the best odds of vanquishing toenail fungus, here are five options that you may not know about—use one or more of these methods…

TREATMENT #1: **Vicks VapoRub.** Dabbed onto the affected toenail once or twice daily, this over-the-counter (OTC) topical cough suppressant often reduces—and sometimes cures—fungus in five to 16 months. It's one of VapoRub's "inactive" ingredients—thymol, a derivative of thyme used for its scent—that helps fight fungus. Other ingredients, including camphor, eucalyptus and menthol (all cough suppressants), may help combat fungus, too. You can apply it at night and then go to bed with or without socks.

Scientific evidence: When 18 adults with toenail fungus applied Vicks VapoRub daily for 48 weeks, the condition improved or was eliminated in 15 of the study participants, according to research published in *Journal of the American Board of Family Medicine.*

TREATMENT #2: **Nail file and OTC topical antifungal.** For an early-stage fungus called white superficial onychomycosis, topical medication applied to freshly trimmed nails may help. This fungus appears as tiny

(a couple of millimeters in diameter) circular or oblong spots. Because it rests on top of the nail bed, rather than inside or underneath the nail, this infection may respond well to topical treatments.

What to do: File the nail as low as possible using a single-use emery board. This will remove some of the fungus-infected nail and deprive the remaining fungus of its preferred food source—the nail itself.

Caution: Never dig under the nail with instruments. Doing so can loosen the nail from the nail bed, making it easier for fungus to enter.

Next, apply an OTC topical antifungal product containing *tolnaftate*, *ciclopirox* or one of the -azole medications (*clotrimazole*, *miconazole* or *ketoconazole*) daily. Although OTC antifungals marketed for athlete's foot, such as Lotrimin AF (which contains clotrimazole), have only been FDA-approved for use on skin, they can be safely used off-label for onychomycosis.

Important: While the fungal-infected nail grows out, avoid nail polish for at least a few months. Conventional nail polishes act like paint, trapping and essentially protecting lingering fungus. In fact, many patients first notice white superficial onychomycosis at the end of the summer when they stop getting regular pedicures and there's no polish hiding the spots.

If you do wear nail polish, choose a nontoxic formula that is free from chemicals such as formaldehyde and toluene. These versions are more "breathable" than traditional nail polishes, so they're less apt to trap fungus underneath. For added protection, try a product (such as daniPro) that contains antifungal compounds to help prevent toenail fungus. Men, or women who wish to avoid color, can use a clear version.

TREATMENT #3: **Lasers.** With the power to vaporize and disable toenail fungus, lasers are one of the more effective treatments. As the nail grows, healthy nail should begin emerging from the base, indicating that the fungus is being killed. Lasers are painless, require no aftercare and improve the majority of cases. Laser treatment for toenail fungus, which is performed by a podiatrist, is typically administered once a month for at least three months.

Note: Laser therapy for onychomycosis is FDA-approved, but is not covered by insurance because it's considered a cosmetic treatment. In some cases, the treatment may be covered if it's medically necessary—for instance, if you have diabetes or are immuno-compromised. Ask your insurer. The fee varies widely—a course of treatment may cost up to $1,000.

TREATMENT #4: **Oral antifungals.** For patients whose onychomycosis is stubborn and affects more than half of the nail plate, oral antifungals may be the most effective option. For years, the standard protocol called for 250 mg of Lamisil, a costly prescription antifungal, once a day for 90 days. The treatment is effective in about 60% of cases, but side effects can include gastrointestinal upset, headache and liver toxicity. Liver damage occurs in less than 1% of patients who use the drug but is potentially fatal.

A new, safer option: A less expensive generic version of Lamisil, *terbinafine hydrochloride*, is now widely available and can be prescribed via an equally effective, more liver-friendly "pulse dosing regimen"—four cycles of 500 mg (two pills) daily for seven days each month (a total of 56 pills over four months). Pulse therapy was as effective at treating onychomycosis as the conventional daily regimen with the brand-name medication (typically one pill daily for three months), according to a 2019 study published in *Journal of Fungi.*

Note: Most insurers only cover terbinafine, the generic medication, and not the brand-name version.

TREATMENT #5: **Sanitized shoes.** The fungus in your toenail is most likely living in your shoes. That's why it's smart to invest in an ultraviolet (UV) light shoe sanitizer. The SteriShoe Essential, for example, is a small device that you place in your shoes (closed-toed or even sandals) and plug in so that UV light can kill the fungi that can lead to toenail fungus. This product, which has the American Podiatric Medical Association Seal of Acceptance, sanitizes shoes and turns itself off in 45 minutes. It's available online for $99.95 at SteriShoe.com. Even though it's unlikely that socks will spread fungi when doing laundry, it's best to wash socks in hot water and use bleach to be safe.

Clean Your Smartphone!

Your smartphone is among the germiest things you own. The germ count is closely tied to how often something is touched, and smartphones are touched very frequently… even in the bathroom. A British study found that one in six phones was contaminated with fecal matter. To kill germs, lightly swab phones daily with alcohol wipes.

Miryam Wahrman, PhD, professor of biology at William Paterson University, Wayne, New Jersey, and author of *The Hand Book: Surviving in a Germ-Filled World.* WPUNJ.edu

Petting Zoo Precautions

Petting zoos can spread antibiotic-resistant germs. A recent Israeli study of 228 petting zoo animals found that 12% carried strains of bacteria that are resistant to antibiotics and capable of infecting humans. Children who cannot yet be trusted to keep their hands out of their mouths should not directly touch the animals or go to petting zoos. Everyone else should wash their hands vigorously and repeatedly after touching these animals.

Howard Smith, MD, a pediatric ear, nose and throat physician and former radio talk show host, broadcasts the weekly podcast "Dr. Howard Smith OnCall." DrHowardSmith.com

Credit Cards Are Just as Germy as Cash

According to a recent study, germs found on credit cards included Staphylococcus aureus, the cause of staph infections...and Salmonella enterica, a source of food poisoning. Consumers tend to imagine, incorrectly, that their cards are cleaner than cash because they don't pass through as many hands. Periodically use alcohol wipes to disinfect cards. Wash your hands or use hand sanitizer between handling cards and eating.

Timothy E. Riedel, PhD, assistant professor of practice in College of Natural Sciences at The University of Texas at Austin. CNS.UTexas.edu/fri

Superbugs in Cosmetics

Ninety percent of cosmetics were found to have superbugs ranging from staph to E. coli. Makeup sponges carried the most bacteria—more than mascara, eyeliner and lipsticks—because they're rarely washed, even after being dropped on a bathroom floor. Protect yourself by washing them with soap and hot water weekly and discarding sponges every two months.

Amreen Bashir, PhD, lecturer in biomedical sciences at Aston University in Birmingham, England, and lead researcher of the study of used makeup published in *Journal of Applied Microbiology.*

Bat Bites and Scratches

Bat bites and scratches can be hard to see and easy to overlook. Some people have been bitten while asleep without knowing it. If you suspect that you may have had a bat bite...or wake up and find a bat in your room...or have a close encounter with a bat behaving oddly—such as being unable to fly or being active during daytime—see your doctor to discuss whether you should get treated for possible rabies exposure. Bats are the leading cause of the disease in the US. Of 89 cases reported between 1960 and 2018, 70% were caused by bats.

Data from Centers for Disease Control and Prevention, Atlanta, reported in *University of California, Berkeley Wellness Letter.*

Chapter 10

KIDNEY, BLADDER AND LIVER HEALTH

What You Don't Know Is Harming Your Kidneys

The early stages of chronic kidney disease (CKD) cause no symptoms. In fact, 90% of people with the condition don't know they have it. But even if your kidneys are still healthy—so far—you could be doing things that harm them without realizing it.

Kidneys are critical to the health of the whole body. They filter waste, balance body fluids, maintain blood pressure, control the production of red blood cells and regulate electrolytes and minerals, such as potassium, sodium and magnesium. When kidney health declines, waste builds up and causes health issues—including high blood pressure, anemia and metabolic bone disease (such as osteoporosis). The final stage is kidney failure and the need for regular dialysis or a kidney transplant.

The Greatest Danger

Thirty million American adults have CKD, which is the ninth-leading cause of death in the US, according to the Centers for Disease Control and Prevention. Chronic kidney disease is more common in women (15%) than men (12%). One factor that drives the prevalence of this disease is that people who are at risk often don't realize it…so they're less likely to get tested…take necessary precautions to protect their kidneys from further damage…and/or take steps to reverse early stages of damage.

People with diabetes and high blood pressure are at especially high risk. Together, these two conditions are responsible for two-thirds of CKD. Other risk factors include age (being 60 or older)…having a family history of kidney failure…being of non-Caucasian descent (African-American, Hispanic, Asian, Pacific Islander and/or Native American)…obesity…lupus…and cancer.

If you have risk factors for CKD, you should be tested with a Kidney Profile annually. The profile combines a urine albumin-to-creatinine ratio (ACR) test and an estimated glomerular filtration rate (eGFR) blood test.

The Threat from the Drugstore

Healthy kidneys are able to filter out medications and supplements without harm to the

---

Joseph Vassalotti, MD, chief medical officer of the National Kidney Foundation, Kidney.org. His research has been published in peer-reviewed journals such as *American Journal of Nephrology, Kidney International* and *American Journal of Kidney Diseases*.

kidneys themselves. However, drugs and supplements can cause kidney damage or other side effects. *If you take any of these worst offenders, check with your clinician and be sure to get an annual Kidney Profile...*

• **Nonsteroidal anti-inflammatory drugs (NSAIDs).** The kidney danger from long-term use of NSAIDs, such as *ibuprofen* (Advil, Motrin) and *naproxen* (Aleve), is well-known, but few people realize how easy it is to do harm. A recent large study published in *JAMA Network Open* that looked at nearly 800,000 active young and middle-aged adults found that using eight or more doses a month put them at a 20% higher risk for kidney damage compared with not taking any NSAIDs.

• **Proton pump inhibitors (PPIs).** Heartburn/reflux/GERD drugs such as *omeprazole* (Prilosec), *esomeprazole* (Nexium) and *lansoprazole* (Prevacid) pose a risk to the kidneys if taken long-term. A recent study published in *Scientific Reports* found that compared with people who took other antacids, those who took PPIs (including over-the-counter versions) were 28.4% more likely to develop CKD.

• **Herbal and dietary supplements.** Since supplements are not regulated in the US, there is no guarantee that ingredients and amounts listed on a supplement label are what is actually in the bottle. Even if the label is accurate, "natural" herbs and supplements can be toxic to the kidneys, especially in large amounts.

For instance, kidney injuries have been reported from using the herbs Chinese yew extract, St. John's wort and wormwood. Talk to your doctor about the health risks of any herbal and/or dietary supplements you take—ideally, before you use them.

• **Prescription medications.** Patients who know they have CKD with decreased kidney function should make sure all their doctors are aware of this. Dosages for some drugs may need to be adjusted for these patients—and some medications, such as *metformin* (Glucophage), used to treat diabetes, and the muscle relaxant *baclofen* (Lioresal), may need to be avoided. But people who don't

know that they have CKD are in danger of getting harmful dosages of certain drugs, including beta-blockers used to treat high blood pressure...antimicrobials...antifungals...and insulin.

• **Insomnia.** Chronic insomnia has been associated with kidney damage. One study of more than one million veterans found that insomniacs were 2.4 times more likely to develop kidney failure than those who slept normally. Poor sleep is linked to high blood pressure and vascular disease, which may in turn lead to kidney disease. People who already have CKD also are at higher risk for sleep disorders, such as sleep apnea and restless legs syndrome.

• **Too much protein.** Low-carb diets that emphasize fat and protein, such as Keto or Paleo, may jeopardize the health of people at risk for CKD—particularly if they heavily consume processed red meats. White meat, fish and dairy protein do not seem to carry the same risk. Vegetable proteins may actually be protective. The research as to whether excessive amounts of protein also are harmful for people who aren't at increased risk for CKD is not conclusive.

• **Processed foods and phosphorus.** Our bodies need some phosphorus for strong bones, and healthy kidneys are able to remove any excess so that toxic amounts don't build up in the body. However, not all phosphorus is the same.

Organic phosphorus occurs naturally in many protein-rich animal and plant foods and is only up to 60% absorbed by the body. There is little danger of consuming too much plant-based phosphorus, as long as the kidneys are healthy. Inorganic phosphorus is an additive used to improve the shelf life and/or color of processed foods, such as processed cheese and sodas. Inorganic phosphorus is more than 90% absorbed...and too much can easily accumulate in the body. Excessive phosphorus throws off the body's delicate calcium balance. It can lead to calcium being drawn from the bones and dangerous deposits of calcium accumulating in blood vessels, the lungs, the eyes and the heart. Because our diet is so

Antiperspirants Dangerous?

The amount of aluminum that is absorbed by the skin from antiperspirants is tiny—especially compared with the amount of aluminum people are exposed to naturally from water and soil.

Recommended: If you have kidney disease, ask your doctor if you should stick with plain deodorants that don't contain aluminum. —Joseph Vassalotti, MD

heavily processed, most of us get up to twice the recommended dietary allowance of 700 mg/day for adults. Check the ingredients list before buying packaged foods—phosphorus additives have "phos" in the name. Or better yet, stick to whole, fresh foods.

•**Air pollution.** A major study of almost 2.5 million veterans published in *Journal of the American Society of Nephrology* estimated that air pollution causes nearly 45,000 new cases of CKD in the US each year. Other research compared county levels of air pollution with the incidence of CKD among one million Medicare patients. The researchers found that diagnoses of CKD were highest in counties that had the highest levels of air pollution. Further studies are under way. But for the time being, it makes sense to avoid or limit exposure as much as possible.

Bladder Not Cooperating?

Jill Rabin, MD, professor of obstetrics, gynecology and women's health at the Donald and Barbara Zucker School of Medicine at Hofstra/Northwell in Hempstead, New York. Dr. Rabin is coauthor, with Gail Stein, of *Mind Over Bladder*.

We've all heard of overactive bladder —that "gotta-go" feeling that so often strikes at the worst possible times. It's annoying—especially when it leads to embarrassing dribbles (incontinence). But there could be a hidden side to this problem that you and your doctor are overlooking.

For some people, those too-frequent trips to the bathroom occur because of "underactive bladder," in which sufferers don't empty their bladders completely when they urinate, so they soon make additional trips to the toilet.

About half of women and one-third of men in the US suffer from underactive bladder at some point in their lives. *Key facts to know…*

What Goes Wrong

Under normal conditions, urine, which is made by your kidneys around the clock, trickles into your bladder all the time. A well-functioning bladder stores the fluid until it gets full enough to send a "time to go" signal to your brain.

Ideally, you heed that sensation and get to a toilet. Then your brain sends signals back to the bladder, causing it to contract and squeeze out urine. At the same time, the brain tells several sets of sphincter muscles to relax, allowing urine to pass through the urethra. The process is the same in men and women, even though the anatomy is slightly different. *When the waterworks do not work, symptoms of underactive bladder might include…*

•**Feeling that you need to go again right after you pee,** resulting in frequent trips to the toilet.

•**Weak urinary stream.**

•**Urges to strain, push and bear down to empty your bladder.**

•**Swelling, tenderness or pain below your belly button.**

If the problem becomes chronic, partial emptying of your bladder may allow urine to collect bacteria, leading to recurrent urinary tract infections.

Finding the Root Cause

Underactive bladder is largely due to two main culprits—obstructions and impaired bladder contractions.

Some causes of obstruction…

•**Weak pelvic floor muscles.** In women, multiple vaginal deliveries can damage or weaken pelvic structures and nerves, leading to a sagging bladder and/or uterus, which can interfere with bladder function. After menopause, the decline in a woman's estrogen levels causes the pelvic floor to thin and weaken. These muscles may be weak in men due to prostate removal. (Also, an enlarged prostate often causes problems for a man.)

Note: Research on supplemental estrogen has been mixed. Kegel exercises that strengthen pelvic muscles can help women—and men—who need to build up these muscles to improve their bladder control.

If Kegels are new to you, here's the basic idea: While sitting or standing, tighten the muscles you would use to stop your stream of urine and those used to keep from passing gas for three seconds (without clenching your abdomen or buttocks), then relax for three seconds. Repeat in sets of five, starting with just a few sets at a time. Slowly work up to 10 sets of five per day.

•**Fibroids.** These benign tumors in the uterus can obstruct the neck of the bladder.

•**Constipation.** In both men and women, hard, impacted stools can press on the bladder and urethra, interfering with the bladder's ability to empty.

Among the causes of impaired bladder contraction…

•**Years of holding in your urine.** This was once called "schoolteacher's bladder," because schools used to forbid teachers to take bathroom breaks except at lunchtime. As a result, the bladder can "forget" how to function.

•**Conditions that involve nerve damage,** such as stroke, Parkinson's disease, diabetes and multiple sclerosis.

•**Medications,** including muscle relaxants, sedatives, antihistamines, tricyclic antidepressants, such as *amitriptyline* (Elavil), and decongestants.

How to Get Relief

If your no-go symptoms haven't become so severe that they are significantly interfering with your life, just improving a few bathroom habits can help. *Here's what to try first…*

•**Urinate at least every two to three hours during the day,** even if you do not feel the urge.

Helpful: Use a smartphone timer to remind yourself to go on this schedule. If you feel much more frequent urges, try to stretch out your bathroom visits by at least 15 minutes at a time, which will train your bladder to wait.

•**Do your best to find private bathrooms if you are prone to "bashful bladder,"** which occurs when you need to urinate but aren't able to do so in the presence of another person.

•**Don't push or strain to urinate…but try shifting your position.** For example, some women and men find that it helps to lean forward or press a hand gently against the lower abdomen to help push urine out of the bladder.

•**Try double voiding.** Urinate, then wait a minute and go again. That can help drain the bladder and prevent the feeling that you need to go again the minute your pants are zipped.

To Get More Help

If you're still struggling after trying the steps described above, talk to your doctor, and be clear about what's bothering you. A good workup will include a lab check of your urine to ensure that you don't have a urinary tract infection…and—after you return from giving your urine sample—a simple ultrasound test to see how much urine is left in your bladder. There will always be some, but more than 100 to 150 milliliters, depending on your age, indicates a problem.

Be sure to ask your doctor if any of your medications could be contributing to your problem.

Important: Never discontinue a prescribed drug without checking with your doctor.

If you have a medical condition that increases your risk for underactive bladder (such as those mentioned earlier), be sure to get proper treatment for it. In other cases, you may have an underlying cause that requires surgery, such as pelvic floor reconstruction for a sagging bladder. Or the doctor may refer you to a physical therapist or other professional who will help you with behavior changes that give you more control over your bladder function.

Also helpful: In some cases, you may be asked to try using a disposable strawlike catheter to empty your bladder several times a day. It's easier than you might think and is sometimes the best way to get on with a normal life.

Implantable Device for Overactive Bladder

People with overactive bladder experience pain, burning and frequent urination—and current treatments aren't ideal.

In development: An implantable device that uses light to sense bladder overactivity and automatically reduce the need to urinate.

Nature

Too Busy to Pee?

Jonathan Vapnek, MD, clinical associate professor of urology, Icahn School of Medicine at Mount Sinai, New York City.

There is a common misperception that "holding it" for too long can be harmful, but there's never been any solid data to support the theory. An adult bladder can often hold at least two cups of urine, if not more, comfortably. In most cases, the worst consequence of waiting to use the bathroom is likely to be temporary discomfort.

Most people urinate about four to eight times in a 24-hour period. A change in the frequency of urinary habits, including getting up more than twice a night to urinate, or an increase or decrease in the amount that a person urinates, warrants attention.

Be sure to watch out for symptoms of a urinary tract infection (UTI). These can include a burning sensation when you do urinate, or sudden urges to use the bathroom. If your urine is darker than straw-colored, foul smelling and/or looks cloudy, these symptoms also can signal a UTI. It's worth noting that UTIs may be more common in people who do not void frequently because the bacteria that are normally flushed out with urination have a chance to build up.

Consistently holding in urine also can potentially weaken bladder muscles, which can lead to urinary retention—a condition that prevents you from being able to fully empty your bladder.

If you develop any symptoms, consult your doctor about getting a urinary flow rate assessment, a noninvasive test that measures the rate of flow of voided urine, and a post-void residual measurement to determine if the bladder is completely emptying.

9 Ways to Love Your Liver

Robert S. Brown, Jr., MD, MPH, the Gladys and Roland Harriman Professor of Medicine and clinical chief in the division of gastroenterology and hepatology in the department of medicine at Weill Cornell Medical College, New York City, and a member of the National Medical Advisory Committee for the American Liver Foundation. LiverFoundation.org

You probably give your liver little thought, but your body's largest internal organ is a multitasking miracle, filtering toxins, working with your immune system to fight off infection and storing and releasing nutrients from food so that your body can access and use them to function.

If you don't protect and nurture your liver—or worse, out-and-out ignore it—it can get overtaxed, and the spillover affects your entire body. Liver disease is on the rise—30 million Americans suffer from some sort of liver disease that can, if untreated, lead to scarring (cirrhosis), organ failure or even death. The problem is most people don't know it, because liver disease is silent.

The good news is that loving your liver isn't complicated. It benefits from many of the same healthy habits you already know to do (but maybe aren't yet doing) for your heart and your body as a whole. *Here, nine easy ways to love your liver...*

1. Brew a pot of coffee. Aside from coffee's ability to help you get up and go in the morning, it has many health benefits, including boosting liver health. A study at Southampton, University, UK, of 430,000 people found that consumption of two cups of coffee a day was related to a 44% lower risk for liver cirrhosis.

Note: The benefit isn't related to the caffeine, so you can enjoy decaf if you would rather. Coffee beans contain hundreds of antioxidants and other compounds that offer protection from liver disease and cancer.

Tip: Green tea is another source of antioxidants that are good for the liver, though it is not as well-studied as coffee.

2. Eat oatmeal for breakfast. Your digestive tract loves all fiber, of course, but you can show your liver extra TLC with foods that help move toxins through the body and out of your system. That lightens the load your liver needs to process. If you don't like oatmeal, other top fiber sources are oat bran, barley, flaxseed, beans, apples and citrus fruits.

Also: If you replace starches and simple carbs with these high-fiber foods, you'll eat fewer calories and feel less hungry.

3. Avoid high-fructose corn syrup. If you make only one change to your diet, eliminate all sugar-sweetened beverages, especially those with high-fructose corn syrup (HFCS).

As you probably know, HFCS has been associated with a greater risk for obesity, diabetes and heart disease, but you may not be aware that HFCS has a direct impact on your liver. It raises your risk of developing non-alcoholic fatty liver disease (NAFLD), a very common disorder affecting nearly one in three people. In human trials, consuming HFCS was found to be more likely to contribute to NAFLD than dietary fat. NAFLD can lead to liver damage and the more serious condition nonalcoholic steatohepatitis and ultimately cirrhosis. Also, HFCS fails to activate the body's normal signal to stop eating when full—your appetite isn't satisfied, so you continue to eat, putting even more stress on your liver.

While there has been a push in recent years to remove HFCS from foods and beverages, read all labels carefully because it is still hidden in many packaged products such as ketchup and salad dressing.

4. Lose weight. Carrying extra weight is toxic to your liver. NAFLD occurs in about 15% of nonobese patients but its prevalence increases along with your body mass index (BMI). Obese (BMI of 30.0 to 39.9) and extremely obese (BMI of 40 or more) patients have a prevalence of 65% and 85%, respectively.

Livers don't need fancy or quick weight-loss diets. A healthy, balanced eating plan that you can stick with for life, such as the heart-healthy Mediterranean diet, is the best way to lose weight and support your liver. Focus on good fats, such as olive oil, nuts, fish and avocado, and more vegetables than animal protein.

5. Add strength-training to get your liver in fighting shape. While better muscle tone is the obvious benefit of strength training, having more muscle mass boosts health in many ways that you can't see, including reducing fat in the liver. Though the exact mechanism isn't yet known, a three-month study at Tel Aviv Medical Center found that three strength-training sessions a week led to reduced fat in the liver. Another study found that doing just push-ups and squats, three sets of 10 reps of each exercise, three times a week over six months lowered markers for liver disease.

6. Know your liquor limits. You think you know how much is "too much," but safe alcohol limits are probably lower than you realize—just one drink a day for women… two for men. One drink means 12 ounces of beer (5% alcohol content), five ounces of wine (12%) or 1.5 ounces of hard liquor (40%). Getting one generous pour, ordering beer by the pint or sharing a full bottle of wine with a friend can put you well over that limit. That's fine for special occasions, but steady drinking damages your liver even if you don't have an alcohol-use disorder, also known as alcoholism. The number of deaths from cirrhosis is on the rise across the country, especially among adults ages 25 to 34.

Important: Saving up during the workweek for a Saturday night splurge is not a safe plan and does not keep you within the week's alcohol limits—overindulging is always toxic to the liver.

7. Limit your liver's exposure to *acetaminophen*. Most people think of acetaminophen (Tylenol) as safe, but it's often overused. In fact, overdoses account for about 50,000 emergency room visits, 25,000 hospitalizations and nearly 500 deaths a year, half of them unintentional. A total of 12 regular-strength, 325-milligram (mg) pills per day is considered safe. Beyond that, the risk increases. At 25 regular-strength pills a day, it's toxic.

Important: To avoid getting a double dose by mistake, always read a medication's ingredients list because acetaminophen is in many other over-the-counter remedies such as cold medicines.

8. Boost liver health with CoQ10, an enzyme that helps generate energy in your cells, and n-acetylcysteine (NAC), a powerful antioxidant. Both are found in many foods, such as spinach, legumes and certain fish—but it may be hard to get enough in your diet. That's where supplements can help. Studies have found that 600 mg of NAC twice a day improved liver function. Between 100 mg and 300 mg a day of CoQ10, also known for heart health, did this as well. Ask your doctor or nutritionist if either or both of these may be helpful to you.

9. Have your liver enzyme levels checked. Your blood pressure and cholesterol are taken by your doctor at every doctor's visit, but you probably have no idea about your liver enzyme levels. Liver enzymes are the proteins needed for the liver to do its work. They're also markers of liver health. When the liver has to work harder than normal or is damaged, higher levels of enzymes show up in your blood. Unfortunately, the basic blood tests done at wellness visits may not include checking liver enzyme levels. For that you need what's called a comprehensive metabolic blood test. An elevated number could be the only early warning sign of liver problems.

Important: Some general practitioners might not think that mildly elevated enzymes, such as *alanine aminotransferase* (ALT), warrant investigation, but if your enzymes are at all high, you should be checked to see if fatty liver disease or another condition is the cause.

Liver Donors Are Saving Lives…

Koji Hashimoto, MD, PhD, director of living donor liver transplantation and pediatric liver transplantation at Cleveland Clinic. His research has been published in *Annals of Surgery, Liver Transplantation* and other leading medical journals.

Deciding to have major surgery is never easy. So imagine how tough the decision might be if the surgery meant giving up a piece of the largest organ in your body, entirely for the benefit of another person—someone whose life might well be saved by your generosity.

The quandary is real for increasing numbers of Americans. That's because doctors are urging more and more people in need of liver transplants to seek out living donors, just as many kidney transplant patients have done for years.

Faced with uncertain odds of getting a timely transplant the old-fashioned way—by waiting for an organ from a deceased donor—patients whose livers are failing due to life-threatening conditions, such as cirrhosis, viral hepatitis and primary liver cancer, are reaching out to family, friends, faith communities and sometimes even strangers on social media.

What's at stake: About 14,000 Americans each year need a new liver, but only about 8,200 get one. Many remaining patients become too ill to qualify for a transplant or die waiting.

Living donation is possible because the liver is the only human organ that can regenerate. That means the person who gives up part of his/her healthy liver will have most of the organ's original size again within two months—and so will the recipient.

The procedure, developed over the past three decades, has continued to evolve over the years and now offers improved surgical techniques and postoperative care. As a result, living liver donations work at least as well as a transplant from a deceased donor with one-year survival often exceeding 90%. And it often means patients get their transplants at earlier stages in their illnesses. But that does not mean the decision to donate is simple.

Who Can Donate a Liver?

Most transplant centers will accept donors between the ages of 18 and 55 or 60. Older adults have increased surgical risks, and younger people are not considered mature enough to give informed consent.

Most living liver donations are "directed"—meaning you offer to donate to a particular patient who has reached out for potential donors among family, friends or strangers. The baseline for consideration is whether you have a blood type that matches or is compatible with the blood type of the patient.

If you think you'd like to be considered as a living liver donor, you can start the process by calling the patient's transplant center. During the initial phone call, a staff member will ask a few questions about your overall health and your reasons for considering donation. If you and the transplant team agree that you might be a good candidate, you will go to the transplant center for a couple of days of tests and interviews.

You can expect a thorough examination of your physical health, including blood draws…tests of your heart and lungs…scans of your liver…and a psychological evaluation to ensure that you understand the risks and that there has been no coercion to participate in a living liver donation. Some people, including those who are significantly overweight and at risk for fatty liver disease, may be asked to undergo a liver biopsy.

If you have certain health problems, including bleeding or clotting disorders or a history of alcoholism or drug addiction, you won't be able to donate. But some common conditions, such as mild high blood pressure that is well-controlled with medication, will not disqualify you.

If the transplant team believes you are a good candidate, a separate donor advocate team, including a physician, social worker, bioethicist, coordinator and psychiatrist, will review the decision with your interests in mind.

Important: If you are accepted, you can change your mind at any point. The final decision is always yours.

What Will I Need to Do to Prepare?

If you are accepted and decide to donate, you usually will have a few weeks to get ready—though in some cases, a patient is in such desperate need that surgery is scheduled within a couple of days. If you do have a waiting period, the transplant team will encourage you to limit or avoid alcohol, which is hard on the liver…eat a healthful diet… and avoid putting on weight, which can lead to fat buildup in the liver.

You also will want to use this time to talk to your family and, if need be, your employer about the support you will need after the surgery.

What Happens During the Surgery?

You and the recipient will show up for surgery on the same day, in adjoining operating rooms. During an operation that can last about six hours, surgeons will remove a portion of your liver—15% to 70% of the volume, depending on the needs of the recipient. Children need the smallest amount of tissue.

At some transplant centers, all donor surgeries are done with a large abdominal incision, shaped like a hockey stick that extends across half the belly and up the chest. Elsewhere, some surgeries are now done with smaller laparoscopic incisions, reducing postsurgical pain and recovery time.

What Are the Risks?

The donor faces a risk for death of about one in 500, according to the best available data. That's comparable to the risk faced by anyone having major abdominal surgery. Other risks include wound infection, hernias, excess bleeding and leakage of bile, a digestive fluid made by the liver. A leak can temporarily cause pain, nausea and vomiting. The rate for a major complication, such as a bile leak, incisional hernia or liver failure, varies by transplant center, but typically is below 10%.

What's the Recovery Like?

Most donors need to stay in the hospital for five to six days after the surgery, but you may be able to leave sooner after a laparoscopic procedure. If you live far from the transplant center, you may be asked to stay nearby for another week or two to be monitored by your caregiver for fever, shortness of breath or other symptoms that might indicate a complication. Recovery can take time due to the fatigue and pain caused by a large incision, which is commonly used. If you have a desk job, you may be able to return to work in two

months or less...someone with a physically demanding job might need three months after conventional surgery.

While no long-term health risks have been found, you will be asked to return to the transplant center for periodic checkups and to continue yearly physicals with your primary care physician at home.

What About Costs?

The recipient's insurance will cover the cost of your surgery and medical care related to any complications from the donation, but not the cost of travel, lodging and time off from work. You should talk with your employer to determine whether your time off can be covered by vacation, sick time or disability pay.

Help with travel, lodging and meals away from home is available to some donors through certain charities or the National Living Donor Assistance Center (888-870-5002 or LivingDonorAssistance.org). While a donor cannot benefit financially from the donation, the recipient and his/her family may be able to help you with some related expenses as well. A transplant center social worker will walk you through the help that is available.

Is "Death Fat" Clogging Your Liver?

Alan Christianson, NMD, a naturopathic medical doctor who specializes in natural endocrinology. He is founder of Integrative Health (IntegrativeHealth Care.com) in Scottsdale, Arizona, and author of four books, including *The Metabolism Reset Diet*.

If you follow a typical American diet, the answer to that headline question is likely "Yes!" Sadly, you're endangering one of your most vital organs and shortening your life.

The liver handles a huge workload—removing toxins from blood...storing and distributing fats, vitamins and hormones... regulating blood sugar...and a lot more. However, a sedentary lifestyle, poor sleep and especially diets heavy in fat, processed carbohydrates and sugar can lead to excess triglycerides, a type of lipid (blood fat) that clogs the liver with fat.

Signs that your liver is clogged…

• **You are overweight, fatigued and/or have food cravings.** A healthy liver easily regulates weight, energy and appetite.

Note: You can have a fatty liver without being overweight, so be aware of the symptoms below.

• **You have a chronic disease such as heart disease,** diabetes, arthritis, lung disease and/or autoimmune disease (such as rheumatoid arthritis).

• **You have high triglycerides.**

• **You have elevated alanine aminotransferase (ALT),** a liver enzyme measured during a complete blood count test or liver panel.

If you think your liver may be fatty—putting you at risk for liver inflammation, scarring (cirrhosis) and even liver failure—consider trying this four-week liver-cleansing diet…*

What to Eat

Studies show that replacing two meals a day with a protein shake burns liver fat, reduces body fat and curbs inflammation while sparing muscle. Many people lose five to 15 pounds and several inches around their waist—a sign that the diet is working. If you shouldn't lose weight, add an extra daily meal. *The shake should include…*

• **A protein powder that contains about 23 g of protein per serving** and does not have artificial ingredients (toxic to the liver) or refined sugar (it turns to triglycerides). Good choices are pea powder or blended-vegetable protein powder.

• **Resistant starch (RS),** a fiberlike carbohydrate found in such foods as potatoes, green bananas, legumes, raw oats and cashews. RS boosts liver function, regulates blood sugar, reduces deep abdominal fat and helps build muscle mass.

Suggestions: Two tablespoons to one-quarter cup of one of the foods above or aquafaba (the liquid left from canned or cooked legumes, such as chickpeas).

• **Liver-supporting superfoods.** Add one cup of greens (spinach, kale, arugula, watercress, etc.)…one tablespoon of milk thistle seeds…one teaspoon of spirulina…one teaspoon of cacao powder…and/or one teaspoon of maca powder, according to preference.

• **Flavoring.** As desired, use stevia, xylitol, cinnamon, ginger, food-grade essential oils such as lemon or wild orange, and natural extracts of vanilla, almond and chocolate.

Place the ingredients in a blender. I recommend a high-powered one such as a NutriBullet, Vitamix or Blendtec. Add enough water to make about 16 ounces and blend for one minute.

More liver-cleansing diet tips…

• **Snack healthy.** Phytonutrient-rich, low-calorie foods such as carrots, bell peppers, broccoli, celery, tomatoes and zucchini support liver function and don't add extra fat. Have at least three such snacks of one or a combination of these foods daily between shakes and after dinner.

• **Power-pack dinner.** When consumed together, cruciferous vegetables (including broccoli, cauliflower, cabbage) and apiaceous vegetables (including carrots and parsley) trigger the liver's fat-clearing process.

• **Lean proteins.** Good dinner proteins include poultry, fish, lean grass-fed beef, cottage cheese, legumes, high-protein grains (quinoa and amaranth), nuts, seeds and soy foods.

Note: After completing the diet, ask your doctor about repeating your blood work, including the ALT test.

---

*Check with your doctor before starting this or any new diet program, especially if you have a chronic disease or take medication.

Chapter 11

NATURAL HEALING FOR WOMEN

7 Natural Immune-Boosting Tricks to Stay Healthier This Winter

"The north wind doth blow, and we shall have snow…" and a runny nose, stuffy head, sore throat, achy muscles and fever, too! With the new coronavirus that originated in China inundating the US, let alone the millions of Americans who are sickened by colds and influenza every year, you may feel more like hiding in bed with a box of tissues than frolicking in the snow. And while remedies abound in the marketplace, the greatest gift you can give yourself is health—specifically, immunity health that's found naturally. *Here are seven simple tricks to build up your body's defense system…*

1. Try a Myers Cocktail.

Not to be mistaken with the hot toddies floating on cocktail trays around your holiday party, the Myers Cocktail is a surefire way to ensure you're getting the nutrients you need—or shortening an illness that has already struck. Pioneered by the late John Myers, MD, these ultra-nourishing blends of key vitamins—from magnesium and calcium to B complex and vitamin C—are delivered intravenously, packing a potent punch that can be felt immediately. Numerous clients come to my clinic for this nutrient therapy whenever they're beginning to feel under the weather. Others use it as a way to accelerate their recovery time from jetlag. The science is there to validate the Myers Cocktail, too. Research demonstrates that it can alleviate a number of symptoms associated with winter illnesses, including fatigue and nasal congestion. Data also shows that it can mitigate the effects of seasonal allergic rhinitis and tension headaches—the very thing that arrives when you see that "OMG" line at Target.

2. Take Turkey Tail (no, not the one you're prepping to eat).

Technically called Coriolus Versicolor, turkey tail is a medicinal mushroom whose healing uses date back to the Ming Dynasty. Then, it was used to bolster energy and reduce phlegm—precisely what you need when the mercury drops and germs are in the air. Since gaining recognition in Western medicine in the 1960s, the mushroom has been

---

Laurie Steelsmith, ND, LAc, medical director of Steelsmith Natural Health Center in Honolulu. She is author of *Natural Choices for Women's Health, Great Sex, Naturally* and *Growing Younger Every Day* and writes the "Natural Healing Secrets for Women" blog at BottomLineInc.com. DrSteelsmith.com

noted for its ability to improve immunity and stave off infections. Turkey tail is available in supplement form. It can also be consumed, such as in tea—add turmeric and lemon for an extra dose of immune power.

3. Add More Zinc to Your Diet.

Emergen-C may be your go-to whenever you feel those chills and sweats coming on. Which is all well and good—vitamin C enriches immunity—but you ought to add zinc to your regimen too. The essential trace element acts like an antioxidant in the diet, thus protecting you from free radical damage. It plays a vital role in a number of biochemical pathways and possesses antiviral properties. A zinc deficiency, on the other hand, may harm immunity and increase your susceptibility to infection.

Women 19 and older should aim for 8 mg of zinc per day; men within the same age category should get 11 mg daily. Supplements that have been chelated (meaning, they're bound to a compound to enhance the mineral's absorption) can help certify that you're getting adequate amounts. Be sure to pair zinc with copper, as excess zinc could affect copper levels in your body. (An optimal combo is 15 mg of zinc to 1 mg of copper.) Additionally, fill your plate with zinc-rich foods, such as pecans, peanuts, wild rice, green peas, yogurt, oysters and pork loin.

Already suffering from a cold? Zinc supplements (syrup, lozenges or tablets) can reduce the length of it—especially when taken within the first 24 hours of exhibiting symptoms.

4. Dodge the Dessert Table.

Gingerbread cookies at the office, eggnog at home, peppermint bark at your beloved coffee shop—it seems that tempting treats are everywhere during the winter months. As tantalizing as they may be, it's more important than ever to pay attention to your diet during winter. Not only do fresh fruits and vegetables brim with immune-boosting antioxidants, but sugar—which is ubiquitous this time of year—can wreak havoc on your ability to combat sickness. As nutritionist Monica Reinagel wrote in *Scientific American*, "Eat-

ing sugar may put your white blood cells into temporary coma"—meaning that fudge your neighbor made may suppress your immune response and decrease its ability to respond to challenges. Whether you have a yen for something sweet or need to use sugar in a recipe, call upon alternatives for the same fix: Stevia and monk fruit are excellent substitutes.

5. Prioritize Sleep.

The holiday season is ripe with wonder and excitement—but it's also marked by countless to-dos that can leak right into your sleep schedule. Sleep, however, is as fundamental to your capacity to fight off infections as hydration and exercise. The National Institutes of Health reports that a lack of sleep not only reduces immunity but also produces changes in both circulating immune cells and cytokines—a category of signaling molecules that help moderate immunity. In other words, when the clock strikes midnight as you're still signing Christmas cards, ask yourself if it's worth the toll that burning the candle on both ends takes. Your holiday spirit will be brighter—and you'll be able to knock off more of your tasks faster—if you get eight hours of quality slumber per night.

6. Plunge into Hydrotherapy.

On an icy winter's night, the last thing you'll likely want to do is take a chilly shower—and yet the last place you want to find yourself on Christmas morning is huddled under the covers. Hydrotherapy—wherein you alternate between hot and cold water—is a mainstay in naturopathy, physiotherapy and occupational therapy for good cause: According to the *Journal of Advanced Pharmaceutical Technology & Research*, the technique, formerly known as hydropathy, "boosts the immune system by its efficient functioning and also improves internal organs by stimulating blood supply." The journal also goes on to say that "Conclusively, it can be elucidated that in the future hydrotherapy will become a major tool for stress relieving, improving body function, and preventing illness." For best results, take a super-hot shower, flip to the coldest temp at full blast for 10 to 20 seconds, return to hot for one minute, and back to cold for another 10 to 20 seconds. Perform this three times per day—and always end your shower on cold. (That's what warm, fluffy towels are made for!)

7. Indulge in a Warming, Herbal Tea.

We all know that herbal teas can offer a cornucopia of health benefits, thanks to their inclusion of unique antioxidants called flavonoids. Winter chills, in particular, can be soothed with a warming, nourishing homemade tea. Add two inches of sliced, raw ginger, one cinnamon stick, one teaspoon of clove, and a pinch of black pepper to eight ounces of water. Simmer on low heat for 20 minutes and serve. (Add a dash of almond milk for more flavor.) The ingredients in this recipe honor Traditional Chinese Medicine's belief that warming herbs such as these increase circulation during cold, damp weather. What's more, ginger's rich phytochemistry provides an anti-inflammatory affect (and antimicrobial benefits), while cloves can enhance immune responses. The scent of the tea itself will evoke this festive time of year—and give you even greater motivation to stay on top of your health.

For Better Health, Balance Your Hormones with Food

Neal D. Barnard, MD, FACC, adjunct associate professor of medicine at George Washington University School of Medicine, president of Physicians Committee for Responsible Medicine and founder of Barnard Medical Center, all in Washington, DC. He is also author of 20 books, including, most recently, *Your Body in Balance: The New Science of Food, Hormones and Health.* PCRM.org

Most people equate hormonal imbalances with hot flashes and mood swings in menopausal women. But scratch the surface, and you'll see that out-of-whack hormones also can set the stage for a wide range of conditions, including cancer, diabetes and depression.

Now: A growing body of evidence shows that potentially dangerous hormonal imbalances respond quickly to changes in diet.

Why Hormones Matter

Most people don't realize the crucial role that hormones play in overall health. You can think of it this way—it's your hormones that provide the "operating instructions" for every organ in your body to work effectively.

Secreted by one of many endocrine glands—from the pineal gland within the brain, to the testicles and ovaries of the reproductive system—hormones speed and slow your metabolism…determine how you store and burn fat…control reproduction and sexuality…affect your moods…and more.

Research shows that compounds in certain foods are the single biggest factor in balancing hormones to create clear instructions within the body.

Hormone-Balancing Foods

The hormone-balancing diet I recommend is plant based, consisting of four primary food groups—vegetables, fruits, whole grains and legumes (beans, lentils, peas). As both research and clinical experience show, this vegan diet works in many ways to balance hormones.

While you might imagine that a vegan diet is challenging to follow, it turns out to be surprisingly easy. It is simple to have bean chili instead of meat chili or to enjoy a tasty tomato-based sauce on your pasta instead of a meat or cream sauce. For complete nutrition, get vegetables, fruits, whole grains and legumes…and add a B-12 supplement (at least 2.4 mcg daily).

Here's how to select the foods you need to help prevent, control and even reverse these hormone-related conditions…

Breast Cancer

Breast cancer is a serious condition. A combination of treatments is often necessary, so you should see your doctor and follow his/her guidance. Even so, hormone-balancing foods can play a vital role.

Excess estrogen is a common driver of breast cancer. For example, women with higher levels of the estrogen estradiol in the bloodstream have twice the cancer risk as women with lower levels.

In breast cells, estrogen can damage DNA—turning a healthy cell into a cancer cell. Once a cancer cell arises, high levels of estrogen can stimulate it to multiply. *To balance estrogen…*

• **Cut the fat.** There is evidence to suggest that any type of fatty food increases estrogen. And fat cells themselves are hormone factories, producing even more estrogen. Avoid animal fats, as well as coconut and palm oils, which are also high in saturated fat. Skip margarine and butter, too. Go easy on vegetable oils, including olive oil.

Instead, use non-oil cooking methods, such as steaming, boiling, baking or sautéing in vegetable broth. For an alternative to oily salad dressings, try lemon juice. For packaged foods, check the label and favor those with 3 g of fat or less per serving.

• **Eliminate dairy.** Research on dairy's link to breast cancer has been mixed. However, recent evidence has increasingly found that it plays an important role in how women do after a breast cancer diagnosis. For example, women previously diagnosed with breast cancer who consumed one or more daily servings of high-fat dairy products had a 49% higher risk of dying of their cancer compared with breast cancer patients who ate fewer servings of full-fat dairy or low-fat dairy, according to a study published in *Journal of the National Cancer Institute*. If you really love milk or yogurt, choose non-dairy varieties, such as almond milk or soy yogurt.

• **Boost fiber.** Fiber helps protect against breast cancer. Women with breast cancer who ate at least five servings a day of fiber-rich fruits and vegetables (and were also physically active) cut their risk of dying from the disease by 50%, according to a study published in *Journal of Clinical Oncology*. Aim for 40 g of fiber a day—daily servings of beans, vegetables, fruits and grains will get you there.

• **Add soy.** Soybeans contain isoflavones that reduce the risk of developing breast cancer and, for women who have breast cancer already, improve cancer survival. In numerous studies, women in Asian countries who consume the most soy (about two servings a day) have about a 30% lower risk of developing breast cancer than those who consume less soy. Good choices include tofu, miso soup and soy milk.

Diabetes

Blood sugar (glucose) is transported into your cells by insulin, a hormone made in the pancreas. If you have type 2 diabetes, your insulin isn't working right—a problem called insulin resistance. From a dietary perspective, the culprit is fat—beef fat, chicken fat, fryer grease, you name it.

Here's why: Dietary fat turns into microscopic fat particles that block insulin action in muscle and liver cells, interfering with insulin's ability to work. *To balance insulin…*

• **Skip animal products such as meat, fish, poultry, eggs and dairy products.** Limit vegetable oils, too.

• **Avoid plant-based foods that are high in fat.** It turns out that any type of fat can interfere with insulin action—even "good" fats. This includes nuts, peanut butter, seeds and avocados.

• **Eat more raw foods, such as fresh fruits and salads.** They promote weight loss—and fat loss. Certain vegetables—such as broccoli and kale—are hard to digest raw. But others, such as carrots and salad greens, are easier.

• **Don't exclude healthy carbohydrate-rich foods, such as sweet potatoes, beans and fruit.** Remember, the cause of insulin resistance is fat buildup—carbohydrates from whole plant foods are not a problem. In my approach to balancing hormones in diabetes, there are no limits on healthful carbohydrates, but I recommend avoiding high glycemic-index foods that cause blood sugar to spike.

Examples: Instead of wheat bread, opt for rye and pumpernickel, which have less effect on blood sugar. Instead of cold cereals, choose old-fashioned oatmeal.

Depression and Norepinephrine

The scientific link between hormones and depression is intriguing, but not definitive. However, research shows that the hormones that control blood pressure—such as norepinephrine (noradrenaline, from the adrenal gland)—also control your emotional state. And low levels of norepinephrine can cause depression. *To balance norepinephrine...*

• **Eat more vegetables.** A study in *Public Health Nutrition* found that people who eat the most vegetables are 62% less likely to develop depression than people who eat the least.

• **Get more soy.** Consuming two to four soy servings per day may have a significant antidepressant effect, according to research published in *Menopause.* This perhaps explains the low prevalence of depression among Japanese people on traditional soy-rich diets. Have two servings per day. A serving would be a cup of soy milk or two to three-and-a-half ounces of tofu.

Tasty Recipes for a Hormone-Balancing Diet

Excerpted from the book *Your Body in Balance: The New Science of Food, Hormones, and Health* by Neal D. Barnard, MD, FACC, with *Menus and Recipes* by Lindsay S. Nixon. Copyright © 2020 by Neal D. Barnard, MD. Recipe text copyright © 2020 by Lindsay S. Nixon. Reprinted with permission of Grand Central Publishing. All rights reserved.

Even though it's not well known, hormone imbalances contribute to a variety of health problems, ranging from breast cancer and prostate cancer to diabetes and depression.

Good news: A plant-based diet focusing on vegetables, fruits, whole grains and legumes can significantly improve the body's hormonal balance, according to an increasing body of scientific evidence.

For a sampling of delicious, easy-to-prepare recipes that incorporate these foods, try the following for...

Breakfast

Green Smoothie Muffins

2 cups flour

½ cup brown or raw sugar

1 teaspoon baking soda

½ teaspoon ground cinnamon (optional)

Zest of 1 lemon

1½ cups (8 ounces) pineapple chunks (fresh or frozen)

2 cups fresh spinach

1-2 very ripe bananas

1 Tablespoon vanilla extract

¼ cup plain soy or almond milk

Preheat oven to 375°F and line a muffin pan with paper liners or silicone cups, or use a nonstick pan.

In a large bowl, whisk together flour, sugar, baking soda, cinnamon and lemon zest. Set aside. In a blender, combine pineapple, spinach, bananas, vanilla and milk. Blend until creamy. Pour wet mixture into dry ingredients and stir until just combined. If the batter is dry, add 2-4 tablespoons milk. Spoon batter evenly into muffin cups.

Bake 20-25 minutes or until an inserted toothpick comes out clean. Let cool completely before serving.

Makes 12 muffins.

Per muffin: 124 calories...3 g protein... 27 g carbohydrates...10 g sugar...0.5 g total fat...2% calories from fat...1 g fiber...113 mg sodium.

Sandwich or Wrap

BBQ Bean Tortas

8 (6-inch) corn tortillas or 4 hamburger buns

1 (15-ounce) can low-sodium black beans, drained and rinsed

½ cup barbecue sauce

½ cup chopped pineapple

1 cup fresh salsa (or diced tomato)

Guacamole (optional)

If using tortillas, preheat oven to 375°F. Bake corn tortillas for 5-10 minutes or until crisp. If using hamburger buns, toast in oven.

Warm beans with barbecue sauce. Spoon onto tortillas or buns and top with pineapple, salsa and guacamole, if desired.

Makes 4 servings.

Per serving: 293 calories...9 g protein... 61 g carbohydrate...18 g sugar...2 g total fat ...6% calories from fat...11 g fiber...579 mg sodium.

Main Dish

Butternut Pasta

3-4 cups diced butternut squash (about 1 medium squash)

1 cup sliced mushrooms

1½ cups uncooked pasta

4 chopped dry-pack sun-dried tomatoes

1 cup canned low-sodium chickpeas (or navy beans), drained and rinsed

2 cups fresh arugula (or spinach)

¼ cup fat-free balsamic vinaigrette

Vegan parmesan (optional)

Preheat oven to 375°F and line a baking sheet with parchment paper. Place squash cubes in a single layer in the pan. Roast for 20-30 minutes or until fork tender and browning at the edges, turning halfway. Add mushrooms to the pan halfway through roasting the squash.

Cook pasta as directed on package, adding sun-dried tomatoes and chickpeas (or navy beans) to the water with the pasta. Drain and transfer to a bowl. Immediately add roasted squash and mushrooms and toss. Serve over (or mix in) arugula (or spinach) and drizzle with balsamic vinaigrette. Sprinkle with vegan parmesan, if desired.

Makes 2 servings.

Per serving: 642 calories...25 g protein ...126 g carbohydrate...13 g sugar...6 g total fat...7% calories from fat...17 g fiber...351 mg sodium.

Press Here for Better Health

Deborah Flanagan, clinical reflexologist and founder of Center for True Health in New York City. *CenterTrueHealth.com*

Did you know that the answer to your sinus congestion problem might be found in your fingers? Or the cure for constipation found in your feet? Reflexology is based on the concept that our hands and feet contain nerve endings that form a map of the entire body. You can learn to do this safe therapy at home for relief from common health concerns such as back pain, allergy symptoms and even insomnia.

How it works: When you apply pressure to key points on your hands and feet, you activate nerve endings and help your nervous and circulatory systems get your body into better balance. Our nerve endings are connected to spinal nerves as well as to corresponding organs. Each can be reached by a point on the feet or hands. (For instance, the side of your thumb matches up with your spine.)

Reflexology has solid scientific research behind it. Back in 1993, the first US reflexology study published in a peer-reviewed medical journal, *Obstetrics & Gynecology*, studied the effects of reflexology on premenstrual syndrome (PMS). The study showed a 46% reduction in premenstrual symptoms.

More recently, the National Center for Complementary and Integrative Health awarded a second round of funding to Michigan State University researchers to continue studying the impact of reflexology on women undergoing chemotherapy for advanced breast cancer. So far, patients have shown improvement in shortness of breath, as well as in 10 areas of physical activity. Meanwhile, preliminary research out of The Ohio State University's Comprehensive Cancer Center is looking at the effect of reflexology and aromatherapy in women undergoing breast cancer radiation treatment—it suggests that the combo reduces pain by 60% and anxiety by 20%.

As a clinical reflexologist trained in this noninvasive, holistic therapy, I see the benefits in my clients every day. While reflexology generally is very safe, there are a few caveats. If you have unchecked diabetes, a blood clot or foot injuries or sores, you should check with your doctor first. And of course, remember that reflexology is a complementary therapy, not a substitute for medical care.

These are some of my favorite techniques that you can do at home for common health complaints. Relax, take off your socks and get hands-on for better health.

Fix Gut Woes

This move regulates and supports your GI system to help with constipation, gas and indigestion.

Equipment: Golf ball (or other similarly sized hard ball).

How to do it: Interlock your fingers.

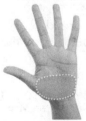

1. Roll the ball around the lower area of your palms, or heels, of your hands. This corresponds to the digestive reflexes for the small and large intestines.

*Credit:*Gettyimages/ sam74100

2. Continue rolling the ball for one minute.

Rx: Do this once or twice a week for two weeks. Then, as needed.

Roll Away a Bloated Belly

Rolling the soles of your feet is great for gastric distress and relieving bloating in particular. This is one of my personal favorite self-help techniques.

Equipment: Wooden foot roller.

How to do it: Roll underneath your arches on the soles of your feet with a wooden foot roller.

Rx: Do this after a big meal when you're feeling puffy. Do this for one to two minutes on each foot.

Beat Insomnia

This technique is great if you're having trouble sleeping. You press a point on your thumb that is the reflex for the pituitary gland. The pituitary gland oversees the entire endocrine system (especially the adrenals, which are involved with cortisol levels and stress), so this is a really important point to help the body balance itself.

Equipment: None.

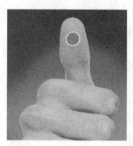

*Credit:*Gettyimages/alvarez

How to do it…

1. Find the middle of the whorl of your thumbprint. This is the reflex for the pituitary gland.

2. Using the side of one thumb, press that thumb's nail firmly into the center of the whorl of the other thumbprint and hold for 45 seconds. How do you know if you found the right spot?

Here are some clues: It might feel like a little metal ball under the skin. Or it might feel like you stuck a needle in your thumb. This area might feel more sensitive if you've had trouble sleeping lately.

3. Repeat with the other thumb.

Rx: Press this spot on both thumbs two to three times a day to sleep more soundly on a regular basis. And next time you wake up in the middle of the night, you'll know what to do.

Relieve Allergy and Sinus Congestion

The fingers contain the reflexes for the head and sinuses. This move alleviates any kind of congestion—and the best part is that it often works right away.

Equipment: Just your hands!

How to do it…

1. Turn your hand palm-up. Press and rub from the base of each finger to the tip.

2. Switch hands, and repeat until you've done all 10 fingers.

Rx: Do this on each finger on both hands a few times, and repeat three or four times a day or as needed.

Banish Back Pain

When you frequently have a sore back, it's hard to find DIY solutions that help ease the pain, so this move is a great one to know. Since this reflex area covers your whole spine, this trick helps alleviate upper- and lower-back pain.

Equipment: None.

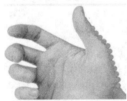

Credit: iStock.com/GCapture

How to do it…

1. The outside of the thumb down to the wrist contains the spine reflex. Starting with the left hand, press there with the right thumb, inching along from the top of the thumb down to the wrist.

2. Repeat on the right hand using the left thumb to press. Anywhere tender? That's normal if you're experiencing back pain. Spend more time on tender areas, but don't apply a lot of pressure if it hurts. "No pain no gain" doesn't apply with reflexology!

Rx: Do this on both hands, go down this area three or four times, and repeat three or four times a day.

Treat PMS or Menopause Complaints

This move, the Wrist Twist, helps women with symptoms such as cramping from PMS and hot flashes during perimenopause and menopause. The reflexes for the ovaries and uterus are on the sides of the wrist. Just don't expect instant relief—addressing hormonal imbalances and reproductive issues takes time, usually three months of weekly sessions. I also use the Wrist Twist on men who have issues with their testes or prostate.

Equipment: None.

How to do it…

1. Using your right thumb and forefinger, create a loose bracelet around your left wrist. Rotate your left wrist and forearm.

2. Do the same on the right wrist.

Rx: Rotate each wrist 20 times or so, two or three times a day.

Religion: The Health Booster No One Talks About

Harold G. Koenig, MD, professor of psychiatry and behavioral sciences, associate professor of medicine and senior fellow in the Center for the Study of Aging and Human Development at Duke University in Durham, North Carolina. He is author of *Medicine, Religion and Health, Spirituality in Patient Care* and *Religion and Mental Health.*

Whether you're being urged to get more exercise, eat better or take your medication, physicians dole out plenty of advice on ways to improve your health. But when is the last time your doctor told you to attend religious services? Most likely, never.

But for people who want to do everything possible to stay healthy, this is a recommendation worth considering.

Even though there's been a steady flow of research linking religious observance to everything from lower blood pressure and less cardiovascular disease to better immune function and higher levels of overall well-being, religion's health-promoting benefits don't get much attention.

Why does religion promote good health… and how can people tap into this remarkable benefit? To learn more, we spoke with Harold G. Koenig, MD, a renowned authority on religion and health.

Do the health benefits linked to religion apply only to certain faiths?

No. Studies finding health benefits have included people of many faiths and spiritual traditions, including Christians, Jews, Muslims, Hindus and Buddhists.

Does it matter how often someone attends services?

Definitely. People who attend services once or more each week see more health benefits than those who attend less frequently. In fact, that's one of the strongest and most consistent findings in studies of religion and health, according to an important research review published in 2017 in *Current Directions in Psychological Science.* One study cited in the review found that regularly attending religious services over the course of a lifetime translated into about seven additional years of life. Other studies suggest that the effects on longevity are as strong as those seen for cholesterol-lowering drugs.

Do some people seem to benefit more than others?

Yes. Studies find stronger associations between religion and health in women and older adults compared with men and younger adults. We also know that women and older adults in the US are more likely to attend services, to pray and to say that religion is important in their lives, according to data from the Pew Research Center.

However, some people with strong beliefs become more distraught if their illness persists or worsens. They may even lose faith if they feel that their prayers have gone unanswered.

How does religion help people deal with chronic illness?

Some of the benefits are social. That's because people who belong to a religious institution have a reliable source of social connection and support—one that will not disappear when, for example, someone becomes too ill to work or participate in hobbies and recreational activities. It helps, too, that most religions put a high value on helping others in distress and have systems in place to assist members in times of need.

People with strong religious beliefs also may find it easier to see meaning and purpose in their illness. They may view it as part of a larger plan and believe that their suffering will be rewarded or will reveal new life lessons. Religious scriptures, from many traditions, provide role models for such fortitude.

Many religious groups also encourage healthy lifestyles—such as not smoking or abusing drugs or alcohol. There is one downside, though, to all those social hall suppers—religious people are more likely than others to be overweight, according to research.

What role does prayer play?

No clear link has been established in the scientific literature between prayer and longevity, though the research could be skewed by the fact that people already battling health problems may tend to pray more. But prayer can be a powerful coping strategy.

One theory is that people who pray may gain an indirect sense of control over their stressful circumstances—by believing that a higher power is in control and that praying can lead to change, the believer may feel more internal control than someone who feels all the power is in the hands of other people, such as doctors.

Should I discuss my religious beliefs with my health-care providers or keep them private?

In an ideal world, your medical providers would ask you about your religious beliefs. One big reason is that your beliefs may affect the decisions you make about your care. You cannot have honest discussions with your doctors if they do not know your values. Your care providers also should know where you get social and practical support. If that includes a house of worship, it should be part of the conversation.

They should also know if you have unmet spiritual needs—and would, for example, like to receive visits from a hospital chaplain. So if religion is important to you, but your providers do not bring it up, you should definitely speak up. That said, don't let any health-care provider try to impose his/her religious views on you.

Is religion ever used as part of formal treatment?

Yes. When patients want such help, some mental-health providers now offer a technique called "religiously integrated cognitive behavioral therapy." The idea is to combine a patient's religious beliefs with evidence-based cognitive behavioral therapy (CBT) techniques to relieve depression or other forms of psychological distress.

When chronically ill patients who were Christian, Jewish, Muslim, Hindu or Buddhist received psychotherapy that incorporated their religious beliefs, it was as effective as conventional CBT in treating depression, according to research published in *The Journal of Nervous and Mental Disease.*

As in other forms of CBT, the goal is to identify and change unhealthy patterns of thinking and behavior. The twist is that therapists ask clients to use passages of scripture from their religious traditions to reinforce those healthier ways of thinking and behaving.

Helpful: If you're interested in religiously integrated CBT, speak to your therapist about using workbooks (for Christians, Jews, Muslims, Hindus and Buddhists) that are available for free from Duke University's Center for Spirituality, Theology and Health. Go to SpiritualityAndHealth.Duke.edu.

What about nonbelievers—can they also get benefits from religion?

Belief in a higher power is not necessary to tap into some of the elements of religion that help people deal with a chronic medical condition, pain, disability, financial strain and the other burdens that can come with illness. Many people can benefit from building strong social connections and doing good for others. Meditation is not exactly the same as prayer, but it can help reduce pain and produce other health benefits, such as reducing anxiety, lowering blood pressure and improving sleep problems.

Likewise, studying philosophy can be as uplifting for some as studying scripture is for others. And of course, adopting healthy habits, such as not smoking, not drinking too much and getting plenty of exercise, requires no religious faith. However, current studies do show that religion offers additional benefits to those who follow these health-promoting practices.

New—and Natural— Ways to Power Up Your Energy Levels

Jacob Teitelbaum, MD, a Kona, Hawaii–based board-certified internist and nationally known expert in chronic fatigue syndrome, fibromyalgia, sleep and pain. He is author of numerous books, including From Fatigued to Fantastic. Learn more at Energy AnalysisProgram.com

Are you in an "energy crisis"—with a bad diet, poor sleep habits, too many commitments and too much stress causing you to feel exhausted and depleted? You don't have to live that way! *Here are seven natural, easy-to-do energy hacks that can dramatically restore your vim and vigor…*

HACK #1: **Check your magnesium— you're likely deficient.** Low magnesium is linked to low energy and even to chronic fatigue syndrome (CFS). Magnesium is essential to many body functions (especially muscle function), regulates heartbeat and helps convert food into energy. Since the mineral is not produced in our bodies, we need to get it from dietary sources. The typical heavily processed American diet does not provide the daily Recommended Dietary Allowance of magnesium—420 mg for men and 320 mg for women.

Power up: Cut back or eliminate processed food. Stick to fresh foods or foods with less than five ingredients on their labels. Good dietary sources of magnesium include leafy greens, seeds, nuts and whole grains. Also consider taking a 150-mg to 200-mg magnesium supplement daily.

Bonus: Taking the supplement at night can help improve sleep quality.

Note: Magnesium supplements are generally considered safe but can cause diarrhea in some people. If that happens, cut back the daily dose to 75 mg. Magnesium glycinate and magnesium aspartate are good forms to take. Check with your doctor before starting magnesium if you take medication or have a chronic medical condition.

HACK #2: Get more D-ribose.

D-ribose, a type of sugar produced by the body, plays a key role in production of *adenosine triphosphate* (ATP), the primary molecule that provides energy to every cell in the body. Our bodies manufacture some D-ribose naturally, but you may need more.

Power up: D-ribose supplements are available in a powder that can be stirred into coffee, tea or a smoothie. Look online or in health-food stores for brands with "Bioenergy Ribose" on the label, such as Doctor's Best Pure D-Ribose Powder, NOW D-Ribose Powder or my own brand, SHINE D-Ribose. Bioenergy Ribose is formulated to be more bioavailable—other kinds may not offer the same results.

Typical dose: 5 g every morning.

Note: D-ribose can lower blood sugar, which may affect dosing of diabetes drugs.

HACK #3: Cut out or minimize toxic relationships.
Being around people we enjoy or engaging in activities that bring us pleasure gives us energy. Doing things we loathe, or being with angry, abusive, manipulative or pessimistic people, depletes our energy levels.

Power up: Keep healthy boundaries. If spending time with a particular friend, colleague or family member drains you, find ways to limit or cut out interactions with that person. Of course, it may be easier to cut off a strained friendship than a relative. Simply learn to say "no" to interactions that feel bad. This can often be done without disconnecting from the person.

Simple trick: For difficult people whom you would like to (or need to) keep around, focus only on aspects of them that make you feel good and ignore the rest. After about eight weeks, it's very likely that only those aspects will show up in your relationship—or the person will no longer be part of your life.

HACK #4: Hydrate with cold water.
According to the Natural Hydration Council in the UK, symptoms such as fatigue and lack of energy account for one in five doctor visits… and for one out of 10 of such patients, dehydration is the primary culprit. Afternoon energy slumps are especially common—partly because we get busy and forget to drink…or a heavy lunch can put our parasympathetic nervous system into "rest and digest mode."

Power up: When you feel your energy dipping, drink 12 ounces of cold water. Or splash cold water on your face. The cold temperature stimulates adrenaline receptors in your skin, which signals your heart to pump harder and drives an energizing blood flow to your brain…while the water hydrates you.

HACK #5: Check your medications.
Statins, such as *atorvastatin* (Lipitor), *rosuvastatin* (Crestor) and *simvastatin* (Zocor), lower cholesterol…but also lower levels of coenzyme Q10 (CoQ10), a vitamin-like substance that helps maintain energy levels. Proton pump inhibitors (PPIs) for heartburn, gastroesophageal reflux disease and ulcers, such as *omeprazole* (Prilosec) and *esomeprazole* (Nexium), cut stomach acid production. But long-term use impairs absorption

of key energy-producing nutrients, including magnesium, vitamin B-12 and iron.

Power up: If you need a statin, ask your doctor about taking a CoQ10 supplement as well. A typical dose is 200 mg per day taken with a meal that contains fat to boost absorption. If you take a PPI, ask your doctor if you can switch to an H2-blocker, such as *ranitidine* (Zantac) or *cimetidine* (Tagamet). Research shows that they are far safer. These drugs reduce stomach acid but don't block it as completely as PPIs do, so nutrient deficiencies are less likely to occur.

HACK #6: Caffeinate...strategically. Caffeine is considered to be an adenosine blocker. (Adenosine triggers sleep and is not the same as energy-producing ATP.) Caffeine attaches to the same receptors in the brain that adenosine attaches to and prevents the drowsiness that occurs as adenosine levels rise during the day. But coffee also can cause a jittery, wired feeling and stomach upset.

Power up: Green tea is gentler than coffee, with about 25 mg of caffeine per cup versus 100 mg to 200 mg for coffee—enough to still kick your energy up a notch. According to a review of nearly 50 studies, just 40 mg of caffeine is enough to provide stimulating effects. Green tea is also rich in theanine, an amino acid that promotes calm alertness and improves deep sleep.

HACK #7: Wind down wisely. You've probably heard a lot of sleep-hygiene advice, such as powering down electronics an hour or two before bed and sleeping in a cool room. *Also try...*

Power up #1: Soak in a warm bath with two cups of Epsom salts added an hour before bedtime. The magnesium from the Epsom salts soothes tired muscles and eases stress, promoting a good night's sleep.

Note: Soaking in a warm bath can lower blood pressure and might make you feel light-headed. Be careful getting out of the bath, especially if you already have low blood pressure.

Power up #2: Eat a small protein-rich snack, such as a hard-boiled egg or a few tablespoons of cottage cheese, before bedtime to prevent blood sugar drops that often wake people up in the middle of the night.

Why Sunlight Can Be Good for Your Eyes

Marc Grossman, OD, LAc, doctor of optometry and licensed acupuncturist in New Paltz and Somers, New York. He is coauthor of *Natural Eye Care: Your Guide to Healthy Vision*. A holistic eye doctor, his multidisciplinary approach uses nutrition, lifestyle changes and Traditional Chinese Medicine to tackle eye problems. NaturalEyeCare.com

You think you take good care of your eyes. You wear sunglasses outdoors and get regular eye exams. But did you know that exercise, stress and even mindfulness practices can impact eye health? Holistic optometrist Dr. Marc Grossman suggests 10 natural ways to show your eyes some love—and see your way to healthy vision for years to come.

• **Pay attention to your posture.** The eyes are extensions of the brain and part of our central nervous system. Signals and messages are sent from the eyes to the visual cortex in the brain, which processes and sends the information down the spinal cord to the rest of the body. Poor posture can disrupt these connections and lead to blurred vision, and conversely, visual strain can result in poor posture. To avoid this, when sitting, keep your chest up, shoulders back and weight over your seat so that both eyes are at task level and an equal distance from what is being seen. Always sit upright while reading or watching television instead of lying on your back, side or stomach.

• **Seek out sunlight.** Walking is one of the best things we can do for exercise, and depending where you walk, it has another benefit—natural sunlight. The eyes are light-sensing organs. It's important to get enough sunlight so that your eyes operate optimally. In fact, a recent study published in *JAMA Ophthalmology* found that increased exposure to sunlight reduces your risk for myopia (nearsightedness). Aim for at least 20 minutes of natural sunlight a day—just be sure to wear sunglasses that provide 100% UV protection and filter out both UVA and UVB rays.

• **Go Mediterranean.** The health-promoting effects of the Mediterranean diet—which emphasizes eating mostly vegetables, fruits, legumes, whole grains, nuts and seeds...and limiting animal products and sweets—are well-known. Yet few people realize that adhering to this eating plan also can greatly reduce their risk for age-related macular degeneration (AMD), the leading cause of irreversible vision loss and blindness after age 50. Most recently, a large-scale European study published in *Ophthalmology* investigated the connection between genes and lifestyle on the development of AMD and found that those who ate a primarily Mediterranean diet were 41% less likely to develop AMD than those who did not. Interestingly, it wasn't any of the specific components that lowered AMD risk. Rather, it was the overall pattern of consistently consuming a nutrient-rich diet that mattered.

• **Cut back on sugar.** Sugar is lurking in so much of what we consume—from beverages to processed foods to desserts—and it's not just bad for your teeth and your weight. Higher sugar intake also is associated with an increased risk of developing—as well as worsening—most eye conditions, such as cataracts, glaucoma and AMD. In the case of cataracts, high blood sugar levels limit the ability of the eye to keep the lens clear. High blood sugar also can cause the blood vessels in the eye to narrow, creating a buildup of fluid that can lead to glaucoma. And people with type 2 diabetes are at risk for a condition known as diabetic retinopathy. Their blood sugar levels have to be carefully regulated with the right amount of insulin or the blood vessels in the eye can leak, which may cause spots in their vision that can lead to severe impairment or blindness.

• **Get moving.** Aerobic exercise not only benefits your heart, it also has been linked to improved retinal health and prevention of eye disease. Exercise raises oxygen levels in the cells and increases lymph and blood circulation. This increased circulation is a prerequisite for good vision. In addition, research published in *The Journal of Neuroscience* has found that moderate aerobic exercise may be able to delay the progression of AMD by preserving the structure and function of the nerve cells in the retina. Get 20 minutes of aerobic exercise daily by walking, swimming or doing any other activity that you enjoy.

• **Don't forget about vision fitness.** Simple eye exercises will ease discomfort and support healthy vision. *Try figure eights to increase the flexibility of your eye muscles in a relaxed way...*

• Stand or sit with your feet shoulder-width apart, hands at your sides.

• Imagine a horizontal figure eight (as wide as is comfortable) about 10 feet away.

• Without moving your head, trace the figure eight with your eyes in one direction, then in the opposite direction. Remember to breathe normally and blink your eyes regularly as they move along the figure eight. Repeat several times. Do this for two minutes twice a day.

• **Change focus.** Don't keep your eyes locked on a computer or television or any other screen for a sustained period of time. Doing so causes tension on the visual system. We don't blink as much when we're staring at something, which dries out the cornea and exhausts the eye muscles. To change your focus when you're doing close-up work, look up and away often—such as out a window—to give your eyes a break.

Try the 20-20-20 rule: Every 20 minutes, look at something 20 feet away for 20 seconds.

• **Relax your eyes.** Relax the muscles around your eyes, and bring healing energy to your eyes through increased circulation and energy flow with a technique called palming. This is especially useful after long periods of computer use. *How to do it…*

• Remove your glasses or contact lenses, and sit leaning forward with your elbows resting on a table and your eyes closed.

• Place the palm of your left hand over your left eye, with your fingers on your forehead, the hollow of your palm directly over your eye (but not touching it), and the heel of your hand resting on your left cheekbone.

• Do the same thing with your right palm over the right eye and the right fingers crossing over the fingers of your left hand and the heel of your hand resting on your right cheekbone.

• Remain this way for three minutes, remembering to breathe normally.

• **Go the distance.** The eye muscles are most relaxed when using our distance vision because that's what they were designed for. Nowadays, to keep your eyes in top shape, make an effort to perform outdoor activities that require seeing at a distance, such as playing golf or tennis, riding a bike or just walking. When walking, keep your head up and scan the horizon. Indoors, do reading, writing or close-up work with an eye-to-activity distance of roughly 14 to 16 inches for adults. Watch TV from a distance of about eight to 10 feet for most large-screen TVs.

• **Be mindful.** It's no secret that mental stress affects the immune and respiratory systems and causes inflammation throughout the body. But did you know that stress-reduction techniques can have a specific impact on glaucoma? Your body can't deliver essential nutrients to your eyes if stress is impairing circulation and digestion. Destress by practicing proven mindfulness techniques such as meditation, deep breathing and yoga. Inversion poses in yoga, such as downward dog, also benefit vision because they increase blood flow to the head (consult your doctor first if you have glaucoma or high blood pressure).

An intriguing new study published in *Journal of Glaucoma* found that meditation in particular may be especially helpful for glau-coma patients. Hour-long, daily mindful-meditation sessions for just three weeks resulted in a significant reduction in eye pressure and in levels of the stress hormone cortisol, helping to minimize optic damage. Even five to 20 minutes a day can be very helpful.

Use Your Sense of Smell

Alan R. Hirsch, MD, board-certified neurologist and psychiatrist specializing in the treatment of smell and taste loss, and neurological director of Smell & Taste Treatment and Research Foundation, Ltd., in Chicago. He has published hundreds of studies on smell in journals such as *Neurology, Headache* and *International Journal of Aromatherapy.* SmellAnd Taste.org

W e've all heard that smell is our "most powerful" sense—touching our hearts with the fond memory of the aroma of Grandma's famous lasagna or Mom's perfume or bringing us the heady whiff of new-car leather. Beyond triggering memories, scents and aromas actually can affect our energy levels, improve memory and even enrich relationships.

It's not surprising that people tend to be happier and more optimistic in environments that smell pleasing to them. Most everyone can smell, and with a little guidance, you can tap into scents' true potentials. *Here's how to use scent to your advantage…*

To Improve Your Love Life

Did you know that purposefully inhaling certain scents may help fuel your libido? Perhaps not surprisingly, sweet scents are associated with arousal in both men and women.

As odd as it sounds, however, it is a combination of donuts and black licorice that increased male sexual arousal, boosting penile blood flow by more than 30%, per research from the Smell & Taste Treatment and Research Foundation. For another sexy combo, try pumpkin pie and donuts. These scents combined increased penile blood flow by 20%.

Women also are affected by black licorice. A blend of the scents of Good & Plenty licorice candy and banana-nut bread enhanced female sexual arousal by 18%. Oddly, a lone vegetable makes it onto the sexiest scents list—a combination of cucumber and Good & Plenty stimulated women.

Scientists theorize that these odors work by reducing anxiety, which in turn reduces inhibitions. That can lead to enhanced sexual desire.

To Resist Cravings

Go ahead and breathe in those freshly baked smells at the grocery store. A 2019 University of South Florida study found that smelling indulgent foods such as pizza or cookies for an extended period of time actually can help ward off cravings. Subjects who were exposed to these ambient scents for longer than two minutes while in a supermarket were less likely to purchase "unhealthy foods," compared with those who shopped with no ambient scent or in the presence of a "nonindulgent food–related ambient scent" such as strawberry or roast turkey.

Scientists hypothesize that the brain may derive sufficient sensory pleasure from the aroma of the food alone, without even tasting it. In essence, you can fool the brain into thinking that you have eaten the goodie already.

Helpful idea: If you're trying to avoid sugary indulgences at an office meeting or party, just wait a few minutes before you lift anything to your lips. The first 30 seconds will be hard—the study showed that a very brief whiff of the cookie scent left subjects more likely to want to eat a cookie. But after that, it became easy to ignore the cookies.

Don't want to stick your nose in a cookie platter or get that close to tempting treats? Study authors theorize that using a cookie-scented extract or cookie-scented candle (or any other indulgent scent) might be just as effective at beating those cravings.

To Ease Stress

Many people know that lavender is a major de-stressor, hence it often is used to scent candles, body lotions, fabric softeners and more. The mere smell of lavender increases alpha-wave activity in the brain, indicative of a more relaxed state. A 2018 Japanese study suggests that the calming effect may be due to linalool, a fragrant alcohol compound that gives lavender its distinct aroma. The calming qualities also improve sleep—a study published in *Journal of Alternative and Complementary Medicine* found that study participants who slept with a chest patch imbued with lavender essential oil for five consecutive nights (Noctilessence, 10 patches for $24.99) experienced better overall sleep quality, compared with people wearing unscented patches. Even more impressive, the sleep benefits remained after two weeks of sleeping patch-free.

But a much more surprising de-stressor can be found right in your laundry basket or on your closet floor. Try breathing in a piece of clothing recently worn by your romantic partner to help calm your nerves. Recent research from University of British Columbia, published in *Journal of Personality and Social Psychology,* showed that women who were asked to smell a shirt recently worn by their partner (without being told that it had been worn by their partner) felt less stressed both before and after a challenging math test or mock interview.

To Wake Up

You know that a cup of coffee can help you wake up in the morning. But did you know that you may be able to derive just as much of an energizing effect from sniffing it as you do from sipping it? Simply smelling coffee can make you feel more awake.

Helpful idea: Program your coffee maker to start percolating 10 minutes before your alarm is set to go off if you want to wake up feeling energized before you've even had your first cup of Joe.

Whether or not you're a coffee drinker, the next time you need to perform at your best—while taking an exam, for instance, or before a job interview—inhale a deep whiff of coffee beans to feel instantly more alert.

To Improve Your Memory

Rosemary oil contains several compounds shown in test tube studies to facilitate activity of the chemical messengers in the brain that are involved in memory.

In a British study, people over the age of 65 were divided among three rooms. One room was scented by placing four drops of rosemary essential oil on an aroma diffuser that ran for five minutes before participants entered…one was lavender-scented…and one was unscented. The participants were presented with a series of challenges designed to assess prospective memory—the type of memory that helps us plan for the future, such as mailing a letter after seeing a mailbox. Rosemary's woody aroma improved prospective memory by 15% across the tasks.

Note: When purchasing essential oils, don't be fooled into thinking that more expensive means more effective. In my experience, more costly brands typically perform on par with less expensive ones. Surprisingly, artificially created oils also perform similarly to ones labeled "natural."

How to Improve Your Sense of Smell

Sense of smell declines with age, but it may be possible to retain it—or even regain it—by purposefully inhaling potent odors several times a day for three months. A 2009 study found that when 40 anosmic volunteers sniffed "Sniffin' Sticks" of rose, eucalyptus, citronella and clove twice a day for 12 weeks, nearly one-third of them ended up with improved olfactory functioning overall. Subsequent studies have replicated the effects. It may work with age-related smell loss, as well as with individuals who have lost their sense of smell from head trauma, a virus or another condition.

What to do: Choose three odors that you currently have difficulty detecting—cologne, cinnamon, roast chicken, for example—and sniff them (one at a time) three times per nostril, four times a day, for three months.

Note: Many medications used for hypertension, high cholesterol, cancer and depression can cause smell loss because they affect your taste receptors…or cause dry mouth, which in turn can diminish your sense of smell. If you are experiencing a loss of smell, talk to your doctor about whether it is a possible side effect of your current medications. You may be able to take a lower dose or a different drug. Smell typically resumes within a few months.

Homemade Sore Throat Remedies from Your Kitchen

Carrie Runde, ND, naturopathic physician, Charm City Natural Health, Baltimore. She is an active member of the American Association of Naturopathic Physicians, where she served on the organization's board of directors for five years. CharmCityNaturalHealth.com

Your throat is so sore that it's agony just to swallow…yet you can't bear the thought of trekking to the drugstore for medicine to ease the pain…

Good news: There's no need to leave the comfort of home—just head for your kitchen. Chances are that your pantry or fridge contains what you need to soothe your poor sore throat…safely, naturally, effectively and economically.

Here is what Carrie Runde, ND, a naturopathic physician in Baltimore, often recommends for her own patients with sore throats…

Four Fixes for Throat Pain

You can use any or all of the following remedies (depending on the supplies you have at hand) in any order you like and as often as you like…

•**Licorice root tea.** Licorice root reduces inflammation, which gives some immedi-

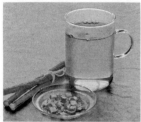

ate relief from a sore throat. Consuming the herb in tea form also helps keep you hydrated and temporarily speeds up the movement of mucus, alleviating the nasal congestion that forces you to mouth-breathe and makes your throat dry and scratchy. In addition, licorice root stimulates the immune system and has antiviral properties that help your body combat the cold, flu or other ailment that's causing your throat pain.

Though licorice root is available in various forms, the easiest thing to do, Dr. Runde said, is to keep licorice root tea bags on hand (find them in health-food stores and many grocery stores). Steep the tea bag in eight ounces of very hot water for five to seven minutes, keeping it covered to preserve the active constituents that vaporize. Then sip.

Caution: Do not use licorice root if you have high blood pressure.

•**Carrot poultice.** You'll need one or two large carrots or the equivalent in smaller carrots…a dry cotton handkerchief, cheese-

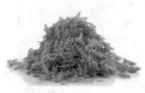

cloth or similarly sized thin cloth… plastic wrap…and a scarf. (It's best to wear an old shirt in case it gets stained orange.) Finely grate the carrot using a food processor or hand grater. Place the grated carrot in the center of the handkerchief, then fold the sides of the cloth up and over to create a packet (like a Hot Pocket) about two to three inches wide and five to six inches long. Lie down and position the packet horizontally against the front of your neck so that the single thickness of cloth is against your skin. Secure the poultice in place by wrapping (not tying) a layer of plastic wrap around your neck—loosely enough

that you're comfortable but snugly enough that the poultice doesn't fall off. Then wrap the scarf around your neck and leave everything in place for 20 to 40 minutes.

What does it do? When you're sick, white blood cells collect viruses and bacteria, then travel to your lymph glands to be filtered out. Carrots have a "cleaning" action on lymph glands. Dr. Runde said, "The carrot poultice increases circulation of blood and lymph fluid to the throat, bringing more healing oxygen, nutrients and white blood cells to the area and helping to clear away toxins."

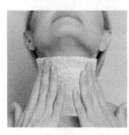

•**Washcloth hydrotherapy.** All you need for this remedy is a washcloth and the kitchen sink. Wet the washcloth with cold tap water, and wring it out so it's not dripping. Place the wet cloth over your throat and rest, sitting or lying down, for 30 minutes. Initially this remedy helps ease the pain by cooling the entire area…then, as your body heat warms the cloth, there's an increase of healing circulation to the throat.

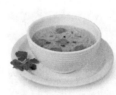

•**"Bone broth" chicken soup.** There are lots of reasons why this is a time-honored remedy. Chicken soup acts as an anti-inflammatory, inhibiting immune system cells that participate in the body's inflammatory response. It also alleviates nasal congestion and throat dryness. In addition, the zinc in the chicken improves your absorption of the nutrients in the soup's vegetables and gives your immune system a boost.

Dr. Runde said that the most effective chicken soup has a "bone broth" base made with chicken bones, vinegar and vegetables such as carrots and celery—all simmered for six or more hours so that the nutrients in the bones and vegetables infuse the broth. (Chicken soup that you buy in a supermarket probably isn't as beneficial, she explained, because valuable compounds in the chicken bones may not make their way into store-bought broths and bouillon cubes.)

Best: Make a big batch of homemade chicken soup, and keep it in your freezer so you'll have it on hand when you need it. If your throat is too sore to handle soup with chunks of chicken and vegetables, you can sip on the broth and still get the healing benefits.

When professional medical help is warranted: Dr. Runde suggested that you alert your doctor immediately if throat pain is severe or is accompanied by a fever of higher than 101°F, headache, stomachache, rash, joint pain and/or trouble swallowing or speaking—you may have an infection or some other condition that requires more treatment. Otherwise, contact your physician if a sore throat lasts for more than three days and is getting worse rather than better.

Peppermint Eases Painful Swallowing

When participants with swallowing difficulties and noncardiac chest pain took two peppermint oil tablets before meals, 73% reported improvement. Of those with just chest pain or swallowing problems, 63% and 53%, respectively, reported feeling better. Participants with swallowing issues took peppermint before every meal and those with chest pain took it during an attack. Peppermint oil, available in health-food stores, relaxes the smooth muscles of the lower esophagus.

Important: Consult your doctor first to rule out obstruction of the esophagus or heart disease.

Mohamed Khalaf, MD, esophageal disorders research fellow, Medical University of South Carolina Health Digestive Disease Center, Charleston.

Restless Legs Syndrome: 8 Best Ways to Get Relief

Brian B. Koo, MD, associate professor of neurology at Yale School of Medicine and director of the Yale Center for Restless Legs Syndrome (certified as a Quality Care Center by the Restless Legs Syndrome Foundation), both in New Haven, Connecticut. He is also director of the Sleep Medicine Laboratory at Connecticut Veterans Affairs Health System.

If you have ever suffered from an irresistible urge to move your legs when, say, relaxing in front of the TV at night—or, even worse, when you're in bed trying to sleep—you know that restless legs syndrome (RLS) can drive you batty.

The condition, which affects up to 10% of people in the US, is so frustrating that some sufferers pace the floor, toss and turn in bed or even consider suicide, according to research recently published in *Sleep Medicine*.

To get relief, many people who would prefer to forgo pharmaceuticals think they have no choice but to turn to drugs that are commonly prescribed for RLS, including medications for seizures or so-called dopamine-agonist drugs mainly used to treat Parkinson's disease. But these drugs can lead to side effects such as nausea and dizziness...and sometimes cause RLS symptoms to worsen (see Step #6).

Good news: You may not have to take medication to relieve RLS. There are lesser-known strategies that can restore your precious sleep...and your sanity. *Eight of the most effective steps...*

STEP #1: Ask to have your ferritin level tested. If it's low or even borderline (still within normal, but on the low end), iron supplements could be all you need to reduce RLS symptoms. Though this has been known for some time among RLS specialists, many primary care physicians aren't aware of it.

Note: Checking ferritin, a protein that stores iron in your body's cells, is not the same as checking your iron level. An iron blood test can still come back normal even after ferritin stores have started to decline.

Some people with an iron deficiency respond best to an iron infusion (through an IV) every few months or even two or three times over a few weeks.

Note: RLS may accompany end-stage kidney disease and peripheral neuropathy, too. Your physician should also check to see if either condition is contributing to your RLS.

STEP #2: **Get a "medication checkup."** A number of medications can make RLS worse. These range from over-the-counter (OTC) antihistamines and sleep aids, such as melatonin, to prescription antidepressants, antipsychotics and antinausea drugs. If you take one of these, you may sleep better without it, but consult your doctor before stopping a medication. If the drug was prescribed by a psychiatrist, he/she should confer with your RLS doctor to look for alternatives.

STEP #3: **Review your sleep quality and quantity.** You know that getting a good night's sleep can improve RLS, and you may already be practicing good sleep hygiene by keeping your bedroom cool and turning off all electronic gadgets at least an hour before bedtime. Just be sure to get enough sleep—seven to eight hours nightly.

Important: If you snore (ask your bed partner if you aren't sure or set your smartphone to record yourself while sleeping), talk to your doctor about scheduling a sleep study to check for sleep apnea. Correcting apnea often improves RLS symptoms.

STEP #4: **Exercise the right way.** Physical activity can help if it's performed during the day or early evening at the latest. Vigorous exercise, such as running many miles at any time of day, may worsen RLS symptoms. If that's true for you, opt for walking, slower and less intense jogging, slow cycling and/or swimming. Research has also found yoga to be a good option for RLS.

STEP #5: **Reduce stress.** If, like many people with RLS, stress worsens your symptoms, try relaxation techniques, such as a warm bath…massage…acupressure or acupuncture…and/or meditation. These thera-

pies may calm down the brain arousal systems that appear to be overactive in RLS.

STEP #6: **Get help for augmentation.** The same drugs that can help RLS at first, such as the dopamine-agonist medications mentioned earlier, can worsen symptoms over time. The initial dose may become less effective, and RLS symptoms can grow more intense. Called augmentation, this medication-related phenomenon usually happens after six months. When the drug is discontinued, symptoms typically improve. However, you'll need to work with your doctor to identify augmentation and then treat it, often with a gradual switchover to a different drug, such as *gabapentin* (Neurontin).

STEP #7: **Ask your doctor about RLS devices.** Two devices that require a doctor's prescription can be used whenever you're lying down. Both were relatively recently cleared by the FDA and are eligible for FSA/HSA reimbursement. Restiffic is a vibrating foot wrap that exerts gentle pressure on strategic muscles in the foot. The device costs $199 online at Restiffic.com. Relaxis is a vibrating pad that you place beneath your legs for better sleep. It costs about $600 online at MyRelaxis.com.

STEP #8: **Go to an RLS center.** As frustrated as you might feel, RLS is very treatable. If you suffer from this condition on most nights or your symptoms have worsened after using an RLS drug, contact one of the nine Quality Care Centers in the US that are certified by the Restless Legs Syndrome Foundation.*

At these centers, specialists take a comprehensive look at your sensory, motor, psychological and sleep symptoms…do a detailed analysis of factors that could be affecting your symptoms (including sleep, diet and medication)…and then personalize treatment to your unique situation.

Also helpful: Consider joining the Restless Legs Syndrome Foundation to share ideas with other patients in its forums and be in the loop on new developments.

*To find a center, go to RLS.org and click on "treatment."

Prevent GERD

To reduce your risk for heartburn, you may want to drink less during meals. Water—or any other liquids—can dilute the stomach acid and enzymes that are needed to aid food digestion.

Andrew Rubman, ND, founder and medical director, Southbury Clinic for Traditional Medicines, Southbury, Connecticut. SouthburyClinic.com

Natural Ways to Relieve Shingles Pain

Andrew Rubman, ND, medical director of Southbury Clinic for Traditional Medicines in Southbury, Connecticut. He is author of Bottom Line's "Nature Doc's Patient Diary" blog.

If you had chicken pox as a child, you still have the varicella zoster virus in your nerve tissue, which can lead to shingles years later. People whose immunity is weakened by cancer or a chronic health problem, such as diabetes, are more likely to get shingles. The itchy, painful rash and fluid-filled blisters can last for up to six weeks.

Medical doctors (MDs) often prescribe an antiviral, such as *acyclovir* (Zovirax) or *valacyclovir* (Valtrex), as soon as symptoms begin, to shorten the course of the illness and lessen associated nerve pain. Other commonly prescribed medications include over-the-counter (OTC) painkillers, such as *ibuprofen* (Motrin)…numbing topical agents, including *lidocaine*…powerful prescription antidepressants, such as *nortriptyline* (Pamelor)…nerve pain medication, including the antiseizure drug *gabapentin* (Neurontin)…and opioid pain medications.

However: Prescription antivirals do not affect the frequency of shingles recurrence, and drugs used to treat shingles-related pain can have side effects, ranging from liver and kidney damage to opioid-related addiction.

Simple self-care steps I recommend…

• **Wear loose, comfortable clothing until the pain eases.** If the pain is too intense to leave the house, wear a lightweight cotton robe until you get relief.

• **Soak in a lukewarm bath for 15 minutes.** Add to bathwater a cup or two of colloidal oatmeal or baking soda, which can ease pain and itchy blisters.

Important: Avoid bathing or showering in hot water during an outbreak of shingles—heat increases blood flow to the skin, which can worsen pain.

• **Try a cool washcloth.** Soak a washcloth in cool water, wring it out and hold it on the rash for several minutes to ease pain.

• **Use a soothing topical.** Mix two tablespoons of baking soda or cornstarch and one tablespoon of water. Gently apply it to the rash, and rinse off with cool water after 15 minutes.

Also helpful: Freshly squeezed aloe gel, as needed, or capsicum, also known as capsaicin, a popular topical nerve-pain blocker derived from hot peppers.

Beyond self-care: As a naturopathic doctor (ND), I often prescribe natural therapies instead of prescription medications to help ease symptoms and restore the body's self-healing capacities following shingles.

Important: These therapies should not be self-administered. An ND* or other health-care practitioner who is knowledgeable in the use of botanical medicines should be consulted for proper dosing and monitoring.

What I often prescribe for shingles…

• **Chinese liniment (Zheng Gu Shui) or efficascent oil, a Filipino remedy, can be helpful for pain.** (I advise my patients to avoid using either product near the eyes, nose or mouth.) Most NDs can boost the effectiveness of efficascent oil by using an ultrasonic device to help the active components penetrate affected areas more deeply.

• **Lomatium is a potent herbal anti-viral that reduces the risk for recurrence of shingles.** An oral supplement of an isolate

*To find a naturopathic doctor (ND) near you, consult the American Association of Naturopathic Physicians at Naturopathic.org.

of lomatium can be taken…or a few drops of lomatium tincture can be added to an eight-ounce glass of water.

Caution: Lomatium can cause a rash in some people, so a small dose usually is prescribed initially and stopped if there are any signs of a new rash.

Best practice: An MD and ND should collaborate on the most effective therapies for you, based on your age, medical history, chronic conditions and use of any medications. To reduce risk for lingering shingles pain (postherpetic neuralgia), prescription antiviral medication is advisable (within 48 to 72 hours of the onset of shingles symptoms).

Conquer Your Pain with These Ancient Healing Secrets

Catherine Browne, DAOM, LAc, DipLAc, RH, a holistic practitioner in Harmony, North Carolina, who specializes in the treatment of pain, emotional imbalances and opioid dependency. She is author of *Natural Therapies for Overcoming Opioid Dependency: Control Pain and Recover from Addiction.* DrCatherineBrowne.com

Whether it's due to arthritis, headache, an injury or some other agonizing condition, chronic pain is endemic in the US. A whopping 116 million Americans live with this dark cloud—more people than heart disease, cancer and diabetes combined.

Treatment for chronic pain runs the gamut from physical therapy and chiropractic care to powerful—often dangerous—painkillers and even surgery. But one approach that can be highly effective isn't even on the radar of most Americans: Traditional Chinese Medicine (TCM).

How TCM Works

TCM treatments focus on underlying imbalances and blockages that lead to pain. According to TCM principles, pain is caused by stagnation in yin (substance, or blood) and yang (movement, or qi, the body's vital energy).

The natural therapies of TCM treat pain by unblocking qi stagnation, restoring blood flow and enhancing qi. A TCM diagnosis is determined in many ways, including the location of the pain…pulse diagnosis…and tongue diagnosis. The location indicates what acupuncture channel(s) the pain is affecting. The pulse and tongue diagnoses help to reveal the body's internal state of qi. These clues help the practitioner form a treatment plan.

Top TCM Therapies

TCM offers a variety of therapies. *Among the most effective…*

• **Acupuncture.** TCM describes qi as flowing through 20 channels or meridians in the body, most of which are matched with organ systems, such as the kidneys, liver, lungs, spleen and stomach. The meridians are covered by about 400 acupoints, the energy points that are targeted by acupuncture. To resolve stagnation and move qi, an acupuncturist inserts hair-thin, disposable needles at the appropriate acupoints chosen as part of the patient evaluation and diagnosis.

Don't expect immediate results from acupuncture—it is a healing therapy that takes consistent treatment to resolve chronic pain conditions in most instances. An average course of treatment ranges from 12 to 22 sessions, depending on the severity of the chronic condition.

Also, let your acupuncturist know if there's been a change in the intensity and/or frequency of your pain. These valuable clues can indicate that the treatment is working, even if the pain is not yet entirely eliminated.

Compelling research: When scientists reviewed the evidence on acupuncture for chronic pain, this treatment was found to be an "effective, safe and cost-effective" solution for relieving many types of chronic pain, including low back, neck, shoulder, knee and headache, according to a research review published in *Current Opinion in Anaesthesiology.*

Look for a licensed acupuncturist (LAc) who is board-certified through the National Certification Commission for Acupuncture and Oriental Medicine, NCCAOM.org—a process that requires an average of approximately 2,000 hours of training specifically in Oriental medicine.

• **Emotional therapy.** In TCM theory, emotions such as chronic anger—which is very common in our society—create stagnation in the liver, which controls the flow of blood and qi throughout the body.

Liver qi stagnation can cause chronic joint pain, headaches, muscle spasms and generalized aches and pains. Many other chronic negative emotions—such as chronic worry or depression—also can play a role in chronic pain.

Self-care option: In addition to acupuncture, you can use herbs such as yellow dock root, bupleurum root or milk thistle seed—all of which soothe the liver and are available individually online. Bupleurum, however, is more widely found in a combination formula such as Xiao Yao Wan, also called "Free and Easy Wanderer," which is available online as well. Follow the dosage recommendation on the label.

Important: Be sure to consult your doctor before taking any herbal formula—especially if you have a chronic medical condition or take medication.

Kick Gout Out the Natural Way

Jacob Teitelbaum, MD, holistic physician and nationally recognized expert in the fields of pain, sleep, chronic fatigue syndrome and fibromyalgia. He is author of numerous books, including *Real Cause, Real Cure…From Fatigued to Fantastic!…*and *Beat Sugar Addiction Now!…*and the free app *Cures A-Z* (available for iPhone and Android). He is founder of the Practitioners Alliance Network (PAN). Vitality101.com

The pain of a gout attack can feel like tiny shards of glass piercing your big toe. Even the slightest brush of a bedsheet on your skin can be excruciating. Sufferers limp with agony and are simultaneously plagued by fever and chills.

Once called the "disease of kings" because only the wealthy had the means to overindulge in the rich foods that are commonly associated with gout, the disease has since reached mass proportions. Incidence has more than doubled in the last 20 years to more than eight million people according to a study published in *The Journal of Rheumatology*. Gout is caused by a buildup of uric acid, which congeals into sharp crystals causing pain and destroying joints.

Doctors commonly suggest that you lower levels of uric acid and prevent future attacks with medications such as *allopurinol* (Zyloprim, Aloprim). Beware—newer anti-gout drugs such as *lesinurad* (Zurampic) and *pegloticase* (Krystexxa) do not have proven safety records and do not provide more therapeutic benefit than allopurinol.

You can avoid dependence on medication and prevent gout flare-ups with successful natural treatments that can get to the root of the problem—excess uric acid and the inflammation that it causes. Since flare-ups are mainly diet-related, treatment also centers around changes in your diet.

Here's what works best for preventing and treating this disease…

• **Eat plain yogurt.** You may already love yogurt because it is high in protein, calcium and vitamins, but now it has also been associated with lowering gout attack risk. In new research published in *Modern Rheumatology*, Japanese scientists studied 25 people with high uric acid (hyperuricemia) and/or gout. Half the patients consumed daily yogurt drinks rich in the probiotic lactobacillus gasseri, and half did not.

After eight weeks, patients who ate yogurt had lower levels of uric acid. Even though it was a small study, the results were significant. If you don't like yogurt, a probiotic supplement may help.

• **Avoid high-fructose corn syrup.** It may not surprise you to learn that uric acid levels have risen along with the skyrocketing consumption of high-fructose corn syrup (HFCS). In a landmark study published in *Diabetes,* scientists from University of Colorado specifically blame rising uric acid levels on the HFCS found in sodas, juice drinks, candy, ice cream, baked goods (including breads), commercial salad dressings and many other processed foods. Although HFCS consumption seems to have peaked and is starting to fall, Americans still consume unhealthy amounts. Beware of other sugars as well. Fructose-rich fruit is OK to eat, but commercial fruit juices deliver too much fructose—even if they don't contain HFCS.

• **For sweetness, consider using stevia.** You're probably already familiar with the sweetener stevia—made from the leaves of the stevia plant and typically available as a powder or liquid extract. It is a safe, healthy and calorie-free natural sweetener. But now there's a new benefit to using stevia—recent scientific research shows stevia lowers uric acid. There are hundreds of stevia-sweetened products on the market, including sodas, chocolate bars, candies, puddings, jams, etc.

Latest research finding: In an animal study conducted by Chinese scientists and published in *Journal of Food Biochemistry*, a stevia extract lowered fructose-caused high uric acid levels and inflammation. And it worked even better when combined with the prescription drug allopurinol.

• **Add more fatty fish to your diet.** The omega-3 fatty acids in fatty fish such as salmon, trout, mackerel, sardines and anchovies are powerfully anti-inflammatory and can help prevent gout attacks.

Important new finding: Researchers at Harvard Medical School looked at more than 700 people with gout. Those who ate omega-3–rich servings of fish were 26% less likely to have a gout attack.

Note: Many doctors and organizations such as the Mayo Clinic and the Arthritis Foundation routinely recommend that patients with gout avoid purine-rich foods, including seafood, organ meats and wild game. But this recommendation is becoming outdated. The most recent scientific research shows that avoiding purines is unlikely to help you avoid gout attacks and only serves to remove potentially healthful foods from your diet.

Try this: It's better to add anti-gout foods to your diet rather than eliminate healthy foods for a questionable benefit.

• **Take the powerful anti-inflammatory curcumin**—the active ingredient in the spice turmeric.

New research finding: In a study published in *Arthritis Research and Therapy,* Chinese scientists successfully used curcumin to stop inflammation caused by uric acid crystals. Researchers concluded that curcumin is so effective, it could be considered a new "drug" for the treatment of gout. Gout attacks often can be stopped with the curcumin-containing supplement Curamin* from Terry Naturally, which contains a highly absorbable form of the same compound.

Directions: Take two or three capsules two to three times daily until you feel better. For a maintenance dose that can help prevent future attacks, take three capsules daily.

• **Take a tart cherry supplement.** You also can treat gout attacks with the supplement End Pain* from Enzymatic Therapy, which contains an extract of tart cherry (as well as boswellia and willow bark, two anti-inflammatory herbs). During a gout attack, take two tablets of End Pain three times daily. For maintenance to prevent gout attacks, take one tablet three times daily.

New research finding: In a study published in *Current Developments in Nutrition,* researchers had 26 overweight people drink either tart cherry juice or a placebo beverage over a four-week period and then switch—so that each group tried both tart cherry juice and the placebo. Tart cherry juice lowered both uric acid and C-reactive protein (an inflammatory biomarker) by 19%.

Caution: Regular intake of tart cherry juice to prevent or control gout is not recom-

*Dr. Teitelbaum works on the scientific advisory board of the company that makes Curamin, and he designed and sells End Pain. He donates all financial compensation for both products to charity.

mended because it delivers too much fructose, so it is better to use a supplement such as End Pain instead.

Note: Drinking a lot of water every day can dilute uric acid levels by helping you stay hydrated but will not stop an acute gout attack. You also can take supplements of omega-3s and antioxidants—these essential fatty acids are crucial for your body's health, but they won't do as much for gout as actual changes in your diet and lifestyle.

Yoga Breathing: The Surprising Secrets to Its Benefits

Sundar Balasubramanian, PhD, C-IAYT, a cell biologist and assistant professor of research in the department of radiation oncology at Medical University of South Carolina in Charleston. He is also founding director of PranaScience Institute, PranaScience. com, a website dedicated to research and education on yoga breathing. His research has been published in International Psychogeriatrics, Evidence-Based Complementary and Alternative Medicine *and other professional journals.*

Most health-savvy people know that deep breathing has a wide range of mind-body benefits backed by loads of scientific evidence.

But cell biologist and certified yoga therapist Sundar Balasubramanian, PhD, was inspired to investigate further after a realization that he produced an abundance of saliva while practicing controlled yoga breathing exercises collectively known as pranayama. He has since conducted pioneering research into the role that spittle (aka "spit") plays in the healing effects of deep breathing.

Hidden Powers of Saliva

Hundreds of studies have demonstrated the benefits of yoga breathing—ranging from lower blood pressure and less depression to better concentration and improved lung function—but it's not known why saliva is produced so abundantly during pranayama.

Recognized mainly for its role in promoting healthy digestion, saliva is comprised of about 98% water and various other substances, such as enzymes that help break down food. When people go about their daily activities, they produce about 25 to 50 ounces of saliva daily. However, if you're stressed, your mouth becomes dry. So it makes sense that when your body is extremely relaxed—as occurs during yoga breathing—you produce more saliva than you ordinarily would.

But how does that boost in saliva production contribute to pranayama's benefits? It's been established that saliva contains more than 1,000 proteins along with other crucial molecules, such as neurohormones. And it's been shown that the specific makeup of each person's saliva is unique, and it can change from day to day—even moment to moment based on one's emotional and physiological responses. *Saliva is believed to contribute to the healing effects of yoga breathing by...*

•**Increasing brain-boosting proteins.** Through our research published in *International Psychogeriatrics,* we discovered that a protein called nerve growth factor (NGF) increased 10 times more in the saliva of people practicing pranayama for a single 20-minute session compared with study participants who quietly read an article for the same length of time. This is significant because NGF goes straight to the brain, where it encourages brain cell growth. NGF levels are substantially lower in Alzheimer's patients.

•**Elevating cancer-suppressing proteins.** With a study published in *Evidence-Based Complementary and Alternative Medicine,* we confirmed that pranayama not only stimulates saliva production but also elevates levels of proteins with immunity-building and cancer-suppressing properties.

•**Reducing inflammatory markers.** Pranayama also reduces production of inflammatory biomarkers in saliva that are linked to such conditions as pain, depression and diseases, such as scleroderma and post-traumatic stress disorder (PTSD), according to research we published in *BMC Complementary and Alternative Medicine.*

Two Exercises to Get Started

With such varied health benefits—and a new understanding of saliva's crucial role in delivering them—you may be eager to try pranayama.

If you're just starting out with yoga breathing, it's common to worry that you'll "do it wrong." But the truth is, all you have to do is breathe, count and pay attention to how you're feeling. If you don't force an uncomfortable breathing practice or hold your breath for too long, there's nothing about pranayama that you can do wrong.

Important: If you have a respiratory disorder, such as emphysema or chronic obstructive pulmonary disease (COPD), consult your physician and/or a yoga therapist on the right exercises for your condition.

Even though there are numerous approaches to yoga breathing, here are two simple exercises to get you started—for best results, sit up straight, close your eyes and do one or both of the following throughout the day…

• **Beginner humming breath.** Also called "bee breath" because of the buzzing sound you make, this exercise is a good introduction to yoga breathing. It's quick, easy and doesn't require you to hold your breath.

What to do: Breathe deeply and inhale as much as you can comfortably. Then hum as you slowly exhale at a rate that is comfortable for you. Repeat this exercise for a minute or two when you wake up…and before eating breakfast and your other meals or snacks throughout the day to stimulate your saliva flow.

• **Cooling breath.** This exercise promotes copious saliva production by stimulating the glands in your oral cavity.

What to do: Roll your tongue in a U-shape. Inhale slowly through your tongue, then exhale through your nostrils. Repeat for five to 10 minutes. If you can't roll your tongue, in-

hale through your mouth while smiling and exhale through your nostrils.

To learn more about yoga breathing, go to PranaScience.com.

Music as Medicine

Barbara Else, MT-BC, board-certified music therapist and managing editor of *Journal of Music Therapy.* She is a consultant who serves as senior adviser, research and policy, to the American Music Therapy Association (AMTA), based in Silver Spring, Maryland. MusicTherapy.org

It's no secret that listening to a mellow song can calm us or that listening to an upbeat song can make us feel energized. But music's power over our minds and bodies runs deeper than people tend to realize. Music can trigger the release of mood-altering neurochemicals in the brain and activate brain regions associated with memory, emotion and creativity. Researchers have discovered that music can reduce pain…pull people out of depressed moods…spur recall of long-ago events…and more.

But you might not reap the potential benefits of music simply by flipping on the radio. The songs you select matter, as does the way you interact with those songs—participating in the creation of music tends to be more effective than just listening. Don't worry if you can't play an instrument or carry a tune—even humming, singing privately in the shower and/or drumming a couple of pencils on a table can convey the benefits of music creation.

Here are four ways to use music therapy to improve your life…

Use Music to Reduce Pain

In 2016, researchers conducted a meta-analysis of 97 earlier studies that examined the effect music has on pain.

Their conclusion: Preferred music can reduce the pain patients report on the one-to-10 pain scale by an average of more than one point, which is enough to lower someone's pain level from "distressing" to "tolerable." This reduction in pain tends to reduce people's use of addictive opioids and other painkillers.

What to do: If you're experiencing a low-to-moderate level of pain—something closer to discomfort than agony—listen to (or better yet hum or sing) music that you find relaxing. The calming effect that this music has on your brain is likely to lessen your sensation of pain. Which songs and genres to choose varies from person to person—the music someone else finds relaxing, you might find irritating. Still, if you're not sure where to start, you could enter words such as "mellow" or "relaxing" into a music-streaming website or app such as Spotify (Spotify.com, free for the ad-supported version to $9.99 per month for the ad-free premium version) or Amazon Prime Music (Amazon.com, included with Amazon Prime, which costs about $13 a month or $119 a year). Listen to the songs that these searches turn up, and create a playlist of only those that are calming for you.

If you experience substantial pain, instead listen to songs that you consider extremely engaging. These are songs that you cannot help but sing or hum along with every time you hear them—whether it's a show tune such as "Seventy-six Trombones" or classic rock such as The Isley Brothers' "Shout." They're songs that pull your attention away from other thoughts when they come on the radio. These songs are so powerful that they actually can distract your mind from your pain, to a degree. (Relaxing songs tend not to capture the attention sufficiently to overcome substantial pain.)

You probably already know what songs you find especially engaging—they're likely the songs that you've been listening to over and over again for years. There's a good chance that many of them date back to when you were in your teens, 20s or early 30s—the music people listen to during this stage of life can become so deeply ingrained that it has special power over the mind. Create a playlist

of these engaging songs to listen to during painful medical or dental procedures…while waiting for treatment in hospital emergency rooms…while waiting for painkillers to take effect…and during other times of significant pain.

Use Music to Remember the Past

Researchers have determined that among the regions of the brain activated when we listen to or create music are regions associated with autobiographical memories. That's why when we hear a song we heard frequently many years earlier, the song isn't all we remember—we often recall events from our own lives that happened around the time when the song was new to us.

What to do: Couples who have been together for many decades often feel closer to each other when they listen to (or sing or play) songs they originally listened to together long ago. The songs revive memories of experiences and adventures they enjoyed together. This can be especially beneficial when one partner is suffering from dementia—remarkably, music has the power to recover autobiographical memories even for these people who are slowly losing their past. The songs people listened to in their teens, 20s and early 30s are especially likely to be tied to personal memories.

Try this: If you're caring for someone who has late-stage dementia and you need to get a message through, such as "it's time for dinner," see if you can capture his/her attention using the melodies or lyrics you know he loved. They are most likely to be effective.

This music also can be useful for reminiscing about the old days with friends…or when trying to reconstruct family history and life reviews for descendants.

Use Music to Remember Things Later

Music doesn't just help us recall the distant past. It also can help us remember day-today details. A study published in *Memory & Cognition* determined that people are more likely to recall a phrase if it is sung as a song lyric than if it is simply spoken. That finding hints at a useful trick for remembering any detail.

What to do: Rather than tell yourself to remember, *The car is parked on 12th Street*, as you walk away from it, sing that line to yourself a few times—any melody will do. And if there's something you chronically misplace or forget to do, create a habit of singing about it.

Example: If you frequently misplace your car keys, you might sing, "I'm hanging my keys on the hook by the door," each time you enter your house.

Use Music to Improve Your Mood

A 2011 study published in *Nature Neuroscience* found that listening to music can stimulate the release of dopamine in the brain—the same mood-lifting neurochemical that gets released when people have sex, use drugs or enjoy a favorite food. In fact, music doesn't just pick us up when we're feeling a little down—it actually can help overcome clinical depression.

Findings: A 2017 analysis of nine earlier studies concluded that music therapy accompanied by other depression treatments was more effective than those other treatments on their own.

What to do: When you hear a song that makes you want to sing…makes you want to get up and move…and/or simply makes you feel good, make note of it—these are the songs that are especially likely to trigger the release of mood-improving neurochemicals for you. Create a playlist of these songs, and listen to it when you feel low. Sing, hum, drum or dance along to these songs—an article in *British Journal of Psychiatry* speculated that the potential physicality of music might contribute to its ability to lift depression.

A board-certified music therapist can provide guidance about how to take full advantage of the benefits of music. To find a music therapist in your area, visit MusicTherapy.org/about/find.

Rock to Sleep

A gentle rocking motion aids sleep. It helps people—even those who are already good sleepers—fall asleep more quickly and have longer periods of deep sleep, during which the mind consolidates memory. A bed that gently rocks all night also preserves sleep continuity—people get up less often.

Editor's note: Rocking bed frames can be found online at RockingBed.com.

Studies by researchers at University of Geneva and University of Lausanne, both in Switzerland, both reported in *Current Biology*.

Try These Medicines Made by Bees!

Jamison Starbuck, ND, a naturopathic physician in family practice in Missoula, Montana, and producer of *Dr. Starbuck's Health Tips for Kids*, a weekly program on Montana Public Radio, MTPR.org. DrJamisonStarbuck.com

---

As a former (and hopefully future) beekeeper, I have a fondness for bees. Beekeeping itself is good medicine—and not that hard to do. I find being around bees and watching their activity to be relaxing and interesting. But there are easier ways to get health benefits from bees. *Bee products with natural medicinal value…**

• **Honey.** I like to use honey instead of sugar as a sweetener because it metabolizes slowly, reducing the "sugar rush" and subse-

*****Caution:*** While allergic reactions to honey, pollen or propolis are rare, consuming these products may not be advisable for those with severe plant allergies. All of these products contain some pollen, which comes from plants. Honey should never be given to children younger than one-year-old due to the risk for botulism poisoning.

quent crash people often experience when consuming "regular" sugar. Also, honey has some nutritional value that sugar lacks—it contains potassium and magnesium, B vitamins, amino acids and enzymes. Both honey and sugar are composed of fructose and glucose, but honey contains the enzymes needed to break down these compounds, making it easier for the body to digest and less irritating to the stomach. Honey soothes respiratory inflammation from a sore throat, cough or bronchitis. Add one teaspoon of honey to a cup of tea (I like slippery elm and mullein for respiratory ailments).

Because of its antibacterial and anti-inflammatory properties, honey also can be used topically for healing wounds, burns and eczema. Simply smooth some honey over a wound, burn or patch of dry, scaly skin, then cover it with dry, sterile gauze. Change the gauze, and reapply honey daily until the area is healed. See your doctor for a deep wound or if you have signs of infection such as redness and/or swelling.

Best types of honey: To get the full benefits of honey, your best bet is to use raw, unpasteurized honey (check the label). For topical use, consider Manuka honey, a type of honey made by bees using the nectar from the wild manuka bush found in New Zealand. Manuka honey is available in most natural-food stores.

• **Pollen** is primarily used to treat mild seasonal allergies. The theory is that ingesting very small amounts of pollen, made from plants to which one is mildly allergic, will improve tolerance to those plants—similar to the way allergy shots or homeopathic allergy remedies work.

To use as an allergy medicine, pollen must be obtained from plants grown in your environment, which you can obtain from a local natural-food store or from a beekeeper directly. I typically recommend taking one-quarter teaspoon of bee pollen granules daily for a month or more before allergy season begins. You can sprinkle it on cereal or toast or add to yogurt or smoothies.

• **Propolis** is a resinlike material that bees produce to protect their hives. It's made from saliva, beeswax and material gathered from trees, including aspen, birch and poplar. I combine tinctures of propolis and slippery elm in a 50:50 ratio to make a soothing sore throat medicine. Spray this mix on the back of your throat every two hours as needed. You can also buy this premade in natural-food stores.

Chapter 12

PAIN AND AUTOIMMUNE DISORDERS

Hidden Cause of Neck and Shoulder Pain: Low Hormones

The patient: Kara, a 51-year-old litigator with debilitating neck and shoulder pain.

Why she came to see me: Kara strode into my office with a confidence characteristic to her profession. Within minutes of our consultation, however, she broke down. Three months earlier, she'd begun experiencing neck and shoulder pain. In recent weeks, it had grown so acute she could hardly fasten her bra. She hadn't been in a car accident or suffered a major injury. As she put it, the persistent pain "seemed to come out of nowhere." Her primary care physician had prescribed *ibuprofen* to little effect, and his next suggested step was a steroid shot in the shoulder. Kara was determined to not only discover the root cause of her pain but to also find a natural route to recovery.

How I evaluated her: Kara and I began with an in-depth look at her personal and medical history. Eight months earlier, she'd experienced her last period. Prior to that, her periods had grown light and irregular, with up to four months between them. Additionally, she'd been suffering from periodic hot flashes, insomnia, fatigue—and more anxiety than she'd had in her life.

Her neck and shoulder pain had started out as seemingly benign—stiffness and aches that she attributed to the long hours she spent at the office and in front of the courtroom. She'd tried a combination of treatments, from purchasing ergonomic office furniture to doing stretches with an app to seeing a well-reputed chiropractor. The pain failed to go away. Indeed, it only grew worse, and most mornings her neck was so rigid she struggled to get out of bed.

Less than a year ago, Kara claimed she'd been living a "much healthier lifestyle"— spending her weekends hiking in the mountains, eating fresh, locally sourced food and working out at the gym three nights a week. But as her work load increased with the arrival of a high-stakes case, and as her symptoms intensified, she'd abandoned her weekend hiking adventures, canceled her gym membership so she could rest immedi-

Laurie Steelsmith, ND, LAc, medical director of Steelsmith Natural Health Center in Honolulu. She is author of *Natural Choices for Women's Health, Great Sex, Naturally* and *Growing Younger Every Day* and writes the "Natural Healing Secrets for Women" blog at BottomLineInc.com. DrSteelsmith.com

ately after work, and resorted to "convenient food," such as premade sandwiches, frozen entrees and Thai takeout. "I feel like I've gone from hero to zero," she said, "and my neck and shoulder pain is impacting every area of my life."

To get to the bottom of Kara's symptoms, I ordered a 24-hour urine test that would check her female hormones and a blood test to evaluate her thyroid hormones and thyroid antibodies. I also did a simple orthopedic exam on her upper back, shoulder and neck...assessed her for range of motion... and examined her patterns of pain and discomfort.

What my evaluation revealed: As we both suspected, our assessment revealed that Kara was nearing menopause, which is defined as going a full year without a period.

The stage she was in was underscored by her lab results: High FSH (follicle stimulating hormone) and low estrogen and progesterone. Further, her thyroid stimulating hormone (TSH) and thyroid antibodies were high, while her T4 and T3 (thyroid hormone) levels were low. All of these are classic indications of Hashimoto's Thyroiditis, an autoimmune disorder that leads to hypothyroidism (underactive thyroid).

Kara's physical exam demonstrated significantly decreased range of motion in her left shoulder and tight muscles in her upper back, anterior and posterior neck, and pectoralis (chest muscles). Kara had what are called "trigger points" scattered over these areas—places where the fascia (our thin connective tissue) had become knotted up and severely sensitive to even the lightest touch. Our exam also showed early warning signs of a "frozen shoulder," which is known in the orthopedic world as adhesive capsulitis and as "the 50-year-old shoulder" in Chinese medicine, in that it frequently occurs in women around menopause.

How I addressed her problem: As I reiterated to Kara, the underlying cause of her symptoms—from pain to exhaustion—was due to a combination of three primary issues: Deconditioned muscles and joints...

low female hormones secondary to perimenopause...and Hashimoto's Thyroiditis. Treating her, I explained, would require a three-pronged approach.

First, I had a long discussion with Kara about the pros and cons of hormone replacement therapy in women between the ages of 50 and 60, or within the first 10 years of menopause. Research demonstrates that taking estrogen during the first decade after menopause may help prevent joint pain and deterioration, support bone health, and decelerate the potential progression towards dementia. And yet, at the same time, it may increase a woman's susceptibility to cancer. Given that Kara had no familial or personal history of estrogen-related cancers, and no history of breast and ovarian cancer, she agreed to try a bio-identical estrogen called Bi-est, which contains a key mix of estradiol (20%) and estriol (80%). I also prescribed natural progesterone. To administer, I asked her to use both as a cream and to apply to her labia, vagina and vulva once a day, as these tissues have a high absorption rate for hormones.

Secondly, we discussed Hashimoto's Thyroiditis. Also called Hashimoto's Disease, the condition—which is the leading cause of hypothyroidism in the United States—occurs when your immune system, in essence, attacks your thyroid. In turn, this interrupts hormone function. While sufferers may go years without symptoms, they can also experience muscle aches, tenderness and stiffness, joint pain, fatigue and sluggishness (among other signs)—in short, the very issues Kara was dealing with. What's more, there is a direct association between frozen shoulder and thyroid malfunction.

In an attempt to remedy this, I put Kara on a natural desiccated thyroid called Nature-Throid, a prescription-only medication that was one of the first available treatments for hypothyroidism. I prefer Nature-Throid over *levothyroxine* (Synthroid) because it contains both forms (T4 and T3) of thyroid hormone. Levothyroxine contains only the inactive thyroid hormone T4. Some people don't convert

T4 to active T3 well, so giving both in Nature-Throid guarantees that the patient will get active thyroid hormone.

I also prescribed 200 mcg of *L-selenomethionine* once a day, which has been shown to improve thyroid function and lower thyroid antibodies. Lastly, I strongly encouraged her to ditch gluten altogether, as increasing research reveals a link between Hashimoto's Thyroiditis and gluten intolerance.

Thirdly, we attacked Kara's most urgent concern—her chronically aching shoulder and neck. To provide immediate relief, I recommended a combination of trigger point therapy and prolotherapy. The injection-based treatments utilize a measured dose of sterile dextrose (a sugar derived from corn), an anesthetic such as procaine and nutrients that include Vitamin B and amino acids. The elixir is then injected into specific areas of the body—those aforementioned trigger points—to stimulate healing, in that they block nerve receptors that release proteins responsible for pain and stiffness. When administered in the joint at high doses, the patient experiences a temporary burst of irritation. This is because prolotherapy operates by generating temporary, low-grade inflammation at the injection site, which "tricks" the body into thinking it's been hurt and rushes a cascade of fibroblasts to the region. The direct exposure to these particular cells ignites new cell growth, collagen deposition and connective tissue repair. (Prolotherapy is also often used for joint inflammatory conditions such as osteoarthritis because it can render joints more flexible, fluid and elastic.) In the end, these treatments would make her tissues stronger and more functional and she would experience less pain.

Trigger point therapy, meanwhile, uses much lower doses of glucose, procaine and nutrients (also B vitamins and amino acids), which are injected into areas of pain and stiffness. In doing so, the technique releases fascial adhesions that may be the underlying cause of one's pain and discomfort. To allay Kara's concerns, I explained that trigger point therapy employs a very small needle (about the size of an acupuncture needle) and has been an effective form of treatment for many of my patients. (Many claim that their chronic upper back and neck stiffness melted away after just a few treatments.) After some consideration, Kara was game. After all, unlike ibuprofen and steroid injections, these treatments stimulate the body to heal itself and don't further weaken the supporting structure and tissues.

Since these treatments are only catalysts for a healing response, I also sent Kara to a physical therapist for strength training. Strength training would help her thwart joint and musculoskeletal problems in the future, particularly further exacerbations of frozen shoulder, in part by developing a layer of muscle over the affected joint. This would then increase joint function, decrease soft tissue and muscle pain, and help inhibit arthritis. Besides, regular exercise bolsters blood and oxygen flow, thus promoting circulation and aiding in the delivery of nutrients to "sore" tissues.

Finally, I referred Kara to an Iyengar yoga class. I see Iyengar yoga as a method of profound self-care—one that combines myofascial release work with mindfulness meditation. (Indeed, I recommend it to all of my patients.) It's also a safe, accessible form of yoga that utilizes blocks, chairs, blankets and other support systems that allow people to learn the practice at their own pace (and, most importantly, without injuring themselves).

The patient's progress: Two months later, Kara returned to my office with her signature confidence—only this time, it remained. "I haven't felt this wonderful in decades," she claimed as she laid out the details of her recovery. Adopting a gluten-free diet was far easier than she realized—thanks in part to the abundance of restaurants in her neighborhood that served gluten-free foods—and strength training had not only relieved her pain but also gave her toned arms. ("I had no idea I had triceps!" she gushed.) Her neck and shoulder pain was "all but gone" and she was far less fatigued. As with many who come into yoga at the right time in their lives, she'd fallen in love with the practice, and attended a class at least four times a week. Her period had not returned and she was still experiencing the occasional hot flash, but she felt ready and keen for what lay ahead. As for that bra she once couldn't fasten? She celebrated with a shopping spree at La Perla.

Surprising Possible Migraine Trigger

Richard M. Davis, MD, associate professor, department of Ophthalmology, UNC, codirector, UNC Center for Diabetes Translation Research to Reduce Health Disparities, University of North Carolina at Chapel Hill, and coauthor of study titled "Association Between Dry Eye Disease and Migraine Headaches in a Large Population-Based Study," published in *JAMA Ophthalmology*.

If you get migraines, you may be at higher risk for also having a certain chronic eye condition—especially if you're a senior. In fact, addressing the eye condition might have a wonderful effect on your migraines. *Here's why...*

A link between migraine, which affects about 14% of the general population in the US, and chronic dry eye disease, which causes a reduction in the quantity or quality of tear production, has long been suspected. However, studies looking into the connection between the two conditions were small and the findings have been inconsistent.

A new study led by researchers at University of North Carolina (UNC) looked at 10 years of records for nearly 73,000 patients age 18 and older who were treated at UNC-affiliated ophthalmology clinics.

Results: After adjusting for confounding factors that can cause dry eye—such as medications and eye surgery—patients who had been diagnosed with migraine headaches were found to be 20% more likely than people without migraines to also have dry eye disease. The association was highest for older patients. Men age 65 and older were nearly twice as likely and women in that age group 2.5 times as likely to also have chronic dry eye.

While this study did not show exactly how migraine and dry eye disease are connected, the researchers suspect that the link is inflammation, which has a significant role in both conditions. It is believed that inflammatory proteins trigger hypersensitive brain cells to produce the painful headaches that are characteristic of migraines. And chronic inflammation is one of the major causes of dry eye disease. (The researchers did note that the stronger association for older patients was not surprising, given that risk for dry eye increases with age, and especially for women because of the hormonal changes of menopause.)

Although the study didn't prove that inflammation from dry eye triggers migraine attacks, the researchers believe that it might... and suggest that diagnosing and treating dry eye in people with migraines may help reduce attacks.

If you have been diagnosed with migraine, ask your doctor to evaluate you for dry eye, especially if you have symptoms—stinging, burning, redness, pain, discharge and/or blurred vision. Treating dry eye, such as with artificial tears or medications to improve tear production, might have the happy "side effect" of fewer or less bothersome migraines!

Coffee Triggers Migraine

While caffeine is known to help relieve headaches and is found in some migraine medications, too much of a good thing can backfire.

New finding: Drinking three or more servings of a caffeinated beverage (one serving is six to eight ounces of coffee or tea or 12 ounces of caffeinated soda) increases the risk for headache that day or the next, according to a study of nearly 100 adults who suffer from episodic migraine.

Elizabeth Mostofsky, ScD, instructor, department of epidemiology, Harvard T.H. Chan School of Public Health, Boston.

Painful Dental Cleanings

Louis Siegelman, DDS, a dentist in New York City who treats patients who fear dental procedures, and clinical assistant professor, NYU College of Dentistry, also in New York City. DentalPhobia.com

There are a variety of strategies that can significantly ease discomfort from dental cleanings.

If your teeth are sensitive, be sure to ask your dental professional to be very gentle. You also can ask for a topical numbing agent (such as *benzocaine*), a numbing oral rinse or an injection of a more powerful anesthetic. Some people find that listening to relaxing music can help, too.

Your teeth become more sensitive when tooth enamel erodes, so it helps to avoid acidic beverages, like sodas, seltzers, fruit juices and tomato juice, which weaken enamel, especially several days before your visit. Using certain over-the-counter (OTC) remineralizing toothpastes, rinses, gels and creams also can help ease sensitivity. Ask your dentist which products he/she advises for you. Taking an OTC pain reliever—*ibuprofen* (Motrin) or *acetaminophen* (Tylenol) —about an hour before the appointment helps to ease discomfort as well.

If these steps don't give adequate relief, you may want sedation, such as laughing gas (nitrous oxide). It can cause nausea and vomiting, so don't eat immediately prior to the appointment, and I don't advise driving immediately afterward. Check with your insurance carrier to see if the cost will be covered.

Also, some dentists now offer a pain-management method called transcutaneous electrical nerve stimulation (TENS) in which pads are placed on the face where the numbing is needed, and the patient uses a remote to control the level of electrical stimulation.

Facial Pain Is Also a Headache Symptom

When nearly 3,000 people with headaches, including migraines and cluster headaches, completed questionnaires about their symptoms, 10% reported facial pain—a previously under-recognized headache symptom.

Takeaway: If you experience facial pain—with or without predominant head pain—be sure to tell your doctor so that you can get properly diagnosed and treated.

Arne May, MD, PhD, professor of neurology and head, headache outpatient clinic, University of Hamburg, Germany.

4 Simple Exercises That Ease Hand Arthritis

Carole Dodge, OTR, CHT, who supervises the occupational hand therapy program at University of Michigan Health System in Ann Arbor. She specializes in osteoarthritis, rheumatoid arthritis, joint replacements and traumatic hand injuries. She is also director of the Michigan Medicine Hand Fellowship program.

If you're struggling with arthritis pain in your hands, you may not want to move them much, but resist that temptation! You need to do exactly the opposite.

Daily exercises that specifically target affected joints can improve pain, range of motion and hand strength by promoting blood flow to damaged cartilage and increasing the natural joint lubrication that occurs with movement.

Try these hand exercises…

•**Make an "O" by touching the tip of your thumb to the tip of your index finger and hold for three seconds.** This will increase thumb stabilization.

•**Handle coins and other small objects to improve pinch and finger manipulation.**

•**Flip and shuffle cards to increase the flexibility of your fingers.**

• **Squeeze putty to strengthen all the muscles of your hand.** This will increase both your grip and pinch strength for opening jars and containers, opening doors and for lifting and carrying items.

My advice: Do these exercises for 10 to 15 minutes, twice daily.

Osteoarthritis Raises Risk for Social Isolation

About 30% of adults over age 65 have the painful joint disease. Because they have difficulty moving around, it is harder for them to stay in social contact with others or make new friends. The pain of osteoarthritis also is associated with anxiety, depression and physical inactivity—all factors contributing to social isolation.

Analysis of data on 1,967 people, all around age 73, from six European countries by researchers from the American Geriatrics Society and published in *Journal of the American Geriatrics Society.*

Beware of Steroid Shots

In a study of nearly 500 patients who received a corticosteroid injection for hip or knee osteoarthritis, the complication rate was 8%—much higher than expected. Serious complications included accelerated joint damage, insufficiency fractures beneath the joint cartilage, bone death and rapid joint destruction that may hasten the need for total hip or knee replacement. Before getting a steroid injection, discuss the risks and benefits with your doctor. Also, ask about getting an X-ray before the injection to determine whether you are at increased risk for complications.

Ali Guermazi, MD, PhD, chief of radiology, VA Boston Healthcare System.

Weight Gain with *Prednisone*

David Sherer, MD, a retired anesthesiologist who now focuses on patient education, writing and patient advocacy. He is author of the blog "What Your Doctor Isn't Telling You" at BottomLineInc.com.

Prednisone is a powerful prescription steroid drug with lots of possible side effects, including weight gain. Used as an anti-inflammatory or immune suppressant, prednisone is commonly prescribed for such conditions as arthritis, ulcerative colitis, psoriasis, lupus, asthma and other breathing disorders.

Like other steroids, prednisone also can cause high blood pressure, headache, nausea, muscle weakness, anxiety and sleep problems. When used long term (typically for more than three months), the drug increases risk for infections, bone loss, cataracts and elevated blood sugar.

The weight-gain side effect can contribute to your back pain. To keep back pain at bay, a good rule of thumb is to stay within about 10 pounds of your ideal body weight. If you are sedentary, getting up to walk for a few minutes every hour will help.

In addition to weight-loss strategies, talk to your doctor about seeing a physical therapist, who can suggest pain-relieving exercises such as stretching. Swimming, yoga and/or massage therapy also can help. Over-the-counter (OTC) topicals, such as capsaicin or arnica, are worth considering as well. Some people report that CBD formulations relieve their pain.

If those steps don't work, ask your doctor about an OTC nonsteroidal anti-inflammatory drug (NSAID), such as *naproxen* (Aleve).

Note: NSAIDs also can cause side effects, such as ulcers and even kidney damage or heart problems. Some people get relief from *acetaminophen* (Tylenol), but liver damage can occur if the dosage exceeds the recommended maximum daily dose. Ask your doctor to identify the safest medication for you.

How Does CBD Treat Pain Versus Opioids... and Is It Addictive?

Diana Martins-Welch, MD, assistant professor of medicine at the Donald and Barbara Zucker School of Medicine at Hofstra/Northwell in Lake Success, New York. Board-certified in internal medicine and hospice and palliative care, she is a member of the Association of Cannabis Specialists, which is dedicated to providing best clinical practices for the use of cannabis medicine.

C annabidiol (CBD) is a chemical found in the cannabis plant and is different from tetrahydrocannabinol (THC), the substance that produces the marijuana "high." We don't yet fully understand how CBD works to relieve pain, but studies show that it is an anti-inflammatory agent. Many painful conditions, such as arthritis and lupus, are inflammation-driven.

Opioid drugs, such as *fentanyl* (Duragesic) and *oxycodone* (Oxycontin), work on different pain receptors in the brain and also release dopamine, the "feel-good" brain chemical that creates a powerful sense of well-being. CBD does not produce an excessive release of dopamine, as opioids do. While pain can diminish drastically with opioids, these drugs can also cause people to feel sleepy, dizzy or "cloudy." CBD's analgesic effect does not result in mental cloudiness.

We don't know why some people become addicted to opioids, while others do not, but a genetic component may affect how the body responds to them. CBD is not thought to be addictive because there isn't a surge of dopamine, so the brain's reward system isn't stimulated, as occurs with opioids. Therefore, there's no craving for CBD, as some people might experience with opioids.

Important: Before trying CBD, be sure to check with your doctor if you have a chronic medical condition or take any medication or supplement.

How to Talk About Your Pain

Seth A. Waldman, MD, director of the Pain Management Division at Hospital for Special Surgery and clinical assistant professor of anesthesiology at Weill Cornell Medical College, both in New York City. He is also the former director-at-large for the New York Society of Interventional Pain Physicians. His scientific articles have appeared in *Anesthesia & Analgesia* and other leading journals in the field of pain and pain management.

W hen you're in pain, it's often difficult to find just the right words to describe it. But it's worth the effort. Accurately describing the "quality" of your pain is one of the most important—yet underappreciated—steps in getting the best treatment.

Now: Pain specialists are giving pain sufferers new methods to help them communicate exactly how they are feeling.

What you need to know...

Beyond the 0-to-10 Scale

It's no surprise that there's huge variability in how pain is experienced. One person's low-back pain, for example, might be "dull and bearable," while another's might be "sharp and unbearable." That's why telling your doctor that you have "low-back pain" is not descriptive. Rather, you must be specific when describing your pain.

While the location of pain is a useful starting point, indicating whether it radiates, what makes it start and stop and describing the quality of the pain are often important clues in determining the source—and planning a way to treat the underlying cause. *Seven key elements to describe...*

• **The intensity of your pain.** The most common way to describe pain intensity is with the classic 0-to-10 pain intensity scale—with 0 being no pain...1 to 3, mild...4 to 6, moderate...and 7 to 10, severe (10 being the worst pain possible). Unfortunately, far too many people rely solely on this pain scale.

This is where your pain description should start, not end.

Both patients and doctors tend to overuse this tool, overlooking more effective ways to verbally describe pain with stories and words (see below). The 0-to-10 scale has only "modest accuracy," according to a study published in *Journal of General Internal Medicine*.

Also, using the 0-to-10 scale leads patients and doctors to both underestimate and overestimate pain. A person with high pain tolerance may say that his/her pain is a "3"—but that pain should be treated. On the other hand, a person who says, *My pain is 30 out of 10*, isn't accurately communicating the level of his pain—he is communicating that he urgently wants the pain treated. What's more, that exaggeration poses a real danger —a well-intentioned clinician might try to help with a pain medication that's stronger than needed.

Interesting recent finding: Researchers from McGill University and University of Toronto conducted experiments that showed that men—not women, as previously believed—are more stressed by pain and more hypersensitive to repeated pain. This study was published in *Current Biology*.

•**What your pain feels like.** Words and stories about pain give your doctor important clues as to the pain's real cause and optimal treatment. In fact, your doctor should ask you to tell your story about your pain—because you most likely have something you want to say…and you want to get better. Telling your story meets both needs.

Example: "I've had an aching back for more than a decade that started after a car accident. Last week, I had a sudden sharp pain in my back—and then the back pain went away! But right after that, I started to have stabbing leg pain." This story tells the doctor that it's likely you have a herniated disk in your spine.

Some of the most descriptive pain words to use in your story include: Burning… sharp…dull…throbbing…sore…stabbing… shooting…aching…cramping…tingling…

stinging…gnawing…dragging…unbearable… intermittent…brief…steady…and constant.

Also, tell your doctor if you have nonpain symptoms that accompany your pain, such as nausea, numbness or weakness. Such symptoms often help clarify the cause of your pain.

•**The location of your pain.** Tell your doctor exactly where the pain occurs…or if it travels from its site of origin to other parts of your body.

Example: Say, "I have a pain in my back that moves into my right buttock, right knee and right foot." Or, "I have a pain on the left side of my neck that goes down into the top of my left arm."

Helpful: Ask your doctor for a "Body Chart" that shows front, back and side views of the body—and make marks on the chart that show exactly where you experience pain.

What not to do: In describing the location of your pain, don't diagnose yourself by saying, for example, *I have sciatic pain or I think I have a hernia*. It's actually dangerous to use words such as "sciatica" that you may have read on the internet or heard from a health professional—they may be wrong and may lead the doctor to a misdiagnosis.

•**The duration of your pain.** Tell the doctor whether your pain has been occurring for days, weeks or months at a time. If it's chronic, does it come and go throughout the day or is it constant? Is it more severe during the week than on the weekend? Has it worsened over time?

•**What makes your pain better and what makes it worse.** This information is very useful to your doctor in creating a personalized protocol to control and relieve your pain.

Examples: I have pain every time I walk on a hard surface. I have pain when I stand up. I always feel better while sitting. My pain is worse (or better) when I—drink alcohol…eat…have a cup of coffee…go out in cold weather…get a massage…feel tense… go to work…exercise…am fatigued…or don't sleep well.

WEEKLY PAIN DIARY

	MONDAY	TUESDAY	WEDNESDAY	THURSDAY	FRIDAY	SATURDAY	SUNDAY
Duration of Your Pain	Start: Stop: Intermittent:	Start: Stop: Intermittent:	Start: Stop: Intermittent:	Start: Stop: Intermittent:	Start: Stop: Intermittent:	Start: Stop: Intermittent:	Start: Stop: Intermittent:
Location of Your Pain (e.g., back, hip, knee)							
Description of Your Pain (e.g., stabbing, dull, throbbing, burning, etc.)*							
Possible Triggers (e.g., missed medication, sleep problems, etc.)							
Intensity of Your Pain (0 to 10)							
What You Did to Relieve Your Pain...and How It Worked (e.g., yoga, massage, ice pack, pain reliever, etc.)	Exercise: Complementary Therapy: Self-Care: Medication:	Exercise: Complementary Therapy: Self-Care: Medication:	Exercise: Complementary Therapy: Self-Care: Medication:	Exercise: Complementary Therapy: Self-Care: Medication:	Exercise: Complementary Therapy: Self-Care: Medication:	Exercise: Complementary Therapy: Self-Care: Medication:	Exercise: Complementary Therapy: Self-Care: Medication:

*__Examples of words to describe your pain:__ Sharp...pounding...pulsing...searing...heavy...radiating...tingling...piercing...squeezing...excrutiating...mild...quivering...crushing...pulling.

Also tell the doctor the environments where your pain occurs—for example, while at work or at home.

• **The psychological impact of your pain.** This tells your doctor what pain means to you—that is, how much it makes you suffer, which can vary significantly in people who have the same type and degree of pain. With this information, your doctor can determine what additional treatments might be beneficial for you, such as psychological or medical support for depression and anxiety (both of which are common in people with chronic pain).

• **The medications you're taking.** Tell the doctor each medication you're taking for pain—the dose, how long you've been taking it and the extent to which each medication helps with the pain.

Also: Be sure to mention any other medication you're taking, which could interact with pain medication.

Keeping a Pain Diary

Keeping a pain diary (see page 251) for at least a week before your doctor appointment is another important way to clearly communicate the details of your pain to your doctor. *You should note the following factors…*

When the pain occurs…where it hurts… what it felt like…what you were doing when the pain hit…how severe the pain was on a 0-to-10 scale…what you did to try to reduce the pain…and the result of what you did.

A common mistake: Logging too many entries. It's important to keep your diary focused. If you describe every incident of pain, hour by hour, day after day, your doctor will have a hard time making sense of your diary.

Better: Set a specific interval for making diary entries about your pain—a few times a day (morning, afternoon and evening) or once a day, for example.

Important: If you have pain, it's always best to start with your primary care doctor. If necessary, he will refer you to a pain specialist.

The Fascia Fix for Chronic Pain

Warren I. Hammer, DC, MS, a chiropractor who has been in private practice in Norwalk, Connecticut, for 60 years. Dr. Hammer lectures internationally on the treatment of soft-tissue problems and is editor of three editions of the textbook *Functional Soft-Tissue Examination and Treatment by Manual Methods.* He is the English editor of *Functional Atlas of the Human Fascial System* by Carla Stecco, MD. WarrenHammer.com

This soft-tissue problem goes undetected by most doctors. You wake up feeling stiff and achy. When you walk, your joints might crackle or pop, and you may even feel a bit uncoordinated. Odds are you are suffering from chronic hip, knee, leg, shoulder or spinal pain.

Most people would be quick to blame an injury or osteoarthritis. But for many of those with chronic pain and immobility, the culprit is myofascial pain syndrome (MPS), a soft-tissue problem that most people—including the majority of those suffering from it—have never even heard of.

With MPS, pain originates within the fascia, the thin, white or nearly transparent connective tissue that covers every muscle fiber, blood vessel, nerve and organ in our bodies. Often, the fascia can stiffen, thicken or lose flexibility due to past injuries, inactivity or mismanaged pain.

Unfortunately, most doctors are unable to diagnose MPS because there is no standard diagnostic criteria or lab test to indicate that you have this condition. It can only be diagnosed with a physical exam that reveals a loss of motion in joints and/or diminished muscle strength related to painful nodules, especially in areas from which pain is referred.

That's why you've probably treated only the symptoms of your pain rather than the root cause. Or perhaps you have simply lived with it. Either way, you need to know that long-lasting relief is possible for people with MPS.

4 Ways to Keep Your Fascia Healthy

If you have MPS, you need to…

• **Do one-minute stretches.** Your brain communicates with an army of receptors in the fascia every time you move your body. Whenever you use your muscles, the fascia receptors must stretch. If pain or injury inhibits that stretch, muscle fibers don't work at full capacity, leading to more stress on the joint.

Stretching is critical to ensure that your muscle fibers continue firing properly. The good news is, just one minute of static stretching (holding the stretch in place) can effectively activate the fascia in an affected area, such as the neck, shoulders, legs and arms.

My advice: To wake up your muscle fibers, start your day with a hot shower. Throughout the day, remember to do one-minute stretches, targeting areas that are particularly painful. For best results, consult a fascial stretch therapist. Some physical therapists, massage therapists and personal trainers are certified in fascial stretch therapy. Check with your doctor or search "fascial stretch therapy" online for a practitioner near you.

• **Move your body.** Immobility leads to stiffness, pain and more immobility. That's why you have to move your body. The specific type of exercise is not that important—just remember to back off when you feel pain. When you move, your body is talking to you. If you listen, you'll be more likely to avoid injury.

My advice: Walking is often the easiest and most convenient form of physical activity. If you've been sedentary, start by doing just five to 10 minutes daily and gradually increase your distance by a quarter mile at a time until you are walking a mile or more daily. Other good exercise options include swimming and tai chi.

• **Try this supplement.** A good way to support your fascia is to get more hyaluronic acid (HA). Our bodies naturally produce this gooey substance to retain water and lubricate our joints, muscles and connective tissues, including fascia. But HA production declines with age.

Up to 80% of my patients experience significant relief after using an oral HA supplement called Baxyl, which should provide relief within the first month.

Typical dose: For the first week, take one teaspoon in the morning and another at night. After the first week, take just one-half teaspoon twice a day.*

Note: For people with bone-on-bone damage and severe cartilage degeneration, HA injections, which are administered by some rheumatologists and orthopedic surgeons, can be given. An injection can provide three to six months of pain relief.

• **Get Fascial Manipulation.** The goal of this therapy is to release restrictions, mobilize areas that are stuck and restore function to your fascia. It is based on myofascial pathways, which are similar to the meridians (energy pathways or channels) of traditional Chinese medicine.

Before treatment, the practitioner (usually a chiropractor, physical therapist or massage therapist) will examine you to find the affected pathways. The practitioner then uses his/her knuckles, elbows and/or hands to manipulate the fascia and muscle using vertical pressure. In some cases, there may be increased pain for a day or two due to the inflammatory process that's needed to heal local fascial points.

Most of my patients show increased mobility after just one or two treatments. Others require three to five treatments before they experience noticeable pain reduction. Check with your health insurer to see whether Fascial Manipulation is covered. For about an hour-long session, the cost will be approximately $125 and up, depending on your location.

To Find a Certified Fascial

Manipulation practitioner: Go to Fascial ManipulationWorkshops.com or FascialManipulation.com/en (for practitioners worldwide).

*Consult your doctor before taking this—or any other—supplement.

Certified practitioners have passed a test after taking the 96-hour Fascial Manipulation course, which originated in Italy and has been taught in 47 countries.

Botox May Treat Heel Pain

Plantar fasciitis is one of the most common causes of heel pain. It happens when the supportive ligament connected to the heel and its surrounding nerves become inflamed. Pain eventually becomes chronic if the condition is not treated. Standard treatments use orthotics, daily stretching and cortisone injections. But some doctors say Botox injections also can relieve the pain and pressure on the inflamed ligament, taking just three to seven days to have an effect.

Caution: Botox is not FDA-approved for this use, not all doctors agree with using it and insurance may not cover the cost, which could be $500 per treatment.

Roundup of neurologists and podiatrists reported at Prevention.com.

Why Is My Bunion Growing So Fast?

Harris H. McIlwain, MD, a board-certified rheumatologist and founder of the McIlwain Medical Group in Tampa, Florida. He is coauthor of *Pain-Free Arthritis*.

A bunion ordinarily takes years to develop, but sometimes in special situations one can develop in a matter of weeks.

As you know, a bunion (the medical term is hallux valgus) is a deformity of the big toe joint. Bunions form when the first bone in the foot shifts outward and causes the big toe to turn inward and rotate toward the smaller toes. The base of the big toe juts out, creating a bony bump at the joint. Bunions can be very painful and make walking difficult.

A variety of factors can increase one's risk of developing a bunion. Age is one of the main risks. An estimated one out of every three adults over age 65 have bunions of varying severity. Heredity also can play a role—a predisposition for the condition is often found in our genes.

People with flat feet and low arches and those who stand a lot or engage in a high-impact physical activity, such as tennis or ballet, also are more likely to develop bunions. Even though wearing too-tight shoes and/or high heels can contribute to a bunion, this is not considered an underlying cause. Not surprisingly, women are at greater risk than men.

The fast-growing nature of some bunions suggests that something else may be going on. It could be linked to rheumatoid arthritis (RA). RA is an inflammatory autoimmune condition that occurs when the immune system mistakenly attacks its own joints, causing pain and swelling. People with RA often develop deformities in their hands and feet.

A rheumatologist can diagnose RA with an imaging test, such as an X-ray or MRI, and a blood test. The condition is typically treated with an over-the-counter (OTC) nonsteroidal anti-inflammatory drug (NSAID), such as *naproxen* (Aleve) or *ibuprofen* (Motrin), a corticosteroid or disease-modifying anti-rheumatic drugs (DMARDs), such as *methotrexate* (Rheumatrex), and/or newer targeted medications, including *tofacitinib* (Xeljanz).

Lifestyle changes, such as maintaining a healthy body weight and eating lots of anti-inflammatory foods, including purple grapes, blueberries and dark cherries, also can help reduce pain and sometimes allow RA sufferers to limit or even avoid medication. If your bunion is linked to RA, it's possible that the RA treatments described above may slow down the bunion's progression.

For the bunion itself, there are various treatment options. If it's not continually painful, simply wearing wider, low-heeled shoes with orthotic inserts will improve foot alignment and provide support. OTC bunion pads may prevent irritation. Using an ice pack for 20 minutes at a time, when needed, and/or taking an NSAID will ease bunion pain after walking or other exercise.

However, if your bunion is large and/or very painful, surgery may be necessary. There are many different types of bunion surgery, which involve shaving the bony bump and/or moving the foot bone into its correct position. Your surgeon will recommend the procedure that is best for you. Surgery is the only way to correct a bunion deformity. To find a foot surgeon near you, consult the website of the American Orthopaedic Foot & Ankle Society, AOFAS.org.

Aching Feet Could Be Arthritis

Kristen Lee, MD, a rheumatologist with the Joint Preservation and Arthritis Center at the NYU Langone Orthopedic Center and assistant professor in the department of medicine at NYU Langone Health, both in New York City. Her research has been published in *Clinical Rheumatology, Arthritis & Rheumatology* and other leading medical journals.

Standing on your feet all day and wearing tight shoes aren't the only causes of foot pain. You might be surprised to learn that the culprit could be arthritis—even if no other joint in your body is achy. There are 100 different types of arthritis (surprising in itself), and many of them can affect the feet, from the toes to the heel and ankle.

Among the most common forms that can trouble your tootsies…

•**Osteoarthritis (OA).** The same degenerative—or "wear and tear"—arthritis that, over time, leads to the deterioration of cartilage in frequently targeted joints, such as hips and knees, also can occur in the feet and ankles. OA might affect just one foot and even just one part of the foot, such as the big toe or the area from the arch to the front of the ankle. This form of degenerative arthritis can develop at the site of a past injury, like a fracture, so if you've ever broken a bone

in your foot, arthritis can strike in that area some years later. OA typically causes pain and stiffness during weight-bearing activities, such as walking or jogging.

•**Gout.** The telltale sign of this inflammatory type of arthritis is sudden and excruciating pain in one big toe, the result of an accumulation of uric acid in the joint. Though gout affects more than eight million Americans, its association with overindulging in food and drink (such as organ meats and beer) leaves many people too embarrassed to seek medical help. But besides having to live with the pain unnecessarily, repeated attacks of unchecked gout can lead to secondary osteoarthritis in the big toe, and the resulting permanent loss of cartilage can cause its own pain, even if the gout is eventually controlled.

•**Rheumatoid arthritis (RA).** This is one of many autoimmune diseases that can affect the joints in the feet, causing them to feel hot and painful, swollen and stiff. An overwhelming 90% of people with RA experience foot pain. In fact, for some, this is the first sign of the disease.

Because RA affects the body symmetrically, you'll feel it in both feet, though the symptoms can alternate, and because RA can attack numerous joints, you may feel symptoms in many of your smaller toes and fingers. RA can lead to joint deformities and cartilage loss within months if severe, and this damage may be visible on an X-ray or MRI.

•**Psoriatic arthritis.** Even though this autoimmune disease is thought to have genetic links to the skin condition psoriasis, psoriatic arthritis can occur on its own in a very small percentage of those who develop arthritis before the psoriasis. Most often, the inflammatory arthritis manifests in people with current psoriasis, past psoriasis or a strong family history of psoriasis.

You may develop plantar fasciitis, which causes pain along the sole or Achilles tendinitis at the back of the heel. But because both of these foot conditions can occur for other reasons, people don't always connect the dots to psoriatic arthritis and attribute their pain to a sports injury or other mishap.

One telltale sign of psoriatic arthritis is a type of inflammation known as dactylitis, the intense swelling of an entire digit, including the joints in one or more toes (or fingers) that creates a sausagelike appearance. Foot pain can be excruciating, and joint damage can set in within a few months.

• **Ankylosing spondylitis.** This is a type of inflammatory arthritis that primarily affects the spine, leading to back pain, but symptoms also can occur in your feet and the heel area, in particular. It can look very similar to psoriatic arthritis. Inflammation can lead to Achilles tendinitis at the back of the heel and/or plantar fasciitis at the base of the heel, with severe pain and tenderness that can limit movement. Ankylosing spondylitis also can lead to sausagelike swelling of the toes.

How to Get Relief

If you're experiencing foot pain, see your primary care physician, a podiatrist or a rheumatologist (if autoimmune conditions are suspected) for an evaluation. You need a proper diagnosis so you can start treatment early enough to help preserve your mobility.

However, getting a correct diagnosis can sometimes be challenging. Testing should include a careful physical exam, along with blood tests and imaging tests, such as X-rays, an MRI and/or an ultrasound. Seeing a rheumatologist sooner rather than later often helps ensure a proper diagnosis.

The types of arthritis described earlier are generally treated with a combination of medication (primarily anti-inflammatory drugs) and physical therapy to ease pain. Specialized drugs, such as disease-modifying antirheumatic drugs (DMARDs), designed to stop or slow the progression of the specific condition, also may be used depending on the diagnosis.

Whatever your treatment plan, make sure that specific foot care is part of it—despite how often feet are affected by these condi-

tions, they're sometimes overlooked in a "big picture" approach.

Here are steps that can help…

• **Make ice your go-to for swelling.** Ice is great for reducing inflammation—alternate 10 minutes on with 10 minutes off until you feel relief. Mold a bag of frozen veggies over the affected part of your foot or simply put your foot in a bucket of icy water.

• **Go shoe shopping.** Arthritic feet will feel much better in shoes with a roomy toe box, a wider width and a lower heel. If you have plantar fasciitis or other soft-tissue involvement, you may benefit from a heel cup or an insert for arch support. See a podiatrist to get a formal biomechanics evaluation of the foot and recommendations for orthotics.

• **See an occupational therapist.** I suggest this to all my patients—there are techniques you can incorporate into your lifestyle to make everyday activities easier to do. Ask your doctor to refer you to an occupational therapist. Insurance typically covers a predetermined number of sessions.

• **Get a handle on stress.** There's a definite link between stress and pain. Diffusing that relationship is helpful whether you do it by practicing deep breathing…working one-on-one with a mental health professional… and/or joining a support group. To find an arthritis support group near you, consult the website CreakyJoints.org.

Healthy Habits That Help

Regardless of which type of arthritis you have, the same good habits will help. *What's most important…*

• **Eat a more nutritious diet.** Obesity, high blood pressure and diabetes often go hand-in-hand with gout and psoriatic arthritis. Rheumatoid arthritis increases risk for heart problems. People with ankylosing spondylitis may also suffer from Crohn's disease or ulcerative colitis, which are inflammatory diseases of the gut. Osteoarthritis is linked to depression. In every case, you'll benefit by avoiding foods that are high in saturated fat and added sugars…and adopting a diet that's rich in fiber with plenty of fruits, vegetables and whole grains.

With gout, you'll also want to avoid foods high in purine, a naturally occurring compound that forms uric acid. These foods include fatty red meats, organ meats and shellfish, as well as beer. Many people with psoriatic arthritis have fatty liver disease and should limit alcohol.

• **Stay active.** Exercise lubricates joints, and keeping ligaments limber and muscles strong reduces the physical load that joints have to bear. Arthritis pain can flare with strenuous activity, so find your personal "sweet spot" when it comes to intensity and duration—do enough to benefit joints without overtaxing them. Many people say strength training that targets the "core" muscles of the abdomen, chest and back makes them feel better.

With osteoarthritis, you might think that your exercise choices are limited because the more you move, the more stress and pain you feel. But listen to your body for ways to adapt, such as switching to low-impact walking if running is difficult.

• **Lose weight if necessary.** For every type of arthritis, carrying around extra pounds means you're putting additional stress on your joints. Losing just 10% of your body weight can make a big difference.

Best Nondrug Ways to Fight Autoimmune Disease

Mark Hyman, MD, director of the Cleveland Clinic Center for Functional Medicine in Ohio. Dr. Hyman is also board president of clinical affairs of The Institute for Functional Medicine and founder and director of The UltraWellness Center, based in Lenox, Massachusetts. He is author of several books, including *Food: What the Heck Should I Eat?* DrHyman.com

Americans are facing an autoimmune epidemic. More than 24 million of us are currently affected by autoimmune disorders, which encompass 80-plus conditions including psoriasis, rheumatoid arthritis, lupus, inflammatory bowel disease and multiple sclerosis.

Conventional medicine attempts to tackle these tricky conditions with treatments such as powerful immune suppressant medications, steroids and over-the-counter anti-inflammatory drugs like aspirin or *ibuprofen* to reduce inflammation and alleviate symptoms such as joint pain, skin rashes, abdominal pain and tingling limbs. But these drugs can be hit or miss and lead to side effects as extreme as bone and muscle loss, diabetes, depression, liver problems and kidney failure. And they don't address the root cause of the problem.

A Much Better Way

Thanks to groundbreaking research in the last decade, functional medicine—which aims to treat medical problems at the root cause—now provides an effective plan to prevent and reverse autoimmune diseases.

The various autoimmune diseases are really just one disorder with countless variations based on a patient's genetic weak link and a common denominator of systemic inflammation that prompts the body to attack its own tissues.

Aside from genetics, most autoimmune diseases stem from environmental or lifestyle triggers, which include hidden infections…allergies or sensitivities to foods…toxins such as chemicals or heavy metals…and physical or psychological stress.

On top of that, the body may be missing factors it needs to regulate itself, such as certain vitamins, hormones, rest and relaxation, and/or exercise. One autoimmune patient's root cause could be chronic stress and a vitamin deficiency while another's might be high mercury levels in the body.

Try these strategies to treat or ward off autoimmune diseases…

• **Make changes to your diet.** Unearthing possible food allergies or sensitivities that contribute to autoimmune problems starts with eliminating grains…legumes…dairy…eggs…nightshades such as tomatoes, potatoes, eggplant and peppers…alcohol and coffee…flour…and processed sugar for six weeks.

Food groups can be added back into your diet one by one while monitoring how your body responds. If you experience symptoms such as fatigue, joint pain, digestive upset, headaches and/or sinus congestion when adding a particular food back into your diet, that food is likely a problem for you and should be eliminated from your diet.

Note: While some lab tests are very helpful in detecting food allergies and sensitivities, the elimination method described here is best.

Beneficial foods for autoimmune disease: Whole and unprocessed foods including vegetables…small amounts of meat and other proteins…and healthy fats such as extra-virgin coconut, olive, avocado, macadamia, walnut and almond oils, organic coconut milk, avocados, fatty fish like sardines, wild salmon, mackerel and herring, nuts (except peanuts) and seeds, olives and grass-fed or clarified butter or ghee.

These foods are nutrient dense with high levels of anti-inflammatory phytonutrients and omega-3 fatty acids.

•**Add these supplements.** Vitamin D, fish oil, vitamin C and probiotics connect with immune receptors to calm the immune response naturally. Also, consider taking a turmeric or curcumin supplement, which research credits with powerful antioxidant and anti-inflammatory properties.

Note: Check with your doctor before taking any new supplement and for the dosage that is best for you.

•**Get more exercise.** Regular physical activity is a proven disease-fighter, largely because it's extremely effective at reducing systemic inflammation. For those with autoimmune diseases, the best types depend on your possible limitations. Cardiovascular exercise such as jogging, biking, hiking or interval training for 30 minutes, six times a week is ideal…but even taking a brisk, 30-minute walk several days a week can make a real difference.

•**Try a variety of relaxation techniques.** We know that stress creates inflammation… so cutting stress is key to fighting autoimmune disorders. Try meditation, massage or even journaling for 20 minutes a day. Yoga can be relaxing as well.

•**Improve sleep.** It's worth a reminder that good immune function and stress reduction are both linked to getting high-quality, deep sleep. To promote optimal sleep, go to bed and wake up at the same time each day, use your bed only for sleep or sex, forgo caffeine after the morning hours, avoid vigorous exercise after dinner, and stop cell-phone and computer use within a couple hours of turning in.

Additional Strategies

From my experience, astoundingly, about 80% of autoimmune disease cases will improve solely by making dietary changes. But if you're not feeling dramatically better within six weeks of making changes to your diet, get tested for other underlying causes of inflammation. *Simple blood tests or other tests can check for…*

•**Infections such as Lyme disease, bacteria, viruses and yeast**

•**Celiac disease**

•**Heavy metal toxicity such as mercury exposure from fish consumption.**

Also helpful: Talk to your doctor about multiple systemic infectious disease syndrome (MSIDS). MSIDS is a persistent illness caused by Lyme disease and/or related tick-borne coinfections, parasitic or fungal infections, allergies, environmental toxicity and compromised immune function. Symptoms can include joint and muscle pain, dizziness and sleep problems.

To access the questionnaire, go to LymeActionNetwork.org and click on MSIDS. If your score is moderate to high, you will be advised to consult your doctor.

Sjögren's Syndrome Update

Alan Baer, MD, a professor of medicine and director of the Jerome L. Greene Sjögren's Syndrome Center at Johns Hopkins University School of Medicine in Baltimore. Dr. Baer, also an associate investigator at the Sjögren's Syndrome Clinic at the National Institutes of Health, is engaged in clinical research studies regarding Sjögren's syndrome.

It's been dismissed as a "nuisance disease" compared with its better known autoimmune cousins such as rheumatoid arthritis and lupus.

Sjögren's (pronounced SHOW-grins) syndrome is far from a minor irritant for many of those affected. Chronic and progressive, it can cause a wide variety of symptoms. Because Sjögren's attacks glands that provide moisture, its symptoms can include dry eyes and mouth, eye pain, blurry vision, burning mouth, loss of taste, rampant tooth decay and difficulty swallowing.

Very often, the syndrome also causes fatigue, joint and muscle pain, rashes and brain fog. Plus, there can be complications, including lung or kidney inflammation. And those with Sjögren's can have a 15 to 20 times higher risk of developing lymphoma, a form of blood cancer, than those without it.

Striking up to 10 in 10,000 people—the vast majority of them women around menopause age—Sjögren's is not only frequently minimized, it's one of the most difficult autoimmune conditions to diagnose and treat.

Diagnostic challenges: An accurate diagnosis can help pinpoint how severely a patient is affected...and estimate the patient's risk for lymphoma. Unfortunately, the symptoms of Sjögren's often don't help with getting a proper diagnosis, as many are common to other health conditions. And no single test can diagnose it. *Useful diagnostic tests that can be underutilized...*

• **An array of antibody blood tests is the best starting point,** since the majority of patients have antibodies that support the diagnosis. However, the antibody tests alone are not sufficient.

• **An eye exam that includes special tests.** The Schirmer test measures tear flow. And the ocular surface stain test assesses damage to the surface of the eye due to dryness.

• **In-office biopsy of the tiny salivary glands inside the lip.** This is an essential test to confirm Sjögren's if the antibody tests are negative. The simple procedure, which involves a shallow incision to remove four to seven glands for analysis, is best done by an oral surgeon with experience in obtaining a good sample for Sjögren's diagnosis.

• **An ultrasound of the salivary glands uncovers changes in the glands caused by Sjögren's and helps define the severity of the syndrome.** For some, this can be a substitute for the lip biopsy.

Best treatments now: A patient with Sjögren's may be seeing multiple specialists, including an ophthalmologist, a dentist, a dermatologist and others, for treatment. A rheumatologist is the best type of doctor to serve as a quarterback of sorts to work collaboratively with all the specialists involved. *The most common Sjögren's treatments now include...*

• **Artificial tears and anti-inflammatory prescription eyedrops**—*cyclosporine* (Restasis) and *lifitegrast* (Xiidra).

• **Cholinergic agonist drugs,** including *pilocarpine* (Salagen) and *cevimeline* (Evoxac), for dry mouth.

• **Prescription-strength fluoride toothpaste to mitigate tooth decay.**

• **Antifungal medications or mouthwashes to treat thrush.**

• ***Hydroxychloroquine* (Plaquenil) for arthritis, fatigue and certain rashes.**

• **Immunosuppressant drugs,** like *methotrexate* (Trexall), *mycophenolate mofetil* (CellCept) and *azathioprine* (Azasan)...the biologic *rituximab* (Rituxan)...and corticosteroids, to reduce inflammation in the body.

•**Pain relievers,** including *acetaminophen* (Tylenol), *gabapentin* (Neurontin) and *duloxetine* (Cymbalta), for joint, nerve and muscle pain. Topical *diclofenac* can relieve pain in large joints.

Sjögren's patients often find that various natural treatments, such as massage, acupuncture and stress-reduction techniques, help their symptoms. An anti-inflammatory diet that includes plenty of whole fruits and vegetables, healthy fats, fiber and moderate amounts of organic meat...and eliminates or reduces trans fats, processed foods, preservatives and red meat may help as well.

Latest research: It's hoped that new clinical trials will discern if existing disease-modifying antirheumatic drugs (DMARDs), used successfully for other autoimmune disorders, might also work for Sjögren's. Arresting inflammation in the moisture-producing glands is the next big goal. To find clinical trials focusing on new treatments, go to info.Sjogrens.org/clinical-trials.

Turning Point for Fibromyalgia

For the first time, researchers have identified metabolic blood patterns that can identify patients with this frequently misdiagnosed (or undiagnosed) condition.

Next step: A blood test for faster, easier diagnosis and the potential for more targeted treatment.

Journal of Biological Chemistry

New Treatment for Crohns?

Immune cells from Crohn's patients contain less of a gut-specific protein found in the cells of healthy patients.

New finding: Infusions of modified cells that produce more of the protein may reduce cramps, diarrhea and other symptoms.

Next step: Clinical trials.

Gastroenterology

Restaurant Food Labeled Gluten-Free May Not Be

Nearly one-third of foods listed on menus as gluten-free contained gluten. Pizza and pasta labeled gluten-free were most likely to contain some gluten. It was present in 53.2% of pizza samples and 50.8% of the pasta that was tested. Restaurants where gluten tests were done were not named, and the amount of gluten found in foods labeled gluten-free was not disclosed. The Food and Drug Administration says foods may be labeled gluten-free if they contain less than 20 parts per million of gluten, but the testing device used in this study was able to detect gluten at levels lower than the FDA limit.

Benjamin Lerner, MD, department of medicine, Columbia University Medical Center, New York City, and leader of a study published in *American Journal of Gastroenterology*.

Rebuilding Powerhouse Muscles Helps Conquer Pain

Eric Goodman, DC, founder and creator of Foundation Training. Based in Carpinteria, California, he is author of *True to Form: How to Use Foundation Training for Sustained Pain Relief and Everyday Fitness* and coauthor of *Foundation: Redefine Your Core, Conquer Back Pain, and Move with Confidence.* FoundationTraining.com

Not surprisingly, all the hunching, slumping and slouching of modern-day life are taking a toll on our bodies. Reading and working on our computers and smartphones...spending large amounts of time in the car...watching TV on the couch. Life in the 21st century is filled with many pleasurable conveniences and one giant modern-day nuisance—chronic pain.

Specifically, the sitting and slumping compress the spine and overtax the joints. Over time, poor posture weakens the muscles along the back of the body known as the posterior chain. These powerhouse muscles—the back, glutes and hamstrings—are intended to do the heavy lifting, working to protect the joints and skeleton.

Excess sitting and inactivity cause the posterior chain to weaken, while the chest and quadriceps overdevelop to compensate. This causes joint degeneration and all of its debilitating symptoms, such as headache, neck, back and hip pain, carpal tunnel syndrome, plantar fasciitis and more. Compression squeezes the internal organs, too, impacting your breathing, your digestion and your immune function.

I created Foundation Training, a series of corrective body-weight exercises that allows you to use gravity to counterbalance the physical changes caused by inactivity. It healed my own chronic back pain, and I've watched as thousands of patients—from former professional basketball players in their 40s to decorated Air Force veterans in their 70s—have experienced great success and eventual pain relief with this system.

When you reactivate and strengthen the chain, your body rediscovers how to move properly, the pain dissipates and, eventually, stops.

Core Movements

Here are four good starter exercises that will help engage your posterior chain and reactivate neglected muscles—without going to the gym or investing in any special equipment.

• **Decompression breathing.** The first of these exercises, called decompression breathing, is present in every future Foundation Training pose. It is the standard way to enter and exit the positions for all of the exercises.

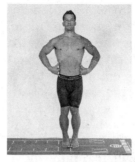

A curled or hunched stance hinders the lungs' ability to expand and contract, leading to shallow breathing, which in turn shortchanges every other organ and process in the body. Decompression breathing works to actively lift and widen the rib cage while simultaneously strengthening all of the muscles that are required to keep the rib cage there.

Stand tall, toes touching, an inch or so between the heels. Place your thumbs on the bottoms of your rib cage, pinkie fingers on the tops of your pelvic bones. Inhale deeply, broadening and elevating the rib cage as much as possible, and trying to increase the distance between your thumbs and pinkies. As your chest lifts up and expands, you begin to experience a widening of the rib cage in all directions. Remember to keep the back of your neck long and shoulders down.

As you exhale, imagine your rib cage remaining in its expanded state. The goal is to maintain that upper-torso expansion when you exhale. Inhale again, filling out even further, using slow and controlled breaths. Breathe in for three to five seconds, and breathe out for five to seven seconds with every decompression breath. Do this for 10 breaths, and you should instantly feel taller and more energized.

• **Supine decompression.** As with the previous move, this is about strengthening and expanding your lungs and lifting your chest so that your internal organs are no longer squished. Begin by lying down on a yoga mat, face up, with your hands resting on your chest and your legs and feet touching each other. Your neck should be long—imagine lots of space between the bottom of your head and the base of your neck. Move your hands to the ground, slightly away from your sides with your palms up.

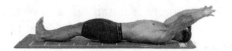

Start to squeeze your knees together, engaging the leg muscles. At the same time, flex your feet so that your toes point toward the ceiling (heels remain on the floor), and press your hands into the ground (try to get every fingernail touching the floor).

Keeping your knees squeezed and feet together and flexed, lift both knees a few inches off the ground—your knees will bend, and your heels will naturally move a few inches closer to your rear end as you do this. Extend your arms above your chest with your fingertips touching, forming a ball. Continue to lift your extended arms overhead with your fingertips still in the ball position, lifting your chest higher with each breath. You should feel tension in your pelvis, shins, arms and neck. Repeat the move 10 times, with the same breath count as you used for the standing decompression breathing.

Reawaken Your Posterior Chain

Even active people can have weak posterior chains—back muscles, glutes and hamstrings—if they spend the majority of their time sitting or have chronic poor posture. Every time they exercise or go for a stroll, they're exercising the wrong muscles. The muscles in the front of the body end up doing the heavy lifting, so to speak, fighting gravity every step of the way. At the same time, the powerful muscles along the back of the legs and hips learn to live in a short, tight, underutilized position.

To shift the burden of supporting your body back to the strong posterior chain, you need to challenge those long-neglected glutes, hams and back muscles with these two very effective exercises…

• **The Founder.** Stand with your feet wide, about three feet apart. Your weight should be in your heels, arms down at your sides, chest up, shoulders down. Your chest should be fully expanded and held high (higher than what might feel natural or comfortable). Face forward and take a deep decompression breath, expanding the rib cage.

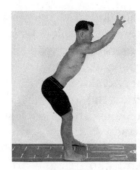

Next, begin to hinge at the hips, knees very slightly bent, extending your hips back behind you, as if you were starting to sit down in a chair. At the same time, reach your arms in front of you, as if you were pretending to touch the top of an imaginary doorway. (You'll be in a pose similar to a chair pose in yoga.) Look straight ahead, keeping your head in line with your spine. Hold for 10 seconds, breathing deeply while keeping your chest elevated. Let your back muscles burn—they're getting stronger! Lift your arms up a few more inches, pointing toward the seam where the wall meets the ceiling. Your gaze remains straight ahead. Hold for 10 more seconds. A few Founders a day will strengthen your muscles. When done well, it's a powerful pose.

• **The 8-point plank.** Begin by lying on a yoga mat, stomach down, head and upper body propped up as if you are in a sphinx pose. You'll be propped up on your forearms, hands flat on the floor, elbows a few inches in front of your shoulders. Your forearms will point straight ahead, and your palms should be flat on the floor. Flex your feet so that your toes press into the ground. Your knees should continue touching the ground.

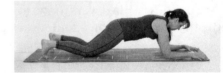

Note: You now have eight points of contact with the floor—two hands, two elbows, two knees, two feet.

Start decompression breathing. With each inhale, feel your ribs expand—you'll feel a lifting sensation in your upper body, almost as if your back is floating up toward the ceiling. Continue pressing your palms, forearms, knees and toes into the ground as your upper back lifts. Eventually, your pelvis will follow, lifting a few inches off the ground.

Note: The eight points all stay on the ground. Allow your head to sag—keep your neck long and your chin back, and gaze at your hands. Continue decompression breathing for five to 10 breaths, then gently lower yourself back down.

Perform several of these planks a day for three to six months to elicit a major shift in your posture, pain and overall health. The exercises will activate muscle connections. Each time you practice, you are improving upon a neurological pattern. You won't just get stronger, you'll get better.

You can find free tutorials for each of the exercises shown in this article by searching "Foundation Training" at YouTube.com.

Roll Away Tight Muscles

Joel Harper, a New York City–based personal trainer whose clients include several Olympic medalists. The creator of the PBS DVD *Joel Harper's Firming After 50*, he designed all of the personal workout chapters for Dr. Mehmet C. Oz and Dr. Michael F. Roizen's YOU series of books and accompanying workout DVDs. He is author of *Mind Your Body: 4 Weeks to a Leaner, Healthier Life* and the Bottom Line blog "Your Personal Mind-Body Coach." JoelHarper Fitness.com

F oam rollers are great for easing muscle tightness and relieving soreness by releasing knots in fascia, which surround the muscles, and increasing blood flow to enhance recovery. *Roll away muscle stiffness and pain in three common tight spots…*

Tight-Muscle Moves

Roll back and forth from the top to the bottom of each target muscle 25 times. Do one set per muscle. Repeat all exercises on both sides of your body. Never roll over joints.

•**IT Band Roll**—for the iliotibial band that runs along the outside of your thighs and helps keep your hips and knees stable. Lie on your right side with the roller under the middle of your thigh. Support your upper body with your right forearm on the ground

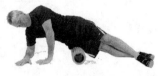

and your left hand on the floor in front of your stomach. Keep your chin up and right elbow pressed back so that you stay on your side and avoid tilting forward with your upper body. Legs are together, ankles crossed. If this is too difficult, cross the top leg over the bottom one and anchor your left foot on the floor for balance. Use your hands and your core to shift your weight and help you roll along the full length of your quad.

•**Lat Roll**—releases tension in the muscles on the upper sides of your back. Lie on your right side, legs together and bent at right angles. Place the roller just below your armpit, perpendicular to your body. Your right elbow is bent in the air, and your right hand is holding your head. Using your left hand as a

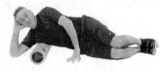

prop, use your hips and legs to roll two inches up and down along the muscles wherever you feel it is most needed. You also can tilt your body forward and back to get a cross-muscle massage as well.

•**Calf Roll.** Sit on the floor with legs straight, and place the roller under your calves (or under only your right calf with your left leg to the side if that is easier), just above the ankle. Lean your upper body back slightly, and place your hands flat on the floor for support, arms slightly bent. Use your hands and hips to help you roll up and down the length of your calves, tilting your legs slightly from side to side as you roll to find the area that needs it most. To add pressure, cross one leg over the other, bending the upper

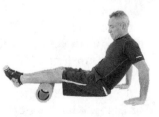

leg so that your foot is on the top of your calf…or for even more pressure, slide your foot down your calf to rest on your ankle. Switch legs and repeat.

How to Make Physical Therapy More Effective

Mitchell Yass, DPT, a specialist in diagnosing and resolving pain and creator of the Yass Method for treating chronic pain. He is author of *Overpower Pain, The Pain Cure Rx* and *The Yass Method for Pain-Free Movement.* MitchellYass.com

If you're suffering from neck, back or knee pain, physical therapy is one of the most commonly recommended treatments. But often, it just doesn't work. There's a good reason for that, though very few people understand what goes wrong.

Typically, when pain is severe and/or chronic, doctors order an MRI, which often identifies a structural abnormality (such as a herniated disk, pinched nerve, arthritis or torn cartilage)—and that structural deviation is usually assumed to be causing the pain.

Here's where things get tricky: Most people—in pain or not—have these sorts of structural variations within their bodies. In fact, research shows that the overwhelming majority of people age 65 and older who are not in pain have some disk degeneration.

Based on my 25 years of treating thousands of patients with neck, back or knee pain, I have found that in more than 95% of the cases, the cause of pain was muscular—and not due to a disk, nerve or some other structural abnormality. Muscular problems often go undetected because they are not visible on an MRI or other diagnostic scans, and there are no medical specialists trained to diagnose and treat them.

Once you're in a physical therapist's (PT) office, he/she is not required to confirm or refute your doctor's diagnosis. If you're diagnosed with a pinched nerve or arthritis when you enter physical therapy, you'll be treated for that condition—even if that's not the real cause of your symptoms.

A complete physical evaluation can identify whether the cause of the pain is structural or muscular. When muscular, the simple tests below will reveal telltale clues to the underlying problem, which often can be corrected with the exercises that follow (typically performed in three sets of 10 reps each, three times a week, resting one minute between sets…until you are pain free).* *Give this information to your PT, who can use it to identify the true cause of your pain and help you perform the exercises…*

Neck and Upper-Back Pain

The likely culprit: Muscle weakness and/or imbalance of the neck and upper-torso muscles will lead to poor posture. Most neck and upper-back pain is felt a few inches away from one or both sides of the spine. However, a structural variation (such as a bulging disk or pinched nerve) would typically lead to a major loss of range of motion (ROM) and cause pain along the spine.

One common offender: The levator scapulae muscle, which attaches from the inside upper corner of each shoulder blade to the upper neck, supporting the head and stabilizing the shoulders. Because of rampant computer and smartphone use, hunched, rounded posture shortens and pulls the chest muscles forward, weakening and overstretching the levator scapulae muscle, causing neck and/or upper-back pain.

Ask your practitioner to…

•**Press on the spot where you typically experience pain.** For many patients, this will be at the top inner corner of one or both shoulder blades, where the levator scapulae originates. If pressing here triggers or intensifies your pain, this strongly suggests a muscular problem.

•**Evaluate your posture.** If your head and shoulders lean in front of your hips when standing, that's another indicator of weak muscles.

•**Check your ROM.** Tight, weak muscles can restrict motion and/or cause pain as you move your head side to side, touch your chin to your chest or lean your head back.

Try this test: Lie on your back on the exam table with your head hanging off the end but

*Ask your PT for guidance on any exercise regimen you take.

supported by the PT. As you completely relax your neck, ask the PT to gently move your head side to side…and up and down.

If your head can be easily and painlessly moved back and forth and up and down, the tight muscle theory is confirmed. If the PT has difficulty moving your head, and it feels like a bone is hitting another bone, this is a sign that a structural variation is limiting ROM and contributing to neck pain.

Exercises to perform to correct the muscular imbalance causing neck pain and poor posture: Lat pulldowns with a neutral grip and a lower trap exercise to strengthen the lower trapezius muscle, which extends from your neck and across your shoulder blade to the middle of your back. (Ask your PT to demonstrate.)

Low-Back Pain

The likely culprit: Tight quads and hip flexors. Hip flexors are workhorse muscles that originate on either side of the lower spine and travel down the front of the pelvis, attaching at the hip joints. Sitting for hours at a time, day after day—at a desk, in a car or in front of a TV, for instance—weakens the hamstrings and shortens and strains the hip flexors. Tight hip flexors, along with weak hamstrings, cause the pelvis to tip forward, creating an excessive arch and back pain… none of which show up on an MRI.

Hint: If you typically need to push on your thighs with your hands to stand fully upright after sitting, you likely have tight hip flexors—your hands are helping to manually lengthen your hip flexors.

Ask your practitioner to…

•**Press on your hip flexors.** Tender? That's one sign they may be causing your low-back pain.

•**Evaluate your posture.** You want just a very mild curve in your lower spine, with the front and back of the pelvis at equal height.

•**Check for dominant quad muscles.** Again, lie on your back on the exam table, this time with your butt at the edge of the table and your legs hanging off. Pull one knee

toward your chest as the other leg dangles. If the foot of the dangling leg is not perpendicular to the knee (less than a 90-degree angle with the foot pointing away from the table), the quad is dominant and overly tight, contributing to low-back pain.

Exercises to resolve the muscle imbalance leading to low-back pain: Hamstring curls, hip extensions and hip abductions. (Ask your PT to demonstrate.)

Note: Perform the exercises only on the painful side—or on both sides if pain affects both sides.

Knee Pain

The likely culprit: People with pain around the kneecap are frequently told they have meniscal tears or "bone-on-bone arthritis," which indicates a complete loss of cartilage in the joint between the base of the thighbone and the top of the shinbone. Both of these conditions limit ROM and can be treated only with surgery. Furthermore, neither of these conditions causes pain around the kneecap. If the real cause of your pain is muscle imbalance (with your quads being far stronger than your hamstrings)—and it likely is—surgery isn't necessary and won't even help.

Ask your practitioner to…

•**Check your ROM when you bend your knee if you've been told you have bone-on-bone arthritis or a meniscal tear.** If either condition is causing your pain, you will have a significant loss of ROM, and the end point of movement will feel like a bone is hitting another bone, preventing further motion. If pain occurs around the kneecap and you have full ROM, this rules out either bone-on-bone arthritis or a meniscal tear as the cause of pain.

•**Watch you negotiate stairs.** A muscular problem causes pain as the knee joint struggles to maintain alignment as you walk up or down stairs—as well as with standing and sometimes with sitting.

•**Check for dominant quad muscles.** (See earlier description.)

Exercises to resolve muscular imbalance and pain around the kneecap: Hamstring curls, hip extensions, knee extensions and quad stretches. (Ask your PT to demonstrate.) Do these exercises only on the side where the knee is painful. If you have pain in both knees, do the exercises on both sides.

Try Pain-Fighting Acupressure for Easy TCM Self-Care

Catherine Browne, DAOM, LAc, DipLAc, RH, a holistic practitioner in Harmony, North Carolina, who specializes in the treatment of pain, emotional imbalances and opioid dependency. She is author of *Natural Therapies for Overcoming Opioid Dependency: Control Pain and Recover from Addiction.*DrCatherineBrowne.com

When it comes to fighting pain, Traditional Chinese Medicine (TCM) offers a variety of therapies—some of which can be used as self-care.

For example, acupressure—in which pressure is applied with the fingers to acupoints (or "energy points")—is a simple, effective alternative to acupuncture, a TCM therapy commonly used to treat pain.

Two acupoints on the wrist—LU7 and LU9 (see below)—can help ease many types of chronic pain.

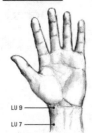

LUNGS (LU)

LU 9
LU 7

What to do: Starting with the left wrist, apply pressure with your thumb or fingers to each point, for one to three minutes. The pressure should be firm but not painful. Repeat on the right wrist. Do this several times daily.

Important: It takes regular, long-term acupressure treatments to affect chronic pain—often for several months. Even though acupuncture is generally considered more "potent" than acupressure, the latter can be an effective and convenient self-treatment option.

Quell Harmful Emotions to Ease Pain

Harmful emotions, such as chronic anger, create stagnation of the liver, which controls the flow of blood and qi (vital energy) throughout the body.

For liver qi stagnation—one of the most common imbalances in Western societies contributing to chronic pain syndromes—use the acupressure points LV2 and LV3 (using the steps described in adjacent article).

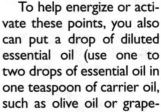

LIVER (LV)

LV 3
LV 2

To help energize or activate these points, you also can put a drop of diluted essential oil (use one to two drops of essential oil in one teaspoon of carrier oil, such as olive oil or grapeseed oil) on the areas that correspond with the liver prior to each acupressure session. Fennel, marjoram and mandarin orange/tangerine essential oil all correspond to the liver acupuncture channel, and you can combine them or choose one that appeals to you.

Note: If you have allergies, test a small amount of diluted essential oil on your wrist before using to make sure there is no reaction.

Credit: Excerpted from *Natural Therapies for Overcoming Opioid Dependency* © by Dr. Catherine Browne, illustrations by Ilona Sherratt, used with permission from Storey Publishing.

Gender Gap with Pain

Boys' pain is taken more seriously than the same pain felt by girls. Women, in particular, rated boys' pain higher—while men rated boys' and girls' pain more similarly. The reason is unknown, but researchers hope that the findings will add insight into the role of gender bias in pain management and health care.

Study in which 264 adults were asked to rate the pain of a child during a doctor's finger-prick test, by researchers at Yale University, New Haven, Connecticut, published in *Journal of Pediatric Psychology.*

Chapter 13

PHYSICAL INJURY AND BONE HEALTH

New Tech for Staying Safe and Independent at Home

New high-tech products, ranging from devices that predict falls to those that provide computer-generated reminders, are making it safer and easier for more people to remain independent as they grow older. *Here are some of the notable new tech devices that can help seniors continue to live safely in their homes and communities...*

Virtual Caregiving

These days, living alone doesn't have to mean there's no one around to help. A number of new tech products can provide some of the oversight and support traditionally supplied by a caregiver when no one else is around—and they can do so without the loss of privacy that comes with an in-home caregiver. *Examples...*

• **CarePredict Tempo** is a behavior-monitoring device that is worn like a wristwatch, but it uses sophisticated pattern-recognition technology to identify the wearer's nascent health issues before they escalate. The system closely monitors the person's move-

ments inside the home—walking speed, the amount of time spent in bed or in the bathroom and the amount of time spent eating, for example—then identifies changes to these patterns that could potentially presage a developing health or fitness concern. When the device spots a troubling change, it notifies loved ones via text and/or e-mail, often before the situation becomes dire. According to the company, a pilot study conducted in assisted-living facilities reduced falls by 25% by identifying the early stages of movement and balance problems. CarePredict Tempo costs $449.99 and $69.99/month for monitoring services. CarePredict.com

• **LifePod from LifePod Solutions,** Inc., is comparable to "virtual assistants" Alexa and Siri, but it's designed specifically to provide support to people of advancing age. LifePod can be programmed to ask its user how he/she is feeling at predetermined intervals, and it reports appropriate replies to loved ones via text message. Caregivers (or seniors themselves) can ask LifePod to provide reminders, such as "It's 10:00—did you take your morn-

---

Laurie Orlov, tech-industry analyst and founder of Aging in Place Technology Watch, a market research company that provides research and analysis about tech designed to help seniors continue to live safely in their homes. AgeInPlaceTech.com

ing pills?" or "It's your grandson Tommy's birthday—don't forget to call him." Like other smart speakers, it also can respond to verbal requests to play music, read audiobooks, check the weather and more. $49/month or $432 for one year. LifePod.com

Fall Detection

Each year, around 25% of people 65 and older suffer falls. Wearable devices that can summon assistance in these situations have been around for decades, but the latest generation of fall-detection tech even can identify a fall and call for help on its own when the wearer is unconscious. *Among the options…*

•**Apple Watch Series 5** can detect that its wearer has fallen and notify a preselected emergency contact if that wearer is unresponsive. Its Emergency SOS feature lets users quickly and easily call 911 and/or notifies emergency contacts via text message when the wearer requires help in other situations. This watch, which is designed to work in conjunction with an Apple iPhone, can monitor heart rate—it even generates electrocardiograms for viewing the results on the watch itself—and serves as an activity and sleep tracker. Non–health-related functions include streaming music, providing maps and directions and making and receiving phone calls and texts. Its price starts at $399 (or $499 for a version that has built-in cellular capabilities so that it can function when the user's iPhone is not nearby). Apple.com

•**MyNotifi** is a fall-detection device that can be worn either as a wristband or with a belt clip. Like the Apple Watch, MyNotifi sends a text to preselected emergency contacts when it detects a fall (unless the wearer dismisses the fall as a false alarm)—but it does not include the other health-monitoring features of the Apple Watch. It costs $199 for a version that works in conjunction with your smartphone…$229 for a version that does not require a smartphone. MyNotifi is compatible with iOS and Android. MyNotifi.com

Medication Management

•**MedMinder Pharmacy** ships prefilled, presorted weekly pill trays to patients, so they don't need to sort out pills on their own…and so they never have to worry, *Did I remember to take my pills this morning?* The prefilled disposable trays are placed in the company's automated pill dispenser—when it's time to take medication a light flashes in the compartment containing the appropriate pills. If pills are not taken on schedule, the device beeps. If that doesn't work, the patient and/or his/her loved ones receive an alert via phone, text or e-mail. MedMinder Pharmacy does not charge extra for this pill-sorting service. It accepts most insurance and Medicare Part D plans, and your co-pays typically are the same as they would be at a pharmacy. There is a monthly fee for the high-tech pill dispenser—prices start at $24.99 per month—but if you want to avoid the added cost, presorted "weekly pill packs" that are designed to be used on their own, without the dispenser, also are available at no additional charge. MedMinder.com

Hearing Assistance

•**Oticon Opn and Opn S hearing aids** also serve as wireless Bluetooth headsets for making and receiving smartphone calls when paired with an accessory called ConnectClip. This accessory clips to the hearing aid wearer's clothing and includes a microphone so that its user can be heard clearly by callers. It works with both Apple and Android smartphones. ConnectClip also can be used to stream music and other audio directly to these Oticon hearing aids…and it can be used as a remote microphone—place ConnectClip directly in front of the person you are speaking with to hear him better in a noisy environment. ConnectClip tends to sell for around $400, while Opn and Opn S hearing aids generally cost $2,000 or more per ear from an audiologist. (The Opn S is the latest generation of the Opn and fares somewhat better in tests of speech understanding.) Oticon.com

Don't Take a Fall

- **Increase lighting in your home,** especially along common paths you travel such as from the bedroom to the bathroom. Motion sensor lights that go on automatically are ideal.

- **Get rid of throw rugs,** or tack them down to avoid tripping. Remove clutter. Clean up spills immediately.

- **Review all your medications with your doctor or pharmacist** to check for side effects such as sleepiness, dizziness and blurry vision that could increase your chance of falling.

- **Get your vision and hearing checked.** If you have the wrong prescription, you may fail to see uneven surfaces. And hearing loss can make you less cognizant of your environment.

- **Improve your sense of balance.** Take tai chi classes, which focus on balance and muscle strength. Studies have shown that tai chi reduces falls significantly when practiced regularly.

- **Be aware of your surroundings at all times.** Don't walk under the influence of your smartphone. Let it wait.

- **For wintry walks, consider adding traction cleats to your shoes' bottoms.**

Kathleen A. Cameron, MPH, director of the National Council on Aging's National Falls Prevention Resource Center in Alexandria, Virginia.

Heart Drugs May Increase Risk of Falls

Taking AFib drugs may increase risk for falls and fainting in older patients.

Latest finding: Amiodarone (Nexterone and Pacerone) was associated with fainting and falls in older people with AFib, in part because it can lead to bradycardia (slow heartbeat). Use precautions—such as rising from a seated position slowly—especially in the first two weeks after starting the medication.

Other AFib drug previously linked to falls: *Digoxin* (Lanoxin).

Frederik Dalgaard, MD, a cardiovascular researcher at Herlev and Gentofte Hospital, Hellerup, Denmark, and leader of a study published in *Journal of the American Geriatrics Society.*

What's Really to Blame for Your Balance Problems

Victor M. Romano, MD, a board-certified orthopedic surgeon in private practice in Oak Park, Illinois, where he specializes in sports medicine. He is also a clinical affiliate faculty member at Midwestern University Chicago College of Osteopathic Medicine and a clinical assistant professor at Loyola University in Chicago. He is author of *Finding the Source: Maximizing Your Results—With and Without Orthopaedic Surgery.* RomanoMD.com

If you feel a little wobbly on your feet, you may chalk it up to the fact that you're simply growing older. After all, when your muscles, joints and vision don't work as well as they once did, it can destabilize you—making a fall more likely.

No one wants to break a hip and end up using a walker or living in a nursing home, so you're probably doing your best to prevent a disabling fall. But are you doing all you can to address the underlying causes of poor balance?

To learn about these hidden culprits, we spoke with Victor M. Romano, MD, a board-certified orthopedic surgeon who diagnoses and repairs ailing bones, joints and muscles. In his practice, he has learned about unexpected issues that can sabotage balance.*

The Misalignment Problem

The medical community has almost entirely ignored two scientific papers published just

---

*Check with your doctor before starting this—or any new—exercise program.

over a decade ago in *Practical Pain Management*, which uncovered a missing link in the role that chronic pain and muscle weakness play in causing poor balance.

The problem: If a joint (where two bones connect) is out of correct alignment, the body unconsciously compensates to restore stability. For example, if one of the joints in the right foot is out of alignment, the body unconsciously overuses the left foot. This "compensation" causes left knee pain, weaker muscles on the right side—and poorer balance. Because there are more than 300 joints in the human body, it can be challenging to find a misalignment—even for an orthopedic surgeon!

Dr. Romano's solution: A series of simple stretches that I have developed and successfully used in my practice over the past five years—called the Romano Stretches—prevent or correct nearly every misalignment that can cause balance problems. By doing these stretches, you will help restore your balance, relieve aches and pains, improve strength and flexibility—and, in turn, prevent falls.

The Romano Stretches

The following stretches address the most common areas where misalignment occurs in the human body, leading to balance problems. *Do the stretches daily—you can complete them all in just a few minutes...*

•**Pelvic stretch.** Restoring pelvic balance improves your side-to-side balance and range of motion of your shoulders. You will feel this stretch in the lower back and buttocks.

What to do: While lying flat on your back, grab your right knee with your left hand and bring your knee across your body toward the left side of your chest. At the same time, stretch your right arm and shoulder to the right, keeping them on the floor. (See right.) Turn your head to

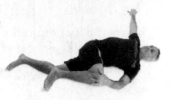

the right for an additional stretch if you desire. Hold for five to 10 seconds. Next, do the exercise on the other side, grabbing your left knee with your right hand, and stretching your left arm and shoulder to the left while turning your head to the left if you desire. Repeat twice on each side of your body.

•**Hip stretch.** This stretch helps restore alignment in the back and neck—and is excellent for reversing loss of balance and restoring mobility of the hip. You should feel this stretch in the top of your thigh, particularly toward the hip.

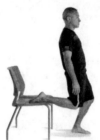

What to do: While standing about six to 12 inches in front of a chair, bend your right leg at the knee so that your foot (toes pointed) and a few inches of your shin rest on the seat of the chair. Lean back to feel a stretch in your right groin. Then slowly bend your left knee slightly to get a deeper stretch. Hold the stretch for five to 10 seconds and return to an upright position. Then do the same stretch with your left leg on the chair behind you, bending your right knee. Repeat twice on each side.

If you feel unstable while doing this stretch: Use a chair with arms and hold onto them as you lean back or stand next to a sturdy counter or desk to steady yourself.

•**Rib stretch.** A misalignment in the ribs can cause pain and weakness in the upper back, neck, shoulders, hands and elbows—all of which can contribute to poor balance. You should feel this stretch in your upper back and ribs.

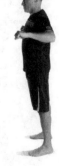

What to do: While standing, bend your arms to a 90-degree angle and bring your elbows out to your sides, parallel to the ground and just below shoulder level. Forcefully and quickly, pull your elbows backward in two short bursts and repeat two to three times.

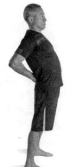

• **Back stretch.** This stretch is excellent for relieving upper and lower back pain. Patients with this problem have impaired balance when moving their heads up or down or turning side to side. This stretch should be felt in your lower back.

What to do: While standing, put your fists against the small of your back and arch your back as far as you can for five to 10 seconds. Relax and slowly exhale while stretching. Repeat two to three times.

Standing This Way Doubles Fracture Risk

Study titled "High Postural Sway Is an Independent Risk Factor for Osteoporotic Fractures but Not for Mortality in Elderly Women" by researchers at University of Eastern Finland and Kuopio University Hospital, published in *Journal of Bone and Mineral Research.*

When you stand still, do you sway a bit? This phenomenon, known as postural sway, affects everyone. But if you rock back and forth like you're riding bumpy waves in the ocean, that's called high postural sway.

Postural sway (which includes side-to-side and forward-backward movements) increases when our muscles become weak and physiologic changes occur in our sensory systems—as we age, for example, and with certain medical conditions such as stroke and multiple sclerosis. Not surprisingly, people with high postural sway don't always have good balance and have been shown to be at increased risk of falling.

To better understand the effects of high postural sway, Finnish scientists decided to take the research a step further to investigate whether this phenomenon increases risk for bone fractures.

To do this, researchers measured postural sway in 1,568 peri- and postmenopausal women and followed up 15 years later with questionnaires and a review of hospital records to see how many of the women experienced a bone fracture.

Study results: Women with the greatest postural sway were twice as likely to have suffered a fracture than women with the least postural sway. This was true for all types of fractures, including those affecting the wrist, spine and hip.

Even worse, the data showed that women with both high postural sway and low bone mineral density—a hallmark of the brittle bone disease osteoporosis and its precursor osteopenia—were five times more likely to have a fracture of any type and 11 times more likely to have an osteoporotic fracture than women with the highest bone density and least postural sway.

Based on these findings, the researchers identified postural sway as a new, independent risk factor for fracture.

Takeaway: Adding postural sway to the current list of risk factors for bone fractures may help health-care professionals identify women who are at increased risk so that steps can be taken to protect their bone health.

If you suspect that you have high postural sway, get evaluated by a health-care provider trained in postural assessment (such as a physical therapist, personal trainer or primary care provider with advanced education in this specialized area). Good posture training and balance exercises may help lower your fracture risk.

Atopic Eczema Increases Risk for Fractures

Having atopic eczema can increase risk for fractures. In a recent study, people with atopic eczema had 13% higher risk for fracture than people without. People with severe cases had at least double the risk for hip, pelvic and spinal fractures.

Caution: Ask your doctor if you need a bone density test, and avoid oral steroids, which increase fracture risk.

Study of more than three million adults by researchers at London School of Hygiene & Tropical Medicine, UK, published in *Journal of Allergy and Clinical Immunology.*

How You Exercise May Be Weakening Your Bones!

Oddbjørn Klomsten Andersen, MSc, doctoral candidate, Norwegian School of Sport Sciences, Oslo, Norway. He competed four years as a semi-professional cyclist and was a national-team cyclist. He is lead author of study titled "Bone health in elite Norwegian endurance cyclists and runners: a cross-sectional study," published in *BMJ Open Sport & Exercise Medicine.*

Cycling is great exercise—especially for your heart and muscles. But new research is finding that cycling and other low-impact activities don't do your bones any favor. There's no need to abandon your favorite sports! Just make sure to add these other activities to your fitness regimen so your bones stay strong and healthy.

Of course, any exercise is better than no exercise. It's well accepted that high-impact activities—such as running, volleyball, basketball and tennis—are good for your bones, particularly by helping to prevent osteoporosis and fractures as we age. It's thought that the repeated pounding against the ground minutely bends bones in the legs, hips and spine…triggering an increase in bone cells that strengthens those bones to withstand future impacts.

Researchers from the Norwegian School of Sport Sciences wanted to look at the effect of low-impact exercise on bones. For their study, they compared the bone mineral density (BMD) of 21 healthy male and female elite runners, ages 18 to 35, with the BMD of a similar group of 19 elite cyclists. Most of the cyclists and five of the runners also did heavy resistance training. The researchers measured BMD for total body, femoral neck (thighbone)

and lumbar spine using dual-energy X-ray absorptiometry (DXA). Both groups also consumed adequate amounts of calcium according to current recommendations.

Results: The cyclists had much lower BMD than the runners. Ten of the cyclists were classified with low bone mineral density, according to American College of Sports Medicine criteria…including one cyclist who had clinical osteoporosis in his spine, despite doing heavy resistance training, which is believed to protect bone. In comparison, none of the runners had low bone mineral density.

While the results of this study may seem to take some of the shine off the exercise halo for cycling, swimming, tai chi, rowing and other low-impact activities—those are still great ways to stay fit. For one thing, such exercises let you work out while sparing your joints. It's also important to note that the lower BMD of the cyclists in the Norwegian study may be because they were elite or professional athletes, who typically keep their weight low to enhance performance during competition. So they may not have consumed enough calories to adequately support bone health. But for the rest of us, if most of your exercises are the low-impact sort, it might be a good idea to take some additional steps to keep your bones healthy. *The National Osteoporosis Foundation recommends…*

●**Get enough calcium and vitamin D.** It's best to get calcium from diet—foods such as milk, cheese, yogurt, collard greens and sardines (with bones) are good sources. Aim for 1,200 mg of calcium daily for women age 51 and older…and 1,000 mg/day for men until age 71, and 1,200 mg/day thereafter. Both men and women age 50 and older should also get 800 IU to 1,000 IU of vitamin D daily. Salmon, oysters, egg yolks and mushrooms are good food sources. Sunlight is another source of vitamin D. You can also get both calcium and vitamin D from fortified foods, such as orange juice. If you don't get enough of these nutrients from diet, talk to your doctor about supplements.

●**Do weight-bearing exercise and resistance training.** While the Norwegian study was not designed to see if weight-bearing exercise helped protect bone (for instance, the cyclists might have had even worse bone health if they hadn't done resistance training), other research has shown that it does benefit bones. The theory is that resistance training—including using free weights, a weighted vest, exercise bands and weight machines—causes muscles to pull on bones, which stimulates them to increase their density. In fact, the National Osteoporosis Foundation suggests that everyone do muscle-strengthening exercises two to three days per week and weight-bearing exercises for 30 minutes most days of the week.

•**Do balance exercises.** Yoga and Pilates can also help protect bones by improving strength and flexibility. But since some positions can put you at risk for fractures if you already have low bone density, be sure to check with a trained therapist to learn which exercises are safe for you.

•**Jump around.** As little as 10 minutes of jumping exercises—such as jumping jacks, jump rope or jump squats—three times a week has been shown to increase bone mass in children and adolescents. Adults may need more jumps to reap these benefits. If high-impact jumping is not an option, perhaps because of arthritis or other joint issues, low-impact weight-bearing exercises such as using an elliptical or stair-step machine will provide some benefit. Aim for 30 minutes on most days of the week.

•**Know your BMD.** A bone mineral density scan lets you and your doctor know what shape your bones are in and your risk for future fractures. The US Preventive Services Task Force recommends screening for osteoporosis with bone measurement testing (such as a DXA scan) for all women over age 65...and women under age 65 who are at high risk for fracture. The National Osteoporosis Foundation recommends a bone density test for men ages 70 and older...and for men ages 50 to 69 with risk factors. Discuss with your doctor how often to schedule additional scans.

Best Way to Walk for Strong Bones

Katarina Borer, PhD, professor emerita, School of Kinesiology, University of Michigan, Ann Arbor, lead author of study titled "Osteogenic Markers in Postmenopausal Diabetics Respond to Higher Mechanical Loading During Exercise After, Rather Than Before, the Meals," presented at the 2019 annual meeting of the Endocrine Society.

For women, risk for bone fractures increases significantly after menopause—even more so if they also have type 2 diabetes. One good way to protect against that risk is weight-bearing exercise, such as walking. Now a new study has found that walking a certain way may make walking even better at fracture-proofing bones.

Researchers at University of Michigan looked at the effect of weight-bearing exercise on bone in postmenopausal women with diabetes. For the exercise, the researchers chose two forms of walking—uphill, which involves working against gravity...and downhill, which involves adding downhill physical force to gravity. And because metabolism also affects bone formation relative to bone resorption (breakdown), they looked at whether eating a meal before or after walking made any difference in markers for bone growth.

Fifteen postmenopausal women with type 2 diabetes were randomly assigned to two of five different tests—walking uphill before eating a meal...walking downhill before eating a meal...walking uphill one hour after eating a meal...walking downhill one hour after eating a meal...no exercise (the control group).

The women who exercised walked twice a day for 40 minutes on treadmills that were set at a six-degree uphill or downhill slope. They wore shoe inserts that measured the amount of pressure being exerted on their feet and had their blood tested periodically to measure levels of two markers involved in bone growth—a marker for bone formation and one for bone resorption. Glucose and insulin levels were also measured. And either before or after exercising, the women ate a meal that contained sufficient calories to maintain weight. (Egg salad with a roll, salad, a piece of fruit, milk, orange juice and four graham cracker squares for the midmorning meal…or a bacon-ham-cheese sandwich, a cup of vegetables, salad, a piece of fruit, fruit juice and ice cream with a cookie for the late-afternoon meal.)

Results…

• **Walking before eating either meal, both uphill and downhill, had no effect on either marker involved in bone metabolism.**

• **Walking after eating positively affected both markers for bone metabolism to varying degrees, depending on after which meal and whether walking uphill or downhill.**

• **The greatest and most effective increase in bone growth changes was shown when walking downhill after the morning meal.**

Bonus: Walking downhill after eating also lowered insulin resistance—47% lower during downhill exercise than during uphill exercise…and 62% lower than during the sedentary trial.

The women in this study had diabetes. However, the researchers have also done another study using healthy postmenopausal women and had similar results. They didn't test walking or running outdoors down actual hills but believe that would be just as effective. No hills near you? Stairs work just as well. In fact, walking down stairs or outdoors may be your best way to get some downhill trekking, since most treadmills can only be set to incline. (*Option:* Put blocks under the back of a treadmill to tilt it downward. But make sure to do it in a way that is sturdy and secure—falling off your treadmill will not help your bones!) And don't forget to have a balanced meal (or at least a snack) that includes carbs, fat and protein before you head out.

High Doses of Vitamin D Don't Help Bone Health

There was no difference in bone strength between people who met the recommended dietary allowance (RDA) of 600 International Units (IU) of vitamin D and people who took 4,000 IU or 10,000 IU supplements—but there was density loss in the tibia with higher doses. For bone health, current findings don't support supplementing over the RDA if you do not have a deficiency.

David A. Hanley, MD, professor emeritus of medicine, oncology and community health sciences at University of Calgary, Canada, and coauthor of a three-year trial of people ages 55 to 70, published in JAMA.

Is a "Slipping Rib" Causing Your Pain?

Cassidy Foley Davelaar, DO, FAAP, CAQSM, division of orthopedics and sports medicine, Nemours Children's Hospital, and assistant professor, University of Central Florida College of Medicine, both in Orlando. She is also clinical care provider for the United States Tennis Association.

The cause of abdominal pain can be hard to figure out, with so many key organs, muscles and skeletal parts located between the shoulders and hips. But if your belly, back or chest hurts when you move certain ways—and other conditions have been ruled out—you might have slipping rib syndrome. Here's what happens… and what to do about it.

You probably think that your ribs expand enough to allow breathing, but they basically stay in place. And that's mostly true. However, your eighth, ninth and 10th ribs are not attached directly to your sternum (the flat bone at the center front of the chest, aka the breastbone). Instead, they are attached to cartilage that attaches to the sternum.

The cartilage itself can weaken because of trauma from activities that involve major movement of the rib cage. Or the cartilage attachments can weaken from unknown causes. The weakening allows one of the ribs to slip from its proper position during normal movements of the abdominal muscles.

Most often, the slipping rib is the 10th one…and 90% of the time it occurs on just one side of the body. The slippage compresses and irritates the intercostal nerve that runs through the tissue between the ribs. This causes pain that comes and goes, often worsening with exercise or certain movements. (More on that below.)

Who's at Risk?

Slipping rib syndrome first came to medical attention about 60 years ago. While the condition is not considered common, it is so often missed or mistaken for other conditions—such as an ulcer, gallbladder disease, kidney stones or appendicitis—that it's hard to know exactly how common it really is. For instance, 54 cases were found at one sports medicine clinic between 1999 and 2014. And a recent study published in *Clinical Journal of Sports Medicine* found that the average person with this condition sees more than two specialists and takes more than 15 months to get a correct diagnosis.

Slipping rib can happen at any age and afflicts more women than men, particularly during reproductive years. (In the sports medicine clinic study mentioned above, 70% of cases were in women.) Certain sports, such as running, rowing, swimming and weight lifting…and conditions that cause chronic coughing, such as asthma or bronchitis, can make slipping rib syndrome more likely. Being hypermobile (the medical term for "double-jointed") also increases risk. About 20% of patients with slipping rib syndrome are hypermobile.

Symptoms and Diagnosis

Upper-abdominal pain unrelated to an obvious injury is the most common symptom of slipping rib. The pain usually starts gradually and is described as sharp, severe or cramping…although over time it may fade to a dull ache. The pain usually is triggered by activities that involve upper-arm movement. However, coughing, getting up from a chair or just rolling over in bed also may cause pain.

Once other conditions have been ruled out and slipping rib is suspected, it's actually not hard to diagnose. This is often done with a simple test performed in the doctor's office called a "hooking maneuver." The doctor hooks his/her fingers under the edge of the lower rib cage and pulls upward and outward to see if that triggers pain. Ultrasound also can confirm the diagnosis.

Treatment Options

Depending on the patient's age, activity level and disability from the condition, treatment usually starts with less invasive treatments—nonsteroidal anti-inflammatory drugs (NSAIDs), Lidoderm patches, chiropractic treatment and acupuncture. Generally, noninvasive treatments are about 30% effective at relieving pain, although some work better than others. *Diclofenac* gel was found to be 60% effective, and osteopathic manipulative treatment (OMT) was 71% effective at relieving pain.

If these methods aren't effective or don't help enough, physical therapy and special home exercises can be beneficial for roughly half the patients who try these therapies.

For patients who still aren't getting adequate pain relief, an ultrasound-guided nerve block can be tried. Injections of numbing medication and/or steroids can provide full relief for several months…and may resolve the pain permanently.

For severe cases of slipping rib, surgery to remove the affected cartilage attached to the problematic rib can relieve the pain. Once healed, pain usually goes away permanently—and the patient can return to normal activities, including sports.

Ankle Weakness Can Linger After an Injury

Luke Donovan, PhD, ATC, assistant professor of kinesiology, University of North Carolina at Charlotte.

Years or even decades after an ankle sprain, some of the symptoms of the original injury can linger, and a person may feel like his/her ankle will give out at times and have cyclic swelling and pain. In fact, about 40% of people who suffer an ankle sprain develop this chronic ankle instability (CAI), which can affect a person of any age.

But aging also can be a primary cause of ankle instability. As we age, there's a natural decline in muscle and tendon function as well as neuromuscular control.

If you're experiencing ankle weakness, simple exercises help. The exercises below are best done barefoot and on both sides of the body. Perform them daily, doing strength exercises and balance exercises on alternating days.

To strengthen ankle-supporting muscles, stand on one foot and roll from heel to toes, then reverse and roll from your toes to heel. Repeat three sets of 10 to 15 reps three to four times a week. Next, walk a few feet just on your heels...then the insides of your feet...the outsides of your feet...and finally on your toes. When muscles start to tire, try to take a few more steps and then work a new muscle group. Balance exercises, such as standing on each leg for 30 to 60 seconds up to three times a day, have been shown to improve neuromuscular control. To make this more challenging, close your eyes.

Note: If you have a balance disorder, check with a doctor before doing these exercises. Also, if any exercise starts to become painful, stop and try another time. And always be sure to stand next to something sturdy that you can grab onto in case you lose your balance.

Helpful: A lace-up ankle brace for support. And if your ankle is painful or swollen, *ibuprofen* (Motrin) or *naproxen* (Aleve) and/

or icing the ankle for 15 minutes can relieve pain.

If your ankle worsens, see a foot and ankle surgeon, who may advise physical therapy or surgery to repair ligaments.

Can Cell Phones Cause Bone Spurs on Your Skull?

David Shahar, DC, PhD, chiropractor in private practice, researcher, School of Health and Sport Sciences, University of the Sunshine Coast, Queensland, Australia. Study titled "Prominent exostosis projecting from the occipital squama more substantial and prevalent in young adult than older age groups," published in *Scientific Reports*.

You might have read—with understandable alarm—the headlines claiming that smartphones cause "horns" to grow at the back of our heads. Before you panic and throw out your smartphone or tablet, here's the real story behind the media hype...and the real message behind the research.

The "horns" the media refer to are bone spurs—the medical term is exostoses—and the research is a 2018 study from University of the Sunshine Coast in Queensland, Australia, that found head and neck X-rays were showing exostoses in a surprising number of younger adults.

Exostoses are not uncommon. They can occur in many areas of the body where muscle attaches to bone. Stress on the spot where the bone grows into the muscle—called the insertion site—can cause the bone to gradually grow an extension into the muscle to strengthen the connection and to spread the load over a larger area of the bone surface. But because exostoses take years to grow, they are more common in older people. An example is a heel spur, which is rarely seen in people younger than age 40.

On an X-ray, the extension can be shaped like a tiny beak or horn, a description the me-

---

Walking's Great...But Watch Out

Pedestrian Deaths Reach New High

Pedestrian deaths reached a new high in 2018. In all, there were an estimated 6,227 fatalities—a 4% increase from the year before. Separate statistics show that the number of pedestrian deaths involving SUVs rose 50% from 2013 to 2017 as those vehicles became more popular. Part of the reason for the increase is that pedestrians are much less likely to survive being hit by an SUV than in an accident involving a smaller vehicle.

Jonathan Adkins, executive director, Governors Highway Safety Association, Washington, DC. GHSA.org

Take Care at Crosswalks

Red-light-running deaths have risen by 31%. The number of people killed—drivers, passengers and people in the vehicle that was hit—increased from 715 in 2009 to 939 in 2017 (latest data available).

Study by AAA Foundation for Traffic Safety. AAAFoundation.org

---

dia apparently latched on to. However, using descriptive terms for anatomical structures is not uncommon. For example, the cochlea of the inner ear is derived from the Latin word for snail shell, which it resembles.

The Sunshine Coast researchers' 2018 study was actually following up a 2016 study they had done that found 41% of 218 relatively young (ages 18 to 30) head and neck X-ray patients had prominent exostoses. And one of the researchers observed in his chiropractic practice that over the past decade, prominent exostoses in younger people seemed to be common. To investigate further, they reviewed skull X-rays for a larger population that included a wider age span—1,200 people ages 18 to 86, including chiropractic patients as well as asymptomatic university students.

Results: Significant exostoses were found in 33% of the total. Not surprisingly, they were found in 25% of patients age 60 and older compared within 5% to 15% of those who were ages 30 to 50. What was surprising was that the group that had the highest rate (45%) were patients ages 18 to 30.

What May Be Going On

The researchers pointed out that the bony growths are not dangerous. While they show up on an X-ray, they aren't visible otherwise. If you have one, you may be able to feel it with your hand at the back of your head just above your neck. And although some very large exostoses have been reported to cause pain, none of the patients in either study complained of pain.

The researchers explained that their study was not designed to look for causes of skull exostoses or why they might be increasing among younger people. The researchers did point out that the posture people adopt when using smartphones and tablets—keeping the head leaning forward and downward—creates the kind of stress that can cause exostoses to develop. In fact, the study did find prominent exostoses to be more common in patients whose habitual posture had a forward projection of their cervical spine. The researchers speculated that the fact that people in the 18-to-30-year-old age group have been using such devices most of their lives could also explain why exostoses are showing up larger and more often in that group.

Bottom Line: Straighten Up!

The hunching over handheld devices connection, however, is only a theory. Further research would need to confirm it. The real takeaway from this study is that it would be wise to pay attention to your posture during all your daily activities, not just when you're using a smartphone or tablet. Slumping at your desk, walking with your chin stuck out or any other bad posture habit affects your body...and may even be affecting your skeleton.

Drowsy Driving

Rachel Salas, MD, sleep neurologist at Johns Hopkins Medicine.

Long drives not only test your patience ("Are we there yet?") but also your driving skills, including your ability to stay awake. The National Highway Traffic Safety Administration estimates that drowsy driving is at the root of more than 70,000 crashes a year—many of them fatal.

By the time a driver feels drowsy, it's likely he/she has already fallen asleep. Your brain falls asleep for one to two seconds, but your eyes are open and you're not aware of it during these microsleeps. If you're driving 65 to 70 miles per hour, that's a recipe for disaster. The solution is to take a break and, if possible, switch drivers. *Before you get drowsy...*

• **Open the window.** A little wind and vibration from the window work as stimulants to keep you awake.

• **Talk to your passengers.** Driving with a car full of snoozers is dangerous. Make sure at least one person stays awake. Having someone talking to you adds stimulation, plus there are more eyes on the road. No passengers? Turn on the radio.

• **Plan ahead for breaks.** If you're on a long, straight drive, there's less stimulation. Add breaks to your itinerary. Get out and move around.

• **Have caffeine at the beginning of your drive, before you get sleepy.** Don't wait until you're already tired—caffeine takes 10 to 45 minutes to kick in.

Crowd Control

Tom Patire, professional bodyguard and personal safety expert, with Antonia van der Meer, former editor, *Bottom Line Personal.*

Here's how to stay safe—at a sports arena, a theater or other big event...

• **To protect yourself from pickpockets,** women should wear a cross-body purse with any openings facing the body. Gentlemen should put their wallets in a front pocket.

• **If you look lost, you risk being a target.** Don't stop in the middle of a crowded sidewalk. Instead, walk near a café or shop, and blend into the building.

• **Stay on the edges of crowds.** There's room to get away if there's a stampede. The worst place to be is in the center. Preplan a meeting place in case you get separated from your companions. Don't rely on cell phones. Service may be bad. Batteries can die.

• **Stay hydrated.** Big crowds suck the oxygen out of the air. You can get dizzy and claustrophobic. If it's 90°F outside the crowd, it can feel much hotter inside the crowd because of body heat—so keep drinking water.

• **Wear tie shoes.** Flip-flops get stepped on. Heels may make you more likely to fall.

• **Go opposite the crowd.** If it goes right, go left. Look for a different way out. You do not have to exit the same way you entered. Choose an aisle seat with good access to exits.

Safe, Affordable Cars

Safest new vehicles for less than $30,000: *Small SUVs*: Mazda CX-5, Subaru Forester, Honda CR-V, Hyundai Tucson. *Sedans*: Toyota Camry, Subaru Legacy, Hyundai

Sonata, Kia Optima. *Pickups*: Ford F-150, Honda Ridgeline.

Analysis of data from Insurance Institute for Highway Safety and CarGurus.com by Kiplinger.com.

Women at Higher Risk for Injury in Frontal Car Crashes

Women are 73% more likely than men to be injured in frontal car crashes while wearing seatbelts. Women also were twice as likely to sustain injuries involving the legs, spine and abdomen.

Study by researchers at Center for Applied Biomechanics, University of Virginia, Charlottesville, published in *Traffic Injury Prevention*.

Driving Hazards

Spotting a second traffic hazard is difficult if you have already seen one.

Recent finding: People were able to detect one difficult-to-notice hazard 70% of the time if it was the only hazard in an image. But if there were two hazards, one being easier to see than the other—say, brightly dressed and drably dressed pedestrians—people saw the harder-to-notice hazard just 30% of the time.

Study by researchers at North Carolina State University, Raleigh, published in *Accident Analysis & Prevention*.

Riskiest State for Seniors Is Florida

That is based on looking at the 50 states plus Washington, DC, and analyzing factors including fraud reported per 100,000 people…monthly housing costs for renters… seniors living in poverty…average annual rate of violent-injury death among seniors…and seniors living alone as a percentage of the state's overall population. The next-riskiest place is New Mexico, followed by Delaware, Nevada, Washington, DC, Arizona, Oregon, Alabama, California and Georgia.

Safest states for seniors, using this methodology: Iowa, Nebraska, South Dakota, Minnesota, Utah, North Dakota, Indiana, Kansas, New Hampshire and Wisconsin.

Analysis of US Census Bureau data by The Senior List.com.

What to Do with a Mysterious Bruise

Eric H. Kraut, MD, professor of internal medicine and director of benign hematology, The Ohio State University Wexner Medical Center, Columbus.

Small bruises on your hands or palms without any known cause are mysterious, especially if the finger above the bruise feels a bit numb. Should you be concerned?

Our hands have so many bones, joints, nerves and tissues that something as simple as bumping into a table or using a tool can cause a bruise or another minor injury. However, if you feel numbness, that complicates matters.

Numbness in the hand (or any other part of an extremity) that lasts for more than a week, warrants a visit to a primary care physician. Hand numbness can signal an underlying condition not related to an injury, such as carpal tunnel syndrome, a pinched nerve or even diabetes, which can damage nerves—especially those leading to the extremities.

To investigate the cause of the numbness, your doctor should evaluate muscle strength and numbness in all your extremities and, depending on his/her findings, perhaps recommend further tests and/or refer you to a neurologist.

If you have only a bruise, you would probably not require medical attention. A bruise is a small bleed into the skin that typically occurs after some kind of physical trauma. Many people bruise easily and don't necessarily recall the injury that caused it.

Older adults tend to bruise more easily—their skin is thinner and blood vessels are more fragile. But people of all ages are often more likely to bruise if they take medications that thin the blood, such as aspirin or anticoagulants, or some supplements like fish oil or ginkgo biloba. Even a vigorous workout, such as weight lifting, could lead to bruising—overtaxed muscles can cause small tears in blood vessels.

It may be helpful to apply ice (a bag of frozen peas works fine) to a bruise for 15 to 20 minutes when it's first noticed. This can help to minimize it. For most people, a bruise takes about two weeks to heal, gradually lightening in color as the leaked blood is absorbed back into the body.

Alexa, Help Me!

Smart home speakers such as Amazon Echo can be designed with artificial intelligence that accurately identifies the irregular breathing that occurs during cardiac arrest—and summon emergency help. Further testing is under way.

University of Washington

Chapter 14

PREGNANCY AND REPRODUCTION ISSUES

Trying to Get Pregnant? Here's the Best Season to Conceive

It's been said that timing is everything. But does that also apply to getting pregnant?

Apparently so, according to recent research led by scientists at the Boston University School of Public Health (BUSPH).

The study, which involved more than 14,000 women in the US, Canada and Denmark who were trying to get pregnant, analyzed data that included details on intercourse frequency, menstruation, smoking, diet, income and education.

Described as a first-of-its-kind study, the researchers focused on fecundability, which is the women's probability of becoming pregnant during a single menstrual cycle. The women were tracked with detailed surveys until they either conceived, initiated fertility treatment or had tried to conceive unsuccessful for 12 menstrual cycles.

"There are a lot of studies out there that look at seasonal patterns in births, but these studies don't take into account when couples start trying, how long they take to conceive or how long their pregnancies last," explained Amelia Wesselink, PhD, a postdoctoral associate in epidemiology at BUSPH.

North Americans in the study were more likely than Danes to begin trying to conceive in the fall (perhaps so the birth would occur in the summer when their work schedules may be less demanding).

Results of the study, which was published in *Human Reproduction*, suggest that seasonal variability does play a role in pregnancy...

In the US and Canada, the probability of becoming pregnant in late fall and early winter was 16% higher than in the spring.

In Denmark, the probability of becoming pregnant in the fall was 8% higher than in the spring.

In all countries, the probability of becoming pregnant was lowest in the spring.

The researchers controlled for other factors that might play a role in fecundability, including frequency of sexual intercourse, frequency of menstruation, smoking, consumption of sugar-sweetened beverages and medication use. These factors did not appear to explain the seasonal variation in fertility.

The study "Seasonal Patterns in Fecundability in North America and Denmark: A Preconception Cohort Study," led by researchers at Boston University School of Public Health and published in *Human Reproduction*.

Even though the researchers do not know why the season appears to affect fecundability, they have some hypotheses that they would like to explore. These include temperature, humidity and vitamin D exposure.

Contraceptive Jewelry?

Family planning could be as simple as getting a new pair of earrings.

New discovery: Early tests show that skin-contact backings on earrings, wristwatches, rings and necklaces can deliver effective amounts of contraceptive hormones for women.

Journal of Controlled Release

Smart Tampon for Fertility

A "smart" tampon that collects endometrial tissue during menstruation can help evaluate a woman's fertility. The tampon, in development, would be used for about two hours, then sent to a laboratory for testing.

Next step: Clinical trials.

Forbes

Pregnancy Exercises That Don't Put Abdominal Muscles at Risk

Stefanie Gordon, Pilates Method Alliance–certified Pilates teacher (PMA-CPT), National Academy of Sports Medicine–certified personal trainer, corrective exercise specialist and STOTT Pilates certified instructor, based in Short Hills, New Jersey. Ms. Gordon is also a pre/postnatal Pilates specialist with The Center for Women's Fitness in Chicago.

It's important to stay fit while you're pregnant. But you need to make sure that how you exercise won't cause *diastasis recti*—a common condition that can leave you with pelvic muscles that don't work properly. You might also be at risk for this common condition because of other factors. The good news is that strengthening the right muscles can help you avert diastasis recti. Below are three exercises that help.

Diastasis recti is the abnormal separation of abdominal muscles. The outer muscle of the abdominal wall is the rectus abdominis, two columns of muscle that run vertically down the abdomen. Between these two columns is the linea alba—a long strip of connective tissue that is an extension of the fascia that covers the rectus abdominis. During pregnancy, pressure from the expanding uterus against the abdominal wall causes the linea alba to widen. Diastasis recti occurs when the space widens more than it should.

Pregnancy is the most common cause of diastasis recti, especially for successive pregnancies, pregnant women over age 35 and pregnancies with multiple births. Genetic tendency and/or excessive abdominal fat can also put you at greater risk...as can rapid changes in weight and intense weight-lifting. The condition can affect men as well as women. Diastasis recti prevents core and pelvic floor muscles from functioning properly and, besides giving you a loose, saggy belly, can cause back pain, constipation and urinary leakage.

Do You Have a Diastasis?

There is a simple way to check for a diastasis...

• **When you are not pregnant (or for men).** Lie on your back on the floor, knees bent and feet flat on the ground, and place your index finger and middle finger about two inches above your navel. Curl your head, neck and shoulders off the ground while gently pressing down with your fingers to feel for the sides of your rectus abdominis muscles. If you feel a gap that is more than two fingertips wide, you probably have a diastasis. (A gap greater than four fingertips is typically considered severe.)

• **When you are pregnant.** When lying on your back and flexing up, a diastasis may look like a visible bulge down your midline where the muscles should be together—often described as "coning." (Your pregnant belly should look rounded…coning looks like a peak.)

Moves to Avoid…and Exercises That Help

While your abdominal wall is already under stress as a result of pregnancy, you don't want to put any more pressure on it. So, avoid crunches, planks, push-ups and other spinal flexion exercises (that is, curling up of the upper torso from a supine position).

What you want to do instead is strengthen your transverse abdominis, the deepest layer of your abdominals. Pilates exercises are one great way to safely work these weakened muscles. But not all Pilates exercises are OK to do during pregnancy, so look for an instructor who has experience with prenatal clients. If you already have a diastasis, perhaps from a previous pregnancy, it's best to consult a qualified physical therapist who has postpartum therapy experience before doing any kind of exercises.

Moves That Safely Strengthen Abdominal Muscles…

•**Transverse abdominis engagement.** Lie on your back with your knees flexed and feet flat on the floor, about six inches away from your sit bones (the part of the pelvis under your glutes). Place your hands on your navel. Inhale through your nose….then exhale through your mouth as you pull your navel toward your spine without tucking your pelvis underneath you. Do 10 reps.

•**Heel drops.** Besides strengthening the transverse abdominis, this exercise also works spinal-stabilizer muscles. Lie on your back with your arms at your sides and both legs in tabletop position (knees bent, legs together and lower legs in the air and parallel to the floor). Inhale and drop your right heel about halfway toward the ground. Exhale while lifting your foot back to starting position. Do the same with your left heel.

Do ten reps for each leg, alternating sides. Make sure to keep your shoulders relaxed and your abdominals engaged and avoid arching your back.

•**Bridging with articulation.** This exercise increases spinal mobility while working the abdominals. Lie on your back, knees bent and feet flat on the ground about six inches away from your sit bones. Inhale…then exhale while slowly lifting your hips towards the ceiling, peeling your vertebrae off the mat until you are supported on your upper back. Avoid putting stress or pressure on your head or neck. Hold the position as you inhale… then exhale while slowly rolling back down to starting position. Do five to 10 reps.

Exercise in Pregnancy Is Good for Infants

Newborns whose mothers did supervised, moderate-intensity, 50-minute exercise sessions three times a week had more advanced motor skills than infants whose mothers did not do the exercise sessions. The effect was more noticeable in girls, who at this age tend to have lower motor-skill levels than boys. The differences were not large, but researchers suggest they could be enough to encourage growing children to be more active in the future. Researchers have speculated that the release of hormones during exercising as well as improved blood flow due to aerobic exercise may contribute to the difference found.

Study of 60 healthy women and their newborns by researchers at East Carolina University, Greenville, North Carolina, published in *Medicine & Science in Sports & Exercise.*

Beware of Smoking Pot During Pregnancy

Pot smoking during pregnancy may raise the child's risk for psychosis. Children exposed to marijuana after their mothers knew they were pregnant had a slightly increased risk for psychosis in middle childhood, around age 10. The study did not prove cause and effect, and the association was not found in mothers who used marijuana before they knew they were pregnant—possibly because the endocannabinoid system, which responds to cannabis, may not be fully developed early in pregnancy. More research is needed.

Ryan Bogdan, PhD, associate professor of psychological and brain sciences, Washington University in St. Louis, and senior author of a study of 4,361 children born to mothers between 2005 and 2008, including 201 exposed to marijuana in the womb, published in *JAMA Psychiatry.*

Vaginal Birth Is Good for Baby's Health

Exposure to their mothers' vaginal fluids may improve the health of babies born via C-section. Vaginal delivery transfers beneficial microbes to a baby during birth. But babies born through C-section are exposed only to environmental bacteria, not the helpful ones from their mothers—these babies may be more prone to immune and metabolic disorders, such as type 1 diabetes, obesity and asthma.

New technique: In vaginal microbial transfer, a mother's vaginal fluids are collected before the birth and swabbed all over the infant within a minute or two of delivery. A small initial study showed that this approach established bacterial colonies on C-section babies that were similar to those from vaginal births, although they still fell short in some areas. Further research is planned.

Study of 18 babies born in San Juan, Puerto Rico, by researchers at New York University, New York City, published in *Nature Medicine.*

Case Study: C-Section Averted When the Baby Didn't Drop

Andrew Rubman, ND, medical director of Southbury Clinic for Traditional Medicines in Southbury, Connecticut. SouthburyClinic.com

The patient: "Suzy," a hard-working occupational therapist, was a patient who originally came to see me many years ago, when in her early twenties. She had since married and was now pregnant. She loved being busy and physically active, both in her work and in her personal life, and was excited about her upcoming delivery.

Why she came to see me: I received a call from Suzy a week before her "due date." Her obstetrician was concerned that the "baby had not dropped as expected" and that a Caesarean section may be necessary. Suzy didn't want to deliver by C-section—she knew that a vaginal birth is generally healthier for both the baby and the mother.

How I evaluated her: Suzy brought in a complete set of her records from her obstetrician that we thoroughly reviewed. Her workup from this doctor was very complete and found no issues with the "pelvimetry" (measurements of the internal dimensions of her pelvis) that might have interfered with a normal delivery. I assessed her pelvic articulations (the joints between her sacrum and her hip bones) and found that her sacrum (the bony structure where the spine connects to the pelvis) was being held in an exaggerated forward-bending, or "nutated," position.

How we addressed the problem: I provided moist heat to her lower back and sacrum area and carefully adjusted the joints between her hips and sacrum. Given her situation literally days away from delivery, this series of adjustments was particularly challenging. Fortunately, I was able to release the sacrum from its "locked forward" position and told her that I felt confident that labor would proceed successfully.

The patient's progress: Suzy's obstetrician assessed her again when she went into labor and assured her that the baby had dropped, and things looked good for a normal delivery. Not long ago, Suzy came in for some follow up physical medicine, and I saw some pictures of happy baby, mom, dad... and, I believe, a happy obstetrician too!

Exercise and Sleep Patterns Different for New Moms and Dads

Sleep and exercise affect new moms and dads differently. Mothers who slept more than average when compared with other mothers reported greater well-being...but fathers who got more than the average amount of sleep reported less well-being and less closeness with their partner and child. Exercise also affected new moms and dads differently. On days when fathers exercised more than usual, the likelihood of an argument dropped...but when mothers exercised more than usual, arguing became more likely.

Possible reason: When mothers spend more time than usual on their own needs, such as exercise, fathers may feel more stress associated with child care, possibly leading to arguments.

Mark Feinberg, PhD, research professor, Edna Bennett Pierce Prevention Research Center at Penn State University, State College, Pennsylvania, and leader of a study published in *Monographs of the Society for Research in Child Development.*

What's Good...What's Bad When You're Expecting

Eat Nuts When You're Pregnant

Eating nuts during pregnancy may boost babies' cognitive abilities. The children of women who reported eating the most nuts while pregnant scored significantly higher on tests of sustained attention, working memory and IQ at ages one-and-a-half, five and eight— compared with the children of women who ate fewer nuts or none at all while pregnant. Researchers speculate that the nuts' high levels of omega-3 and omega-6 fatty acids, as well as high levels of folate, may aid in the development of certain brain regions.

Study of more than 2,200 mother-and-child pairs by researchers at Barcelona Institute for Global Health, Spain, published in *European Journal of Epidemiology.*

...But Avoid Artificial Sweeteners

Eating artificial sweeteners while pregnant or breastfeeding could have consequences for baby. In a rat study, both aspartame and stevia (considered safe low-cal sweeteners) were linked to the offspring's higher obesity risk...impaired glucose control, especially in males from aspartame...and changes in the brain's reward system that influences desire for high-calorie foods, also more from aspartame. Until more is known, limiting sugar alternatives might be safest.

Raylene A. Reimer, PhD, RD, a professor at University of Calgary in Canada and senior author of a study published in *Gut.*

Moms Get a Heart-Health Bonus from Breast-feeding

Moms who breast-feed get a heart-health bonus later in life.

Recent finding: Just six months of breast-feeding led to reduced arterial stiffness and plaque and a lower risk for heart disease. The longer women nursed, the greater the benefit.

Breast-feeding also helps prevent postpartum depression and certain cancers and can help regulate blood sugar. Nursing women have high levels of prolactin, a hormone that lowers the risk for diabetes.

Irene Lambrinoudaki, MD, professor of endocrinology at National and Kapodistrian University, Athens, Greece, and leader of a study of 283 postmenopausal women presented at the European Society of Endocrinology annual meeting in Lyon, France.

Pregnancy Heart Attacks: How to Protect Yourself

Nathaniel Smilowitz, MD, interventional cardiologist, assistant professor of medicine, NYU Langone Health, New York City, and lead author of study titled "Acute Myocardial Infarction During Pregnancy and the Puerperium in the United States," published in *Mayo Clinic Proceedings*.

When you're pregnant, there's a lot on your mind, but you probably aren't giving much thought to your heart health. Recent research suggests that you should—your life could depend on it.

According to the most recent statistics available, the proportion of women in the US who had heart attacks during pregnancy, delivery or the postpartum period (the six weeks after delivery) rose nearly 25% between 2002 and 2014—from seven out of every 100,000 pregnancies to 9.5 out of every 100,000 pregnancies.

If 9.5 out of 100,000 doesn't sound like something to be concerned about, keep in mind that all of the women having these heart attacks are young or relatively young (of childbearing age).

Within this group, older pregnant women are more likely to have heart attacks than younger ones. Pregnant women age 35 to 39 are five times more likely to have heart attacks than pregnant women in their 20s, and women in their early 40s have 10 times that risk. But few people think of their early 40s—or younger—as heart attack age. This is especially concerning as growing numbers of American women are choosing to delay motherhood.

Heart attack is not the only pregnancy heart threat. A separate study found that the number of pregnant women experiencing heart failure—when the heart grows weaker and is unable to pump enough blood and oxygen—is rising, too, by about 4.9% a year during pregnancy and 7.1% in the six weeks following birth.

What's happening: Pregnancy on its own does stress your heart. Your heart pumps more blood each minute to feed the baby, and your heart rate, in turn, increases. And while you might think of heart disease as a problem for women well after childbearing years, you could have heart disease risk factors much earlier in life. Many of the patients in the heart attack study had high blood pressure, high cholesterol and/or diabetes (high blood sugar), each of which is considered a major risk factor for heart attack. High blood pressure is also one of the risk factors for heart failure.

Use these study findings to get proactive about your heart health when planning to become pregnant and while pregnant…

- **See your doctor before you start trying.** All women, especially those in their 30s and up, who want to become pregnant should get an all-clear from their doctors first. Simple screening tests can identify high blood cholesterol, high blood sugar and high blood pressure.

- **Work with your doctor on a plan to reduce your risks.** This plan could include well-known lifestyle changes that you might have been procrastinating about, such as eating healthier, losing weight, exercising and, of course, quitting if you smoke. But medication may be needed if lifestyle changes alone don't get your numbers down.

- **Know the symptoms of a heart attack.** For women in particular, it's not always the typical chest pain depicted in the movies. And yet some of the other symptoms, such as nausea and shortness of breath, are also common pregnancy symptoms.

- **Call 911 immediately if you think you could be having a heart attack.** Many women don't seek attention as quickly as they should because the possibility of having a heart attack isn't on their radar, but it should be.

Heart attacks and other heart issues during pregnancy are rare, but they're also happening more often than they used to. The quicker you get treated, the better the outlook for you and your baby.

Chapter 15

RESPIRATORY CONDITIONS AND ALLERGIES

Is Your Medication Harming Your Lungs?

Maybe you've taken antibiotics to treat a urinary tract infection…or you regularly take medication to combat a chronic condition such as psoriasis or atrial fibrillation. If breathing problems (such as a hacking cough or shortness of breath) occur during that time, would you ever think that the culprit may be a drug you take for something entirely unrelated to your lungs or respiratory tract?

What most people don't realize: Everyday medications—including those prescribed for pain, common infections, heart conditions and cancer—can endanger your respiratory system.

Here's how to protect yourself…

A Bigger Problem Than Thought

Certain medications have been known to cause lung problems, including allergic reactions, abnormal buildup of fluid in the lungs and inflammation of the lung air sacs, but a recent systematic review of 156 research papers found that such complications are more common than previously understood.

New finding: While more than 350 medications have been associated with some type of drug-induced lung problems, a study published in October 2018 in *Journal of Clinical Medicine* implicated 27 drugs that are most often linked to interstitial lung disease (ILD).

What exactly is ILD? It's a fancy term for a group of disorders that cause scarring of the lungs. The culprit might be an irritant (such as asbestos or silica dust)…an autoimmune disease (such as rheumatoid arthritis or scleroderma)…or a medication. While we may think that our lungs are safe when we take medication for, say, arthritis pain or an irregular heartbeat, there's a catch—every organ in the body, including the lungs, has the ability to metabolize drugs.

This means that the lungs can be vulnerable to any toxic effects—even if the drug isn't inhaled. The result can be ILD or another illness such as pneumonia, pneumonitis (inflammation of lung tissue) or pulmonary fibrosis (lung scarring). Shockingly, up to

Jack Fincham, PhD, RPh, professor of pharmaceutical and administrative sciences at Presbyterian College School of Pharmacy in Clinton, South Carolina. He serves as a special appointee to the FDA's Peripheral and Central Nervous System Drugs Advisory Committee and an appointee to the Canadian Institutes of Health Research College of Reviewers.

5% of ILD cases are drug-induced, according to this research, and death rates of 50% or higher for a handful of medications, including the colorectal cancer drug *panitumumab* (Vectibix), were reported in some of the multiple studies reviewed.

A Tricky Timeline

While you might assume that a drug-induced lung problem would show up right after starting to take a medication, that's not always the case. Symptoms of ILD, which can include labored breathing and even general malaise, might develop shortly after starting a new medication (as might occur with an antibiotic, for example)…within days or weeks…or months or even years later—in some cases, even after the drug has been discontinued. This tricky timeline can make it far more difficult for you or your doctor to connect the dots.

Getting a correct diagnosis of drug-induced ILD generally involves a thorough clinical exam, listing all medications taken over the last several years…as well as X-rays or other imaging tests, which might show changes in the lungs. Pulmonary function tests might also be ordered. *In addition to blood tests to measure oxygen and carbon dioxide levels, other tests may include…*

• **Spirometry,** in which you breathe multiple times into a tube that is connected to a computer, to measure your rate of air flow.

• **Pulse oximetry,** in which a probe is placed on your fingertip or a skin surface such as your ear, to estimate oxygen levels in your blood.

Once ILD has taken hold, there's no way to rid the lungs of the telltale lesions that accompany this disease, but you can potentially stop it from progressing. A corticosteroid can reduce inflammation and ease symptoms, but this medication comes with its own potential side effects (such as weight gain, high blood pressure and bone damage) that need to be weighed against potential benefits. Lung transplants are a last-resort option for those who are most severely affected.

Top Threats

If a drug leads to ILD and an alternative medication exists, your doctor may recommend switching. Which medications are the worst offenders? *Watch out for these in particular…*

• **Chemotherapy drugs,** including *bleomycin* (Blenoxane)…*busulfan* (Myleran)…*cyclophosphamide* (Cytoxan)…and *panitumumab* (Vectibix), among others. Biologics used as cancer immunotherapies also appear on the list, including *bevacizumab* (Avastin) and *trastuzumab* (Herceptin).

• **Antiarrhythmic medications,** especially *amiodarone* (Cordarone), which treats atrial fibrillation and is the most common cardiovascular drug linked to lung problems. As many as 6% of people taking this drug develop ILD, and an estimated 10% to 20% of them die from its lung-related complications.

• **Antibiotics,** such as *nitrofurantoin* (Macrobid), which treats urinary tract infections… or *sulfamethoxazole/trimethoprim* (Bactrim), which fights ear infections, bronchitis and other bacterial infections.

• **Vasodilator drugs,** especially *hydralazine* (Apresoline), used for high blood pressure and heart failure.

• **Disease-modifying antirheumatic drugs (DMARDs),** especially *methotrexate* (Rheumatrex, Trexall, Rasuvo), which treat autoimmune conditions, such as rheumatoid arthritis and psoriasis, as well as cancer.

• **Seizure medications,** such as *phenytoin* (Dilantin) or *carbamazepine* (Tegretol).

• **Nonsteroidal anti-inflammatory drugs (NSAIDs),** such as aspirin, *ibuprofen* (Motrin) and *naproxen* (Aleve), used for pain.

Note: An NSAID user's vulnerability to ILD is highly individualized.

• **Beta-blockers,** such as *atenolol* (Tenormin) and *propranolol* (Inderal), for high blood pressure.

• **Statins,** such as *simvastatin* (Zocor) and *atorvastatin* (Lipitor), to lower cholesterol.

Take These Precautions

It's unfortunate that drugs we need might wreak such havoc on our lungs. *But there are smart precautions to take…*

•**Know your baseline.** Be aware of your body's normal "feel" and function, and monitor all symptoms after you begin taking any new drug. Be alert for new or persistent trouble breathing, and consider getting a baseline spirometry test (described earlier) when starting a drug that may lead to ILD.

•**Get vaccinated.** Both the pneumococcal vaccine, which helps prevent pneumonia, and the flu vaccine, which is ideally received each year in early fall, before flu season begins, are important protections against ILD. Why? If you take a pill predisposing you to ILD and are then exposed to bacteria or viruses, it can spell double trouble for vulnerable lungs. By preventing pneumonia or the flu, the vaccines can mitigate any ripple effects from compromised lungs that may contribute to ILD.

Note: The CDC recommends the annual flu vaccine for all adults…and the pneumococcal vaccine for all adults age 65 and older and anyone ages two to 64 with certain medical conditions, such as heart disease, asthma or weakened immunity. Smokers also are advised to get the pneumococcal vaccine.

•**See your doctor promptly if you develop any breathing problems** (such as a cough, labored breathing, shallow breathing or wheezing) that seem acute or last longer than a few days. Bring a list of medications you take, and ask the doctor if your symptoms could be due to one of these drugs.

•**Get monitored.** If you take one of the drugs linked to ILD, ask your doctor to monitor your lungs with one or more of the tests described earlier.

If Your Voice Is Shaky and Weak, Here's the Checkup You Need

Lesley Childs, MD, associate professor of laryngology, neurolaryngology and professional voice at University of Texas (UT) Southwestern Medical Center in Dallas. She also serves as the associate medical director of the Clinical Center for Voice Care at UT Southwestern. Dr. Childs is a classically trained soprano who has recorded songs for Walt Disney Records. Her research has been published in *Laryngoscope, Journal of Voice* and other professional journals.

It's easy to take your voice for granted. A brief bout of laryngitis may even be fun if you enjoy having the raspy sound of Clint Eastwood or Kathleen Turner. Such episodes usually improve in a week or so, and we can blame the problem on a cold or loud cheering for a favorite sports team.

But the culprit behind certain changes in your voice might not be so obvious or fleeting. *What you need to know to figure out the cause…*

Is It Time for a Voice Checkup?

Our vocal cords perform small miracles every day. They vibrate several hundred times per second when we speak—and even more when we sing.

With age, our vocal cords tend to thin and lose flexibility, often causing us to develop chronic hoarseness and/or a weak, shaky voice. But you don't have to live with this. With the right checkup, you can get the treatment you need to improve (or even correct) the problem. *Voice symptoms that should be investigated…*

•**Your voice is hoarse or your sound quality has changed for two weeks or more—regardless of your age.** For example, if your voice is raspy, breathy or shaky or you notice a change in pitch—to a lower or higher range—you should find out what's going on.

•**You feel pain or discomfort when you talk or sing.** Some people with such symptoms are straining their neck muscles to produce sounds.

• **Your voice grows weaker or strained over the course of a day.**

Unraveling the Problem

If your voice problems aren't linked to an obvious cause, such as laryngitis, consider seeing an ear, nose and throat specialist (an otolaryngologist).

If possible, it's even better to seek out a laryngologist, an otolaryngologist who specializes in voice, airway and swallowing disorders. Such doctors often work as part of teams, along with speech therapists, at specialized voice centers. To find a laryngologist near you, consult the American Academy of Otolaryngology—Head and Neck Surgery, ENTnet.org.

When you go for a checkup, you'll be asked to describe what's bothering you. When doing so, mention what—if anything—seems to help or make matters worse. Also describe how you use your voice. Are you a salesperson who is on the phone several hours a day? A teacher in a noisy classroom? Providing this information will help in evaluating your problem.

Your vocal cords will then be examined using a scope equipped with a video camera that passes through your nose or mouth to your larynx (voice box). This test is called laryngoscopy.

The gold standard version includes stroboscopy, an exam in which a strobe light is combined with the camera on the scope. The stroboscopy, which is available at most voice centers, allows for visualization of the vocal cord vibrations, so it provides more detail.

You will be asked to speak so that the camera can capture and record video images of your vocal cord vibrations when you make sounds.

Voice problems can be symptoms of many different conditions, including…

• **Noncancerous growths,** such as nodules, polyps and cysts, on the vocal cords. These often result from trauma caused by using your voice too much or incorrectly without adequate rest. This occurs more often in singers, teachers, ministers and other people who use their voices in their work.

• **Allergies and/or postnasal drip can irritate the throat,** leading to voice changes.

• **Chronic throat clearing and coughing are both traumatic to the vocal cords and expose the delicate vocal cord tissue to undue wear and tear.**

Helpful: Try sipping water instead of throat clearing or coughing.

• **Laryngopharyngeal reflux, in which stomach acid washes up into the larynx.** The condition often improves with weight loss (when needed)…not eating right before going to bed…and other lifestyle changes.

• **Neurological conditions such as a vocal tremor.** However, vocal tremors are not necessarily a sign of a systemic neurological condition, such as epilepsy or Parkinson's disease.

• **Cancerous growths.** If your doctor sees something suspicious on the vocal cords or in the voice box, a biopsy will be performed to determine whether a malignancy is present.

• **Stress and anxiety are sometimes felt in the throat.** For example, someone who is on the verge of tears may feel tightness in the throat.

Getting the Right Treatment

The cause of your voice problem will determine which treatment is most appropriate. *Treatment options…*

• **Speech therapy.** If your problems are caused by misuse of your voice, a speech therapist (ideally, one with special training in the voice) can teach you techniques that will help. By pairing sound production with diaphragmatic breathing, for example, most people speak more efficiently and without straining.

Note: People who are unhappy with the way their voices have changed with age also can work with speech therapists. Over time, changes occur to the vocal cord tissues and the respiratory system, which affect the quality of the sound. Voice therapy helps us optimize how we are producing sound to better adapt to changes that occur over time.

•**Vocal pacing.** This involves being aware of how much you are using your speaking and singing voice in a day. Reducing your "vocal dose" and pacing your vocal demands, such as resting the voice for five minutes for every 30 minutes of use, can help prevent injury to the vocal cords.

Also helpful: Teachers, fitness instructors and other public speakers may be urged to try a personal amplification system for the voice—basically, a microphone that helps them be heard without raising the volume of their voices.

•**Hydration/vocal hygiene.** Water is the best choice for hydration because it helps thin the mucus that then lubricates and protects your vocal cords as they vibrate.

Best practice: Consume 64 ounces of water daily, drinking it throughout the day to keep the vocal cords hydrated.

Important: Avoid too much caffeine and alcohol—both are drying. If you consume these fluids, match with an equal amount of water—in addition to the daily recommendation of 64 ounces.

Also: Chronic use of decongestants is drying, and certain inhaled medications, such as inhaled corticosteroids to treat asthma and chronic obstructive pulmonary disease (COPD), can be irritating to the vocal cords.

•**Surgery.** People with vocal cord lesions may benefit from surgery to remove them. Oftentimes, however, voice therapy is recommended as a first step as most voice-related vocal cord abnormalities are reversible to an extent. If vocal cord surgery is needed, it is usually performed through the mouth with a microscope and under a general anesthetic. If vocal cord cancer is to blame, treatment for the malignancy typically includes surgery and another therapy, such as radiation.

•**Laser treatment.** Some specific types of vocal cord lesions benefit from laser treatments. These can be performed both in the operating room and in the office.

•**Filler injections.** People whose voices have become weaker due to age-related vocal cord atrophy or who have vocal cord weakness may be offered a procedure in which temporary fillers are injected into the vocal cords to help them vibrate more effectively. Often, insurance covers these procedures, which are usually performed in the office. All fillers are temporary and can last up to 12 months, depending on the material used.

•**Botox.** Neurological voice disorders, such as vocal tremors and spasmodic dysphonia, cause the vocal cords to spasm, resulting in a choppy-sounding voice. For these individuals, a vocal cord injection with *botulinum toxin* (Botox) can be used. The treatment can ease spasms that interfere with smooth speech. The effects from these injections in the vocal cords typically last about two to three months. Insurance usually covers these injections, which are performed in the office.

Horehound for Winter Respiratory Ills

Jamison Starbuck, ND, a naturopathic physician in family practice, Missoula, Montana, and writer and producer of *Dr. Starbuck's Health Tips for Kids*, a weekly program on Montana Public Radio, MTPR. org. DrJamisonStarbuck.com

Horehound* might be familiar to some as an old-fashioned candy/cough drop. For centuries, it has been used to treat ailments of the respiratory tract, including bronchitis, colds, sore throat and cough. Horehound is especially useful because it has expectorant and decongestant properties, so it helps the respiratory tract rid itself of mucus or phlegm. Because horehound dries up mucus, you should use it when you are blowing your nose a lot or coughing up or spitting

*As with any herbal medicine, talk to your doctor before trying if you have a medical condition or take medication.

out phlegm many times throughout the day. Don't use horehound if your cough is dry or if your throat is raw. Even though horehound candy has traditionally been used as you would a cough drop, many brands contain a lot of sugar. The tincture, however, doesn't have sugar and it's more potent—thus more effective—for respiratory ailments.

Typical dose: 30 drops, in two ounces of water, taken on an empty stomach, four times a day until symptoms improve. If it's too bitter for your taste buds, stir the tincture into a teaspoon of honey.

Getting Over a Cold or the Flu?

Joseph Feuerstein, MD, assistant professor of clinical medicine at Columbia University in New York City and director of Integrative Medicine at Stamford Health in Stamford, Connecticut. He specializes in family medicine, focusing on nutrition and disease prevention. Dr. Feuerstein is also certified in clinical hypnosis, clinical acupuncture and homeopathy. He is author of *Dr. Joe's Man Diet*.

When you're sidelined by the fever and head-to-toe body aches of the flu or even the endless sneezing and coughing of a cold, it's tempting to want to get back to normal life at the first sign of feeling better. Wait! These illnesses take a toll on your body, and the flu, in particular, can set you up for serious complications.

When flu turns deadly: While the flu itself can quickly lead to lethal respiratory failure if the lungs are overtaken by inflammation, complications of the flu, such as pneumonia or sepsis, are often the actual cause of death. In some cases, being run down from a bad cold can even set the stage for pneumonia.

Whether you're battling the flu or a cold, here's a natural six-step recovery plan that will also help fortify you against serious complications…

•**Get tested.** If you're sure you've got a cold, you might be able to tough it out on

your own. But symptoms of the cold and flu can be similar. The distinguishing characteristics are typically the flu's rapid onset and extreme fatigue, but both illnesses can cause headache, coughing and a runny nose. A fever is more common with the flu, but not everyone with the flu will run a fever.

That's why if you're not sure what's causing your illness—especially if you're over age 65…have had a heart attack or stroke…or have a chronic condition such as lung disease, diabetes or cancer—talk to your doctor about getting tested for the flu. Some nasal or throat swab tests can provide an answer in 30 minutes or less. If you do have the flu, your doctor may want to closely supervise your recovery—in some cases, with monitoring in a hospital if you're frail and/or have a chronic health problem.

Important: Don't assume that a cold is harmless. If it improves but then worsens… lingers for more than 10 days without getting better…and/or causes fever that lasts for more than three days, consult your physician. This could signal a complication such as bronchitis or pneumonia.

If you have a cold or the flu and experience shortness of breath, chest pain or a fever over 103°F, call your doctor or 911.

Caution: Respiratory infections (particularly the flu) are linked to increased risk for heart attack—especially in the week following a flu diagnosis.

•**Stay "horizontal."** There's a reason you're tired and feverish and have no appetite. Your body is forcing you to stop all activity so that it can wage an all-out effort to fight the virus. In most cases, fever is an integral part of the process—it actually stimulates your immune system to work harder than normal. What you need is lots of sleep, fluids (see next page) and bed rest!

Don't let a hectic schedule or guilt over missing obligations keep you from listening to your body. It usually takes about a week to get over a cold, but the flu can set you back for up to two weeks. It may take even longer if you were run down before getting sick or if you're managing a chronic condition, such as lung disease or diabetes, that was already stressing your system.

Important: When you must get up (to, say, go to the bathroom), do so in stages—sit up…swing your feet over the side of the bed…then stand for a few seconds before you start to walk. Prolonged bed rest can lower your blood pressure, which can cause dizziness and even fainting if you stand up too quickly.

• **Consider taking elderberry and echinacea.** Even though some people prefer to take a pharmaceutical such as *oseltamivir* (Tamiflu) for the flu, elderberry and echinacea are worth considering.

While some modern research on these botanicals has been mixed, both have been used for centuries to ease cold and flu symptoms, and a comprehensive 2017 study published in *Journal of Evidence-Based Complementary & Alternative Medicine* found that elderberry and echinacea were effective against cold and flu viruses.

The phytonutrients that give elderberry its deep black-purple color have been found to help stop virus cells from multiplying. Black elderberry extract is available in liquid, tablets and lozenges. Sambucol, Black Elderberry is particularly effective.

Echinacea purpurea (one of various species of echinacea) has been shown to have immune-stimulating properties. It's available in capsule, extract and liquid form.

Note: If you have allergies or asthma, be sure to check with your doctor before trying echinacea.

Some cold and flu products, such as Gaia Herbs' Quick Defense with Echinacea & Elderberry…and Solaray's Echinacea & Elderberry, contain both herbs. A combination tea, Echinacea Plus Elderberry, is available from Traditional Medicinals.

Also: To treat your fever, consider alternating the lowest possible dose of *acetaminophen* (Tylenol) and a nonsteroidal anti-inflammatory drug, such as *ibuprofen* (Motrin). This helps minimize the side effects of each medication.

Top Cold and Flu Preventive

With its antioxidant and antimicrobial properties, the herbal remedy American ginseng (Panax quinquefolius) has strong research supporting its use as a cold and flu preventive.*

In a study involving nursing-home patients that was published in *Journal of the American Geriatrics Society,* it reduced the risk for flu by 89% compared with a placebo. The study participants took 200-mg capsules twice daily of a product called Cold-FX, which is usually taken throughout the cold season.

Important: For cold and flu prevention, it's American ginseng that should be used, rather than Asian, Siberian or other ginseng varieties. — Joseph Feuerstein

*Check with your doctor before taking any herbal remedy or supplement—especially if you have a chronic medical condition or take medications.

Zinc supplements have been shown to significantly reduce the length and severity of cold symptoms. For a cold, try zinc lozenges within 24 hours of the start of your symptoms and for the duration of the illness.

• **Drink more fluids than you think you need.** You don't have to force yourself to eat solid foods, but liquids are essential—and you may not realize how much water you're losing when you're sweating from a fever. This can lead to dehydration, another reason for dizziness when you go from lying to standing.

My rule of thumb: Drink enough to make your urine clear. Listen to your body and stick with broth and other soups at first to avoid straining your digestive system.

• **Spice up your chicken soup.** To amp up the healing power of chicken soup, add immune-boosting, anti-inflammatory spices such as turmeric and ginger, along with garlic. Use as much as you can tolerate of each to taste. When you are ready for solid food, start with healthy starches such as oatmeal and whole-wheat toast. It takes more effort for your body to digest raw fruits and vegetables, so try to avoid them until you've recovered.

• **Pace your reentry.** The common rule of thumb is to wait at least 24 hours after your fever is gone before returning to your usual activities, but that can be too soon. Whether it's work, household chores or hobbies, the more physical activity that's involved—even standing for long periods of time—the more gradual your return should be.

As for resuming your exercise regimen, wait until you have gone back to your normal diet...and start with slow-to-moderate walking for 10 minutes. It could take a week or more to get back to your full workout schedule.

Surprising Ways That Winter Affects Your Health

Drew Koch, DO, FACOEP-D, MBA, a board-certified physician in emergency medicine at Guthrie Robert Packer Hospital in Sayre, Pennsylvania, and clinical assistant professor of emergency medicine in the department of clinical sciences at Geisinger Commonwealth School of Medicine in Scranton, Pennsylvania. He is a Distinguished Fellow of the American College of Osteopathic Emergency Physicians.

C old weather is rough on health. Colds and cases of life-threatening flu are rampant. Ice and snow increase the risk for dangerous falls.

Those problems are bad enough. But there also are hidden health dangers of winter that few people know about—problems that can turn you into a seasonal statistic.

Death rates are 25% higher in winter than in summer—with winter triggering more circulatory, breathing, hormonal and digestive problems, according to recent research published in *The Journal of Steroid Biochemistry and Molecular Biology.*

Cold-weather risks to guard against...

• **Dehydration.** It sounds like a summer issue, but dehydration is a big cold weather risk, too, since the problem is less obvious this time of year.

For one thing, sweat evaporates more rapidly in cold, dry air, tricking you into thinking you're not losing a lot of water from your body. But you are.

The body's thirst response is reduced as well when temperatures are cooler, so you may not drink enough water.

Medications play a role, too. People who take fluid-draining drugs, such as diuretics, as well as other medications for high blood pressure, heart disease and kidney disorders are at increased risk for dehydration. *What to do...*

• Drink more water. If you have mild-to-moderate dehydration, marked by such symptoms as a dry, sticky mouth, sleepiness, dry skin, headache and/or dizziness, drink more water!

• Chronic diseases—particularly diabetes, kidney disease and heart failure—put you at higher risk for dehydration year-round. If you have a chronic medical condition, ask your doctor for advice on how much fluid you should drink.

• Call 911. If you have symptoms of severe dehydration, such as extreme thirst...irritability and confusion...feeling faint...little or no urination...sunken eyes...shriveled and dry skin (it lacks elasticity and doesn't "bounce back" when pinched into a fold), this is a medical emergency, and you need to be rehydrated with intravenous fluids immediately.

• **High blood pressure.** When temperatures fall, your body conserves heat by constricting blood vessels—and those tightened vessels can lead to high blood pressure, which increases risk for heart attack and stroke.

Scientific evidence: The average systolic (top number) blood pressure reading was 5 mmHg higher in winter than in summer, according to a study of adults age 65 or older and published in *Archives of Internal Medicine.*

Even though everyone is at risk for cold weather increases in blood pressure, you're especially vulnerable if you've already been diagnosed with high blood pressure. *What to do…*

•Talk to your doctor if you take blood pressure medication. The dose of antihypertensive medication you take in the summer may not be high enough for winter control.

•Dress warmly. To avoid blood pressure spikes when you're outside in the winter, dress in layers and wear a hat, scarf and gloves. (Cold hands alone can spike blood pressure for hours.)

•Keep it toasty indoors. Cooler indoor temperatures have been linked to higher blood pressure, according to a study published in *Journal of Hypertension*. Researchers advise people with high blood pressure to keep indoor temperatures at around 70°F.

•Don't overexert yourself. People with high blood pressure can have a heart attack if they're unfit and try to shovel snow.

Smart step: Ask your doctor to assess your overall health and give his/her OK for such activity before winter starts or initiating any exercise program. And if you do shovel snow, take breaks every 10 minutes or so and make sure you're dressed warmly and are well-hydrated.

•Get your vitamin D-3 level checked. Blood levels of this sunshine-produced vitamin can plummet during the winter—with research published in *Circulation* linking low levels to high blood pressure…and to nearly twice the risk for heart attack, stroke and heart failure. Ask your doctor to test your vitamin D-3 level. If it's lower than 30 ng/mL, take 2,000 international units (IU) of vitamin D daily throughout the winter.

•**Neuropathy.** Cold slows the flow of blood to your hands and feet. With this decreased circulation, there's an increase in symptoms of peripheral neuropathy—prickling, burning nerve pain in the hands and feet, along with numbness. The most common causes of peripheral neuropathy are diabetes and chemotherapy. *What to do…*

•Keep your hands and feet warm. When you're outside in the cold, wear thick gloves and thick socks. Dress in layers and always wear a hat.

•Keep your feet dry. Because peripheral neuropathy reduces sensation, it's sometimes hard to know if your feet are damp and cold. As soon as you get home from being outside in winter weather, remove your shoes and socks, dry your feet and put on a fresh pair of socks and warm slippers.

•Wear sheepskin gloves and sheepskin slippers to bed to help keep hands and feet warm during a long, cold winter night.

•Exercise regularly—indoors. Use a treadmill or stationary bicycle to exercise regularly. Regular aerobic exercise will improve your circulation, and core-strengthening exercises will help prevent falls.

Helpful: Get an exercise prescription from a physical therapist.

•**Chronic obstructive pulmonary disease (COPD).** The number of COPD "exacerbations"—worsening symptoms such as breathlessness, requiring corticosteroids, antibiotics and/or hospitalization—double during winter, according to research published in *European Respiratory Journal.*

COPD sufferers take a hit for several reasons. For example, up to 70% of COPD exacerbations are triggered by bacterial or viral infections, which tend to peak in the winter. Low blood levels of vitamin D in wintertime may worsen the disease. *What to do…*

•Wear a scarf or mask when outside in cold, dry air—and avoid exercising outside in excessively cold temperatures.

•Wash your hands several times a day. It's the number one way to minimize your risk for infections from a cold or flu virus. Use warm water and soap. An alcohol-based hand sanitizer is fine if you don't have access to water.

•Get a flu shot. Protection is a must if you have COPD, which makes you far more susceptible to the flu and pneumonia. You should also get vaccinated for pneumonia.

Talk to your doctor about the appropriate vaccination schedule for you.

•Boost your immunity. Load up on whole foods (phytochemicals in vegetables, fruits, beans and other whole foods strengthen the immune system)…and limit processed foods. Consider taking a multivitamin mineral supplement, with immune-strengthening vitamin C and zinc.

•Take vitamin D. A team of international researchers found that daily or weekly supplementation with vitamin D was safe and significantly reduced respiratory infections in people with COPD. Daily doses in research have ranged from 300 IU to 4,000 IU daily. Consult your doctor for the dose that's right for you.

Important: Cold, dry air can trigger asthma attacks, too. If you have a history of asthma, wear a mask or scarf when outdoors and avoid temperatures below 10°F when you're active.

This "Silent" Sleep Problem Stumps Even Some Doctors

Steven Y. Park, MD, assistant professor of otolaryngology at Albert Einstein College of Medicine in New York City. Dr. Park's research has been published in *Journal of Sleep Research* and other professional journals. He is author of *Sleep, Interrupted.* DoctorStevenPark.com

Ask people to name a disorder that interferes with a good night's shut-eye, and chances are obstructive sleep apnea (OSA) is what you'll hear.

But a little-known condition—often referred to as OSA's "silent sister"—also leads to unexplained daytime fatigue and can even contribute to seemingly unrelated health problems (see below). The problem is, the typical red flags that patients—and doctors—look for when zeroing in on a sleep disorder, such as loud snoring and gasping during sleep, often are missing.

This mysterious sleep saboteur is called upper airway resistance syndrome (UARS). Like OSA, it causes multiple, micro-awakenings that occur when the sufferer unconsciously senses difficulty breathing while sleeping. The person will soon fall back to sleep only to awaken again, seconds or minutes later. This cycle can continue throughout the night—without the sufferer (or bed partner) even realizing it. But there are subtle differences between OSA and UARS. *What you need to know…*

How to Detect This "Silent" Disorder

No one knows exactly how many people have UARS. However, in a study of 527 subjects in a military hospital who had daytime fatigue, the prevalence was 8.4%, according to research published in the journal *Chest*.

Unlike OSA, in which breathing completely stops for tens of seconds at a time, breathing is merely impaired with UARS. The condition can be caused by a naturally narrowed airway (as may occur in a person who is thin)…an ill-positioned tongue (if it relaxes and partially covers the airway)…or loose throat tissues that interfere with breathing.

Some people with UARS go on to develop OSA, but many do not. As a result, these individuals can have UARS for years (or even a lifetime) without it being diagnosed and treated.

When UARS goes undetected, the repeated micro-awakenings cause sufferers to become not only tired and stressed in the daytime but may also make them highly sensitive to emotional triggers, light, sounds and weather changes.

The ongoing anxiety that so often accompanies UARS also can lead to tension headaches and depression. In research published in *Respiration*, the continual stress and lack of restorative sleep that mark UARS have been linked to the development of digestive symptoms, such as irritable bowel disease, and increased cardiovascular risks due to blood pressure spikes that can occur with the repeated micro-awakenings.

Do You Have This Disorder?

If you have daytime fatigue, with or without the health problems that can accompany UARS, consider seeing a dentist or a sleep specialist who is familiar with the disorder—not all physicians are. Before scheduling an appointment, call the physician's office and ask whether he/she treats UARS.

A knowledgeable specialist will inspect the back of the mouth, nose and jaw to see whether the person's airway appears unobstructed to the eye.

A surprising clue: Crooked teeth or a "scalloped" tongue, in which ridges or indentations on the sides of the tongue indicate where it pushes against the molars, can indicate a crowded jaw and partially obstructed airway.

If UARS is suspected, the next step is a sleep study, in which the number and frequency of respiratory effort-related arousals (RERAs) are monitored. These arousals from sleep do not technically meet the definition of apneas (pauses in breathing) or hypopneas (periods of shallow breathing), both of which occur with OSA.

Note: A sleep study performed in a lab is more sensitive to the subtle obstructions that accompany UARS than in-home studies.

If apneas and hypopneas last for more than 10 seconds, they qualify as a sleep breathing event, and more than five such events an hour points to OSA if you have other symptoms such as daytime sleepiness, cognitive dysfunction or high blood pressure. When the patient does not have OSA, a high number of RERAs may suggest UARS.

Recent development: A procedure called drug-induced sleep endoscopy has emerged as a useful technique for diagnosing UARS. With this procedure, which is performed with the patient under sedation, a surgeon will insert a small camera through the nose into the airway to view any blockages that affect breathing during sleep.

3 Self-Care Measures

Even without an official diagnosis, people who suffer from unexplained daytime fatigue and suspect that they may have UARS can take steps to improve the disorder. *For example…*

•**Don't eat within three hours of bedtime.**

Here's why: When a person with UARS has difficulty breathing, stomach juices get sucked up into the throat causing swelling and more obstruction. Meal timing helps prevent this.

•**Choose the right sleep position.** Sleeping on your side or stomach (though this can trigger back pain in some people) helps many individuals with UARS. When sleeping on your back, it's easy for the tongue to fall back into the throat area and partially block the airway.

•**Try simple oral exercises.** Strengthening your airway muscles will help prevent UARS by reducing the odds that the muscles will collapse and impair breathing.

What to do: With an exercise called the "tongue slide," you push the tip of your tongue against the roof of your mouth and slide your tongue backward and forward, repeating the motion 20 times. Do this several times daily while working or watching TV.

When More Help Is Needed

If the steps above aren't adequate, you may need one of the following…*

•**Mouth guard.** If your dentist thinks you may have UARS due to a misaligned jaw, you can be fitted with a personalized mouth guard—known as a mandibular advancement device (MAD)—that slightly pushes the lower jaw and tongue forward to hold the airway open when the throat muscles relax. This prevents the airway from collapsing during deep sleep.

•**Bone-growth appliance.** Some dentists can fit an orthodontic device (known as an

*Most insurers do not cover these treatments unless UARS progresses to OSA.

anterior growth guidance appliance), which can stimulate bone growth by allowing the jaw to expand outward, ultimately providing more space to breathe while sleeping. It is usually worn all day and night for up to two years.

• **CPAP.** Continuous positive airway pressure (CPAP) devices send a constant flow of air pressure into the throat to ensure that the airway stays open during sleep. CPAP is usually used for OSA but also helps relieve UARS.

• **Surgery.** The most definitive treatment for UARS is surgery to physically alter the anatomy of the breathing airway. This may involve, for example, stiffening of loose palate tissue and/or the placement of an implant.

The good news is that people who have been successfully treated for UARS report waking up refreshed, as well as having a better quality of life and a reduced risk for the health problems related to this disorder.

Sleep Apnea Robs Memories

Background: Sleep plays a crucial role in consolidating memories.

Recent finding: More than 50% of people with obstructive sleep apnea (OSA), in which breathing stops intermittently during sleep, had "overgeneral memories"—those that lack specific detail—versus less than 19% of those without apnea, according to a study of 44 adults.

If you have sleep apnea—or are a heavy snorer, a sign of apnea: See a sleep specialist. Treating OSA may promote better retrieval of memories—and can help alleviate symptoms of depression, which is linked to memory loss and OSA.

Melinda L. Jackson, PhD, senior lecturer, Monash University, Melbourne, Australia.

Got Sinusitis That Won't Go Away?

Richard Firshein, DO, director and founder of Firshein Center for Integrative Medicine in New York City, and author of several books, including *Reversing Asthma, Your Asthma-Free Child, The Nutraceutical Revolution* and *The Vitamin Prescription (for Life).* FirsheinCenter.com

Y ou've got a stuffy and/or runny nose… swollen and tender sinuses…and fatigue that just won't go away. Sounds like the classic symptoms of a sinus infection (aka sinusitis), so your doctor prescribes an antibiotic. You take a full course of the medication, but you still feel rotten.

Feeling frustrated, you switch to an over-the-counter decongestant, and then you get another prescription…this time for a steroid. When the symptoms drag on for 12 weeks or more, it's official—you've got chronic sinusitis.

Most doctors are quick to blame this condition—the bane of some 34 million Americans each year—on a bacterial infection, nasal polyps or a deviated septum. The problem is, they're all too often wrong.

Eye-opening statistic: In a landmark study published in *Mayo Clinic Proceedings*, 96% of people with chronic sinusitis were found to have fungus in their mucus—and worse still, the symptoms were exacerbated by mold (a type of fungus) in their environment.

When doctors prescribe antibiotics for acute sinusitis that's not caused by bacteria (a practice that evidence-based medical guidelines do not support), it often leads to chronic sinusitis because these drugs don't eradicate viral or fungal infections or allergic sinusitis—which are the likely root causes.

Here's how to discover whether mold is fueling your chronic sinusitis—and what to do if it is…

The Mold Menace

Most people are scared of mold—but they're not scared enough! Not only is this common environmental toxin (mycotoxin) implicated in a significant number of cases of chronic sinusitis, it also causes or complicates a surprising number of cases seen in clinical practices of allergies and asthma, two conditions that often occur together.

Mold is especially dangerous because it is…

•**Pervasive.** Outside, it's found in leafy piles, dense vegetation and plant debris. Inside, mold is found in damp areas, such as those near leaky roofs and sinks…behind appliances connected to plumbing (such as the refrigerator, washer and dishwasher)… in basements with high humidity…under carpets…and behind walls. You can even find mold in clothing (such as sweaty gym clothes) that's not washed within a few days of use.

•**Invisible and airborne.** Mold spores can easily find their way into your nasal passages and lungs. Mold can then live in your body as a low-grade, ongoing inflammation/infection. Mold spores are insidious—the toxins from mold may cause serious illness even when the mold itself is hidden from view.

•**Highly allergenic.** Millions of people react to one or more types of mold. This can trigger allergic symptoms (including chronic sinusitis)…or cause or complicate cases of asthma.

Defeating Mold

You can detect and remove environmental mold. And you can strengthen your immune system so that your body is more mold-resistant. *Here's how…*

•**Suspect unhealthy levels of mold if there's discoloration or black mold on baseboards, wallboards or wallpaper**…if there are cracks in shower tile or leaks under the sink…if carpet or padding is in direct contact with a concrete slab…if your air-conditioning or heating has been poorly maintained…if you have a damp basement or crawl space…if there are watermarks or mold spots on walls…or if your dwelling has a musty, moldy odor.

Useful clue: If you have chronic sinusitis, mold may be an issue if you feel worse when you're in a building affected by a recent leak or flood, such as your house, apartment, office or vacation home.

Note: These places may also harbor hidden mold, even in the absence of a known flood or leak.

Another clue: You have been treated repeatedly for acute sinusitis…or have multiple infections that never get better.

Helpful: If you can't see mold but have chronic sinusitis, allergies or asthma, buy a mold-detection kit. These kits are widely available online and at hardware stores.

•**Don't expect there to be no mold—like bacteria, it can be found everywhere.** But high levels (as described on the test kit instructions) are a red alert. If the test detects high levels of mold and you subsequently discover a moldy area that covers less than 10 square feet (about three feet by three feet), you can probably clean it yourself.

What the Centers for Disease Control and Prevention recommends: Scrub with a mixture of one cup of laundry bleach and one gallon of water (never mix bleach and ammonia) to kill mold on surfaces. (For a less toxic cleaner, consider using undiluted white vinegar, which is especially effective on porous surfaces.) Use a fan to dry the area. Wear rubber gloves, goggles and an N95 respirator. Be sure also to wash your clothes carefully afterward.

For larger areas of mold or if a mold test you conducted detected high levels of mold but you can't locate the source, consider hiring an experienced mold-remediation professional. (Mold can hide on the backside of drywall, the topside of ceiling tiles, the underside of carpets, etc.) A mold-remediation specialist can be found online, but be careful to find someone who is certified and/or has years of experience.

In addition to addressing any mold in your surroundings…

•**Try immunotherapy.** If you have chronic sinusitis, see an allergist for a skin or blood test to find out if you're allergic to mold. If you are, ask about immunotherapy—allergy shots or drops that can desensitize you to mold.

•**Ask about antifungal medication.** If you have chronic sinusitis and/or asthma, ask your allergist about getting secretions and/or tissue samples from your sinuses tested to see if you have a fungal infection. If you do, your doctor may want to consider treating you with an oral antifungal medication or steroid.

•**Avoid trigger foods.** Avoid mold- and yeast-containing foods, including bread, beer, wine and certain cheeses (such as Brie, Gorgonzola and Roquefort), as well as fermented foods, such as soy sauce, yogurt and pickles. Reduce or eliminate refined carbohydrates, such as white rice, sweets and pasta—mold feeds on the sugars that are produced when refined carbs break down, leading to the growth of fungi in the body.

•**Consider supplements and other natural treatments.** Nutritional supplements that may help battle chronic sinus infections include prebiotics…probiotics…turmeric or its active ingredient curcumin…and natural antifungals, including caprylic acid and artemisia. Follow the dosage recommendation on the label. Once fungal sinusitis is successfully treated with medication, natural treatments can be used, under your doctor's supervision, to suppress fungal growth.

•**Do nasal irrigation.** Using saline or a neti pot (filled with distilled or sterile water) once or twice daily will help clear your sinuses of fungus.

Daily Steroid Inhaler Useless for Many Asthmatics

Stephen Lazarus, MD, professor of medicine at University of California, San Francisco, and director of the university's training program in pulmonary and critical care medicine. UCSFHealth.org

Doctors often instruct patients suffering from mild persistent asthma to use a steroid inhaler every day—but nearly half of those patients receive no noticeable benefit from doing so, according to a recent study published in *The New England Journal of Medicine.*

The study divided asthmatics into two groups—those who had high levels of a type of white blood cell called eosinophils in their sputum (phlegm) and those who did not. High levels of eosinophils are an indicator of a specific type of inflammation, and for patients suffering from this inflammation, the study confirmed that daily steroid use is beneficial. But 73% of the mild persistent asthma sufferers who participated in the study did not have indications of this type of inflammation—and for two-thirds of this larger group, daily steroid use was no more effective than a placebo. What's more, daily steroid use is expensive and can have adverse side effects—including increased risk for bone loss, cataracts and glaucoma.

If a daily steroid is not providing any noticeable improvement, ask your health-care provider…

•**"Can you confirm I'm using my inhaler properly?"** Improper inhaler use is more common than people realize. *If this fails to solve the problem, ask…*

•**"Is it worth trying a different treatment option, such as a long-acting muscarinic antagonist (LAMA)?"** LAMA is traditionally used for COPD. A LAMA inhaler can be effective for some asthma sufferers, with few side effects (notably, dry mouth).

Note: As yet, there is no easy and accurate way to test eosinophil levels—you may just have to try a LAMA and see if it works.

Case Study: IV Nutrient Therapy for Asthma and Allergy Relief

Laurie Steelsmith, ND, LAc, medical director of Steelsmith Natural Health Center in Honolulu. She is author of *Natural Choices for Women's Health, Great Sex, Naturally* and *Growing Younger Every Day* and writes the "Natural Healing Secrets for Women" blog at BottomLineInc.com. DrSteelsmith.com

The patient: "Stephanie," a 40-year-old nurse and avid cyclist.

Why she came to see me: Stephanie was clearly keyed up when she walked into my office for the first time. While originally from Hawaii—where my natural health center is based—she'd spent the last decade working at a hospital in Portland, Oregon. Shortly after returning to Oahu a year earlier, her body, as she put it, "went haywire." High stress was overwhelming her from morning to night. A rash had been breaking out on her face intermittently; the rest of her body felt relentlessly itchy, even her ears. Her eyelids were often swollen. She'd also been struck by either a cold or the flu every two to three months. And while she'd suffered from asthma and allergies for as long as she could recall, they had reached unbearable levels upon her return to the islands. In short, she was exhausted, anxious, itchy, constantly coughing—and incredibly frustrated.

How I evaluated her: I began our work together by striving to get a complete picture of Stephanie's medical history and lifestyle.

Stephanie had worked as a nurse in Honolulu for several years before a chance encounter with a fellow cyclist compelled her to try out a new life in Portland. There, she enjoyed a respite from the asthma and allergies she'd been diagnosed with in her teens, in part by leading a healthy lifestyle with her partner. When she and her partner amicably split, she wanted to be closer to her family and friends in Hawaii. She secured a work transfer, scored a great apartment and came home to start anew.

But the stress of relocating—no matter that she was returning "home"—seemed to have upset her "entire system," she said. Her asthma returned with a vengeance, as did her allergies. Her new primary care physician prescribed at least a year's worth of nasal steroids, inhalers and oral *prednisone* (a corticosteroid medication commonly used to treat allergies, skin diseases, immune system disorders and more).

They proved to be ineffective: Her symptoms only seemed to worsen, and she loathed the idea of relying on a series of medications to merely make it through the day. She had also seen an allergist, who provided "symptomatic relief" but not a cure.

Lastly, Stephanie had seen a dermatologist, who was concerned she may have an autoimmune condition such as lupus. To this end, the dermatologist had done a biopsy of the skin on her forehead. (Fortunately, the pathology report only revealed what appeared to be an allergic response.)

Meanwhile, Stephanie claimed she was getting sicker and sicker—so much so she frequently canceled on friends, called in sick to work, relied upon her mother for assistance and tried to find relief for her consistently itchy skin and asthma attacks by watching Netflix and eating take-out and ice cream inside her air-conditioned apartment—dietary "snags" she tried to undo with copious glasses of lemon-infused water and short sessions on her apartment complex's indoor bike. "I came back to Hawaii to enjoy the beautiful outdoors and restart my life," she said unpityingly, just factually. "And now I'm too uncomfortable and afraid to spend time outdoors. This is no life at all."

To get to the bottom of Stephanie's litany of symptoms, I did a full physical exam. This was followed by a blood test that would evaluate for food allergies and her levels of copper and zinc. I also ordered a stool culture to assess for yeast, bacteria and parasites.

What my evaluation revealed: Stephanie's results demonstrated that she was allergic to a number of foods and compounds, many of which she regularly consumed. These included gluten, dairy, beef, MSG, several food colorings and that lemon she ingested daily.

Her blood test demonstrated that she had a surplus of copper relative to zinc, which can contribute to inflammation and anxiety. She also had low vitamin D levels, which arrived as no surprise, given that she'd spent 10 years in rainy Portland and had willfully sequestered herself inside in Hawaii. (As I told Stephanie, low vitamin D levels impact immunity and the body's ability to fight off infection. It can also exacerbate anxiety and contribute to the health and metabolism of skin.)

Finally, her stool culture revealed an imbalance in her intestinal flora: She had too much yeast, too little "friendly" gut bacteria and a slight overgrowth of a potentially pathogenic flora. In sum, the foods Stephanie was consuming and the products she was using—from sausage on her pizza to her favorite face wash—were triggering a full-body inflammatory response, leaving her with aggravated asthmatic symptoms, anxiety and atopic dermatitis.

Note that Stephanie did not change her diet when she came back to Hawaii. She simply couldn't tolerate certain foods and chemicals anymore. Probably her detoxification systems were overwhelmed, and she most likely had leaky gut leading to excess allergy, increased systemic inflammation and an overwhelmed liver. The stress of the move was probably her tipping point.

How I addressed her problem: To restore Stephanie to the health she'd enjoyed for most of her life, we began with dietary treatment, as it was inarguable that she needed to eliminate any and all potential al-

lergens. In addition to ridding herself of the foods mentioned above—gluten, dairy, lemon, beef, MSG and any food that contained food colorings (to be on the safe side)—I asked her to toss or donate her facial and body care products and start fresh with organic items that were comprised of natural ingredients. (Even the toothpaste she'd begun buying in Hawaii contained a dye that has been linked to hypersensitivity.) I also advised her to be especially careful of tartrazine. Also known as FD&C Yellow #5—and found in many brands of that ice cream she loved—it's been shown to result in hives, swelling, skin rashes and asthma.

Additionally, I prescribed Stephanie a set of dietary supplements to help decrease her allergic reactivity. *These included…*

• **Quercetin,** a flavonoid that has potent anti-inflammatory capacities

• **Zinc,** to help lower her copper levels

• **Vitamin A** to naturally support her immune system and mucous membranes

• **Vitamins B5 and B1,** which organically promote adrenal health and the breakdown of histamine

• **SAMe (*S-adenosyl-L-methionine*),** a sulfur-based compound, to support hormone and cell function (and, thus, overall health).

I further suggested she take a probiotic to re-establish a healthy ratio of intestinal flora, and weekly acupuncture sessions to help her strengthen her qi (or life force).

Perhaps the biggest step I asked Stephanie to take was to sign up for intravenous (IV) nutrient therapy. Presently gaining a great deal of attention for its rapidity and efficacy, intravenous nutrient therapy is favored in hospitals and beyond to treat patients whose immune systems have been compromised. Administered directly into the blood, the nutrients used in these therapeutic cocktails bypass the intestines, which allows for direct and immediate access to cells. What's more, high doses of nutrients that would not be tolerated if ingested can be used, thereby accelerating the healing process and providing profound biochemical shifts that foster healthy change. An example is magnesium—an IV of high dose magnesium doesn't cause diarrhea but taking it orally could have this side effect. Also, glutathione, which is not very stable when taken orally but IV administration allows for therapeutic doses to be administered.

Now used in a variety of settings, the therapy has been shown to be beneficial in a variety of ways, including detoxification, sports recovery (such as pre and post marathon running, or high intensity sports like Iron Man competitions), inflammatory conditions, allergies, supportive cancer care, eczema, chronic fatigue syndrome, autoimmune conditions, chronic tick infections and chronic viral conditions. I personally use it for jet lag and any time I'm in a weakened immune state and I feel like I'm about to come down with a cold. IV nutrient therapy is also used to "pre-condition" patients before surgery or an intense sports event. And it's recommended to expedite healing after a stressful occurrence, such as chemotherapy. I have found IV nutrient therapy has been key towards helping many of my patients restore homeostasis (balance in the body).

In Stephanie's case, the IV bag she would receive during treatments would include high doses of Vitamin C and magnesium with cofactor minerals and B-complex vitamins. This therapy has been shown to be particularly effective against asthma attacks and other disorders. I also added intravenous glutathione. While naturally produced in the body, high doses of this powerful antioxidant help shield the body from free radical damage and clear toxins like heavy metals from the blood and liver.

The patient's progress: Six weeks later, Stephanie was a changed woman. She'd found the dietary changes I'd recommended easier than imagined, exchanging traditional pizza for pies made with gluten-free cauliflower crusts, antioxidant-rich vegetables and dairy-free "cheese"…and swapping milk-heavy ice cream for dairy-free Coconut Bliss. While she still suffered from the occasional bout of atopic dermatitis, her skin was otherwise glowing, thanks in large part to the synthetic-free skincare brand she'd discovered.

Her real breakthrough—as we both noted—arrived with the sixth intravenous glutathione therapy I gave her. At that point, we'd increased her dosage of glutathione from 200 mg to 2,000 mg, which made a tremendous difference in terms of her symptoms. (In traditional naturopathic medicine, treating the liver is the golden chalice to healing from allergies and asthma, and glutathione is famed for its impact on this fundamental organ.) Her eyes had stopped swelling, the rash on her face had completely disappeared and her asthma attacks were far less frequent and destabilizing.

"I feel like my old self again, only even better than before," she said, stating that her fatigue was gone and her vitality had announced itself again. The first thing she planned to do with all that energy? To get outdoors on her bike, of course, and savor the paradise she'd missed.

Inhaler Alert

Primatene Mist, the metered-dose epinephrine inhaler that was recalled in 2011, is now ozone safe, newly FDA-approved and available over-the-counter. However, respiratory health groups, including the American Lung Association, point out that epinephrine inhalers, such as Primatene Mist, are not recommended for asthma by any expert guidelines…and may tempt patients to self-treat rather than get proper medical care. Prescription *albuterol* and corticosteroid inhalers are safer, more effective and longer lasting.

Michael Blaiss, MD, executive medical director, American College of Allergy, Asthma & Immunology, Atlanta. ACAAI.org

The Safe Way to Take NAC If You Have Lung Disease

Andrew L. Rubman, ND, founder and medical director, Southbury Clinic for Traditional Medicines, in Southbury, Connecticut. He is a member of Bottom Line's panel of experts and writes the Bottom Line blog "Nature Doc's Patient Diary." SouthburyClinic.com

The health benefits of antioxidants such as N-acetylcysteine (NAC) have been so widely touted that many people think you can't get too much. However, while research does confirm many of the health benefits, unless NAC is taken in an appropriate dose and in combination with the right supporting nutrients, it can be disruptive and devastating to health.

NAC is found naturally in the body. Research suggests that it protects against DNA damage that results from oxidative stress caused by free radicals—unstable molecules that break down cells, disrupting the cell DNA. Oxidative stress is especially a problem in the lungs, where free radicals can form from lung irritants such as smoking and air pollutants. The resulting cell damage leads to upper respiratory infections, such as chronic obstructive pulmonary disease/COPD (which includes emphysema and chronic bronchitis) and cancer.

Smokers and people with lung diseases such as asthma often take NAC because it helps thin mucus, reduces phlegm and coughing and eases expectoration. NAC is also a powerful detoxifier and is used in hospital settings to help clear the liver from *acetaminophen* overdose. Since NAC helps strengthen immunity, it's also used as a preventive for colds and flu...and for general immune system support.

Lung Cancer Concerns

However, although NAC is beneficial when the body has more free radicals than it can handle, too much NAC creates another problem. That's because NAC helps all the body's cells stay alive longer—including old and damaged cells that are more likely to turn to cancer and that normally would be killed off by the body's immune system, a process called senescence.

In fact, a recent study led by researchers at Hôpital Henri Mondor in France published in *JCI Insight* found that NAC not only can accelerate lung cancer, it can initiate the disease when there was no prior increased risk. The researchers tested NAC on two types of mice—normal aged mice and mice who were genetically altered to have stressed lungs similar to people with COPD. Half the aged mice and half the genetically stressed mice were fed NAC added to their drinking water...the rest just got the usual drinking water.

Results: Mice who got NAC had less emphysema (one of the main types of COPD)... but they were more likely to have lung cancer. Not surprisingly, the NAC-fed mice with genetically stressed lungs, making them already at higher risk for lung cancer, were at highest risk—they were 50% more likely to have lung tumors compared with genetically stressed mice who did not get NAC. Alarmingly, though, NAC-fed normal aged mice also had an increased risk compared with normal aged mice who did not get NAC—they were 10% more likely to have lung cancer.

Safer Way to Take NAC

Taking a NAC supplement in an appropriate dose and in combination with other supporting nutrients, such as vitamins A, C and E, can help you get the health benefits while making you less vulnerable to health risks. NAC is generally regarded as safe, and unsafe levels have not been determined. Research supports that typical doses—500 mg of NAC taken twice daily along with 25,000 IU of vitamin A (as beta-carotene)...2,000 mg of vitamin C (as ascorbic acid)...and 200 IU of vitamin E (as mixed tocopherols/tocotrienols), also taken twice daily—are therapeutic. However, individual dosage levels for these nutrients will depend on a patient's age, lifestyle and history of chronic diseases.

Check with a naturopathic doctor or a medical doctor with nutritional expertise before taking these supplements, especially if you are trying to treat a medical condition—good advice that applies to taking other antioxidants as well!

Plants May Be Better Than Technology for Reducing Air Pollution

They could be cheaper and more effective at cleaning the air near industrial sites, roadways, power plants and oil and gas drilling areas. Restoring plants and trees to landscapes near pollution sources could reduce pollution by an average of 27%. The effect would occur in urban and rural areas, with real-world success rates depending on how much land was available for plant growth and how much pollution was already present. But there was only one specific sector studied—industrial boilers—in which technology would be cheaper for cleaning the air than extensive ecosystem upgrades.

Bhavik Bakshi, PhD, professor of chemical and biomolecular engineering, The Ohio State University, Columbus, and leader of a study published in *Environmental Science echnology*.

You're Never Too Old for a New Allergy

Neeta Ogden, MD, an allergist in private practice in Edison, New Jersey. She is a member of the Medical-Scientific Council of the Allergy and Asthma Foundation of America and a spokesperson for the American College of Allergy, Asthma and Immunology. NeetaOgdenMD.com

You're sniffling. You're sneezing. You're itching. Is it a cold? A rash? You're too old for it to be an allergy, right? Wrong. Kids aren't the only ones who develop new allergies. In fact, adult-onset allergies are more common than you think.

A study published recently in *JAMA Network Open* found that among people who have food allergies, nearly half developed at least one of their allergies during adulthood. Researchers who study allergies are not certain what is to blame for this general trend of growing allergies in both kids and adults. Some have speculated that it could be related to changes in our habits, such as the overuse of hand sanitizers and antibiotics…as well as changes in our diets.

Adult-onset environmental allergies are more common as well, possibly because rising temperatures are leading to larger amounts of pollen in the air. Those pollen rates also are believed to be responsible for increasing rates of environmental allergies among children.

Here's what you need to know about adult-onset food and environmental allergies…

Food Allergies

If you have a bad reaction to shellfish (hives, itching, breathing problems)—even if it has never happened to you before—odds are that you are allergic. In fact, the most common adult-onset food allergy is to shellfish.

Other likely allergens: Seafood, tree nuts, soy and peanuts, among other foods.

Potential symptoms: Food allergy sufferers typically experience itching and/or hives within minutes or up to an hour and a half to two hours after consuming the food. Sufferers also might experience coughing, difficulty breathing, abdominal pain, nausea, vomiting, light-headedness and/or swelling of the lips, face, throat and/or tongue.

Some exceptions…

Recently, an allergy to red meat including beef and pork has been reported—the allergy is to a carbohydrate called *alpha-gal*, which can enter the body from a Lone Star tick bite. When someone who has been bitten subsequently eats red meat, he/she can suffer an allergic reaction that is atypical because it occurs several hours after consuming the red meat.

It's also important to distinguish between an intolerance and an allergy. Symptoms such as cramps, gas, diarrhea and bloating that occur several hours after eating, without itchiness or hives, may suggest an intolerance or your body's inability to digest that food, but you are not allergic to it. Unlike allergies, these digestive issues do not occur because your immune response has misidentified a molecule in the food as something harmful.

Example: Many adults who have consumed dairy products without any issues for their entire lives suddenly start to experience cramping or gas after drinking milk or eating ice cream. These people have not developed a dairy allergy—they have developed lactose intolerance. Their digestive systems no longer produce enough of the lactase enzyme needed to digest a sugar found in dairy foods.

If you experience mild tingling or itching in your lips, tongue and/or throat after consuming certain fruits and vegetables, you might have a condition known as oral allergy syndrome, a very mild form of food allergy that actually suggests that you have a pollen allergy (see below for more about pollen allergies). A protein in the fruit or vegetable is so similar to a protein in pollen that your body is misidentifying it. Causes of common oral allergies include apples, carrots, celery, corn, kiwis, lettuce, oranges, peaches, peppers and tomatoes. *What to do…*

If you have a reaction that includes difficulty breathing, seek immediate medical attention. Many people don't realize that they can fall victim to allergies as adults and may try to convince themselves that it is something else, such as a stomach bug or flu. That can be a dangerous mistake. Call 911. A person having a serious allergic reaction needs *epinephrine* right away to ensure that his airways stay open.

After experiencing any allergic reaction, write down everything you had consumed in the 90 minutes before symptoms appeared, as well as any meats you ate in the five hours prior to symptoms. Do this even if it was a relatively mild reaction that did not require immediate medical attention. If possible, write down not just the names of the food products consumed, but a complete list of ingredients in those products. If appropriate, take digital photos of the ingredients lists on food packaging.

Schedule an appointment to see an allergist approximately one month after your allergic response. Bring your list of suspect foods and ingredients to this appointment. Why wait a month to see an allergist? The allergist likely will conduct tests to determine what you are allergic to, and the odds of inaccurate test results increase during the weeks following an allergic reaction. In the meantime, avoid foods that you suspect might be the cause of your reaction—particularly the most likely culprits, such as shellfish and other seafood, nuts and soy.

Note: An initial mild allergic reaction does not guarantee that future reactions also will be mild—your next response could include potentially fatal anaphylaxis, which can constrict airways and cause a rapid drop in blood pressure.

Warning: Do not try to confirm whether you have the allergy by consuming suspect foods again.

If you do have a food allergy, the allergist likely will recommend that you avoid the food and carry an EpiPen Auto-Injector, a device that can be used to self-inject epinephrine if you were to have a severe allergic reaction in the future. Continued follow-up with your allergist—and yearly blood work—will help confirm if your allergy is persisting or has gone away.

Environmental Allergies

It's no secret that pollen, dust mites, mold spores and pet dander can trigger environmental allergies. But many adults are taken off guard when they suddenly develop environmental allergies, also called seasonal allergies or nasal allergies, in the years following a move to a different part of the country. There might be higher pollen levels in this new place…or different types of pollen than they have been exposed to in the past. Many people are allergic to certain types of pollen but not others. Similarly, their new home might harbor more dust or animal dander.

Potential symptoms: People who have environmental allergies often feel as though they have colds that they can't seem to shake, complete with runny noses, watery eyes and sneezing. But allergy sufferers typically also experience an itchy feeling in the throat and, potentially, in the eyes, nose and/or skin as well. If the allergy is to pollen, there likely will be a seasonal predictability to the symptoms—these people might believe they "come down with colds" every spring or fall, for example.

What to do: Adult-onset environmental allergies are far less likely than food allergies to be life-threatening, though they can be very uncomfortable. People who experience them rarely require emergency medical attention or an EpiPen. It sometimes is possible to control the symptoms of environmental allergies on one's own with over-the-counter medications such as antihistamines or steroid nasal sprays, but speak with your doctor before using these.

Important: If you know that your environmental allergies appear predictably at a certain time of year, start taking these medications approximately two weeks before then. If you wait until the full-blown season to start medications, your allergy symptoms may be harder to get under control.

Resource: Pollen.com gives local allergy forecasts on its national allergy map.

If over-the-counter medications fail to provide relief, see an allergist. The allergist might be able to fine-tune your use of over-the-counter medications or prescribe allergy shots or oral allergy immunotherapy. An allergist also can perform skin tests or blood tests to determine precisely which allergens are causing your problems, and he could suggest other solutions.

Example: Perhaps you are allergic to dust mites, not pollen. If so, your symptoms might be dramatically reduced if you use allergen-proof bedding or a mattress cover,

wash it frequently in water heated to at least 130°F, dust your home frequently using a damp rag, remove carpeting and/or install a HEPA filter air purifier.

What's in Your Household Dust

Gabriel Filippelli, PhD, professor of earth sciences and director of the Center for Urban Health at Indiana University–Purdue University Indianapolis. He is a researcher with 360 Dust Analysis, a new project in which scientists are analyzing the contents of consumers' vacuums and gaining insight into the health dangers of dust, and editor in chief of *GeoHealth*. 360DustAnalysis.com

Scientists define dust as fine particulate matter that is made up of dirt, organic material, pollen and human and animal skin cells. Dust is also produced by mold spores and cigarette smoke. Although dust can enter your home when you open a window, about one-third of household dust is created inside your home.

It's no surprise that a major cause of dust is pets. Dogs and cats shed dander from their skin, which causes allergies for many people. And dust mites, another well-known allergen, feed off pet dander and skin cells shed by people. *Other sources of dust in the home...*

• **Textiles.** Carpets, bed linens and clothing are common sources of dust. The fabrics these items are composed of break down over time and give off chemicals that get absorbed into the dust we breathe. The routine use of flame retardants and surface protectants on textiles stopped when researchers demonstrated that these chemicals made their way into human blood and tissue. But other harmful chemicals, such as Teflon, are still used in textiles and can end up in household dust.

• **Lead.** The federal government banned consumer use of lead-containing paint in 1978. But lead paint is still present in millions of homes, under layers of newer paint, contributing to lead in house dust. Children exposed to lead can experience behavioral and learning problems, slowed growth, hearing problems and anemia.

• **Chemicals tracked in from outside.** Shoes worn outdoors pick up cancer-causing toxins from asphalt road residue, lawn chemicals that can disrupt the endocrine system (glands that produce hormones that regulate many functions in the body) and much more. Also, researchers find that 96% of shoes have traces of feces on their soles.

Other problems: We all know that dust can cause eye irritation, sneezing and coughing. But for people with asthma or chronic obstructive pulmonary disease (COPD), even small increases in dust can worsen symptoms.

Best Ways to Minimize Dust

Sweeping with a broom or using a feather duster just stirs up dust and spreads it around. *To reduce dust…*

• **Vacuum at least once a week using a vacuum with a high-efficiency particulate air (HEPA) filter,** which mechanically forces air through a fine mesh that traps harmful particles such as pollen, pet dander, dust mites and tobacco smoke particles. A HEPA vacuum filter will also trap harmful metals, such as lead, and chemicals in dust. A standalone HEPA air purifier is helpful, too.

• **Run an air conditioner.** Central air-conditioning can filter the entire home, and window air conditioners can help as well. Filters for a central system should be changed at the frequency recommended by the manufacturer. Filters for window units should be washed monthly and thoroughly dried.

• **Before entering your home, take off your shoes.** Change into slippers reserved for indoor use.

• **Make cleaning simple.** Mix one-part white vinegar with nine-parts water, dip a cloth in the mixture and wipe down surfaces. This is one of the most effective ways to get rid of dust, including lead dust, and helps to eliminate bacteria. And it's chemical-free.

• **Don't use antimicrobial cleaning products and hand soaps.** A recent study found that the antimicrobial chemical triclosan, which the FDA banned in antibacterial soaps in 2016 after discovering dangerous side effects, including possible impact on the endocrine system, is abundant in dust, resulting in organisms that can cause antibiotic-resistant infection. Triclosan is still used in consumer products that may not list it on the label. Plus, other antibacterial chemicals are used instead and may have the same impact on dust as triclosan.

• **Wash hands with plain soap and water,** and use vinegar (see above) to clean.

• **Be sure to use dust-blocking covers on your mattresses and pillows,** and when possible, replace carpets with hardwood flooring or tile.

Beware of Sesame Allergy

According to a recent finding, more than 1.5 million adults and children in the US are allergic to sesame—and the condition is often undiagnosed.

Problem: Because the seeds are not included among the eight allergens that the FDA mandates for listing on food labels, consumers could be at risk for potentially serious allergic reactions. Sesame is found in many foods such as ethnic dishes (including sushi) and sauces (including tahini).

Note: Sesame-related ingredients are often identified with unfamiliar terms, such as "benne," "gingelly" or "simsim."

Ruchi Gupta, MD, MPH, director, Science and Outcomes of Allergy and Asthma Research, Northwestern University and Lurie Children's Hospital, both in Chicago.

Chapter 16

STROKE ALERTS

Alert: Pregnancy Strokes Are on the Rise...and They're Preventable!

Stroke doesn't happen just to "old people." Young women are also at risk, particularly if they are pregnant—and the weeks just before and right after giving birth are especially dangerous. Alarming as this sounds, most of these strokes don't have to happen if pregnant women and new mothers—and their doctors—take the right preventive measures.

Stroke is the fourth-leading cause of death for women, in part because even a seemingly healthy pregnancy can raise the risk for stroke. Levels of the hormone estrogen increase dramatically during pregnancy, and estrogen helps blood to clot. Pregnancy also increases the risk for two conditions that can lead to stroke—preeclampsia (characterized by high blood pressure and protein in the urine)...and eclampsia (characterized by high blood pressure, protein in the urine and seizures). Women who become pregnant after age 40 are at highest risk for both these conditions.

According to a recent study led by researchers at the Centre for Surveillance and Applied Research in Canada, stroke during the postpartum period (42 days after delivery) rose almost six percentage points in a little more than a decade—from 10.8 out of every 100,000 pregnancies to 16.6 out of every 100,000 pregnancies. Data from the US Nationwide Inpatient Sample from 1994 to 1995 and from 2006 to 2007 showed a 47% increase for hospitalizations during pregnancy and an 83% increase for postpartum hospitalizations associated with stroke. And a more recent Centers for Disease Control and Prevention (CDC) study published in *Obstetrics and Gynecology* found a 62% increase in strokes during pregnancy or after childbirth over a 17-year period.

Risk for the deadliest form of stroke, hemorrhagic, is highest during the third trimester of pregnancy through 12 weeks after giving birth, according to an American Heart Association study that looked at 3.3 million births over a 10-year period.

Larry B. Goldstein, MD, FAAN, FANA, FAHA, spokesperson for the American Heart Association and American Stroke Association. Study titled "Stroke and Cerebrovascular Disease in Pregnancy," led by researchers at the Centre for Surveillance and Applied Research, Public Health Agency of Canada, published in *Stroke*.

What You Can Do

Among the factors that might be driving the increase in pregnancy-related stroke is that more women are having children at older ages, and older age is a stroke risk factor in itself. But while it may not be an option to choose pregnancy at a younger age, other factors—primarily, high blood pressure—that can make a pregnant women stroke-vulnerable are preventable.

Stroke-prevention steps to take during and after pregnancy...

•**Prioritize pre- and postnatal care.** The American College of Obstetricians recommends that women have a follow-up visit with their doctors within three weeks postpartum. This is an update from their previous recommendation that a follow-up visit should happen six weeks postpartum. If you're at high risk for stroke, you may need to check in even earlier than that.

•**Check your blood pressure at least several times a week.** Even if your numbers stay in the normal range, if there's a significant increase—20 points or more in the systolic (upper) number—you should call your doctor. It's especially important to check your blood pressure regularly if you were diagnosed with preeclampsia or eclampsia during or after pregnancy.

Best type of blood pressure monitor: The American Heart Association (AHA) recommends an automatic upper-arm cuff-style monitor.

•**Make time for your own health.** Now that your baby is in your arms rather than your belly, it may seem as though, along with breast milk, your little bundle of joy sucks up all your time and energy. But you need to find time to take care of your own health, too. Eat a healthful diet (both Mediterranean and DASH diets are excellent for stroke prevention)...exercise regularly... take steps to manage stress...don't smoke and avoid environmental tobacco smoke exposure...and avoid or limit alcohol.

Also, if you have been diagnosed with diabetes, or pregnancy caused your blood sugar to go into the diabetic range, take steps to keep your blood sugar at a healthy level. And if you're overweight, discuss with your doctor safe, healthy ways to control your weight during pregnancy and shed pounds once your baby is born.

•**Be alert to stroke symptoms.** The acronym F-A-S-T, developed by the AHA, makes it easy to recognize the signs and get help immediately. It stands for Facial drooping...Arm weakness...Speech difficulty...and Time to call 911 right away! Also realize that stroke symptoms in women can be different from those in men.

•**Discuss with your doctor whether you should take aspirin.** Low-dose aspirin (81 mg/day) may have cardio-protective benefits for women at high risk for preeclampsia. However, aspirin can also increase risk for bleeding complications, so discuss the pros and cons with your obstetrician.

•**Know your health history.** Preexisting conditions, such as diabetes, heart disease, lupus, rheumatoid arthritis, blood-clotting disorders, atrial fibrillation (AFib) and irregular heartbeat, can increase risk for stroke. So can a history of multiple miscarriages. Be sure to discuss your whole health history during prenatal and postpartum checkups.

Prevent Stroke with Good Oral Hygiene

Nearly 80% of blood clots removed from 75 stroke patients contained DNA from mouth bacteria.

Theory: The bacterium Streptococcus mitis is harmless to the mouth, but when it enters the circulation from infected gums or a tooth extraction, it can bind to platelet receptors, making a person more prone to blood clots.

Important: Brush, floss and see a dentist at least twice a year for cleanings and oral exams.

Pekka J. Karhunen, MD, PhD, professor of forensic medicine, Tampere University, Finland.

These Infections Could Increase Your Stroke Risk

The study "Infection as a Stroke Trigger: Associations Between Different Organ System Infection Admissions and Stroke Subtypes," led by researchers at Icahn School of Medicine at Mount Sinai in New York City and published in *Stroke*.

If you are an older adult with diabetes, high blood pressure, atrial fibrillation, high cholesterol or migraine, you likely know that you are at higher risk for stroke. But did you know that an infection also may boost your odds of having a stroke?

While it's been known by scientists that a nasty urinary tract infection or respiratory infection may increase one's vulnerability to a life-threatening stroke, questions have remained around the specific types of stroke that may be triggered by different infections.

Now: To find out exactly which infections most often preceded three types of strokes, researchers at the Icahn School of Medicine at Mount Sinai in New York City delved further into the data.

Study details: For their study, researchers searched databases at New York state hospitals and analyzed admissions for three types of stroke along with hospital or emergency room admissions for five types of infection.

Ischemic stroke, the most common type of stroke, which is typically caused by a blood clot that blocks blood supply to the brain... intracerebral hemorrhage, due to bleeding into the brain...and subarachnoid hemorrhage, resulting from bleeding in the inner lining of the brain, were the types of stroke studied.

In addition, the researchers looked at five types of infection—skin...urinary tract... sepsis (a life-threatening infection of the bloodstream)...abdominal...and respiratory (including pneumonia and other lung infections). The odds of an infection triggering a stroke seven to 120 days after infection were then calculated.

Study results: Every type of infection included in the study increased the odds of an ischemic stroke. Urinary tract infection had the strongest association, increasing the risk by threefold within 30 days after infection.

For intracerebral hemorrhage, urinary tract and respiratory infections and sepsis increased risk. This time, the strongest association was found with sepsis, which tripled the risk within 60 days after infection.

Only a respiratory infection increased the risk for subarachnoid hemorrhage. This infection tripled the risk in the shortest period of time—within 14 days.

The good news is, with all types of infection studied, the risk for any stroke decreased over time.

The researchers theorized that various factors could be at play. People who develop infections may be more likely to suffer a stroke because the infection leads to inflammation that damages blood vessels...and increased numbers of white blood cells and platelets may contribute to the formation of blood clots. Infections also tend to make people less active, which also may increase the risk of blood clotting.

What this research could mean for you: The study did not analyze whether avoiding infection helps protect people from stroke. However, it's always wise to guard against infection—regardless of one's stroke risk.

During cold and flu season, for example, this includes avoiding illness-causing germs by washing your hands frequently, staying away from sick people and crowds whenever possible—and getting a flu shot and pneumonia vaccine. Warning signs of a urinary tract infection include chills, fever and burning pain when passing urine.

While it's not known whether treating an infection promptly will tamp down any increased stroke risk, be sure to let your doctor know about any symptoms of infection right away.

The 15-Minute Stroke Alert

Getting treated for stroke just 15 minutes earlier could save your life.

Recent finding: For every 1,000 stroke patients whose time from hospital arrival to start of treatment was 15 minutes sooner, 15 fewer died…and 17 more walked out of the hospital without assistance, compared with the average stroke patient undergoing treatment, according to a study of more than 6,500 hospital patients with ischemic stroke (caused by a blood clot). The average time from arrival to treatment was one hour and 27 minutes.

Reza Jahan, MD, professor of neurosurgery, David Geffen School of Medicine, University of California, Los Angeles.

Fit People Have Milder Strokes…and You Won't Have to Exercise as Much as You Think

Study titled "Prestroke Physical Activity Could Influence Acute Stroke Severity (part of PAPSIGOT)," by researchers at Institute of Neuroscience and Physiology, University of Gothenburg, Sweden, published in *Neurology*.

One incentive for exercising is that it cuts the risk of having a stroke. It would be wonderful if exercise eliminated any chance of having a stroke. Unfortunately, strokes still happen. But thanks to a recent study, we now know that if you do have a stroke and you've kept yourself in shape, it still pays off—big time.

The study: Researchers at University of Gothenburg in Sweden studied 925 patients, average age 73, who had had first strokes between 2014 and 2016. Nearly all of the patients had had ischemic strokes, those caused by blocked blood vessels in the brain. The patients were asked to report their general levels of physical activity before their strokes. Then the severity of the strokes in patients who reported light or moderate physical activity was compared with the severity of strokes in patients who reported being inactive.

Results: The physically active patients (both light and moderate activity) were about twice as likely to have had mild rather than severe strokes…to have recovered completely…and among those who had not recovered completely, to have milder long-term disability compared with the patients who were physically inactive. These results held even when the researchers adjusted for other factors that impact the severity of stroke such as high blood pressure, age, gender, smoking history and diabetes. (The only other factor besides physical activity that reduced severity of stroke was younger age.)

The researchers suggest that physical activity may reduce stroke severity and improve recovery because it increases blood supply to the brain, which may protect the brain from at least some stroke damage.

So how much do you have to exercise to get this stroke protection? Light activity was defined in the study as light walking at least four hours per week…and moderate activity was defined as engaging in an exercise program, such as physical training or a competitive sport, at least two or three hours per week. Not so bad!

A Severe Stroke Didn't Stop Him

Ted W. Baxter, a stroke survivor who now volunteers at hospitals and universities, providing his firsthand expertise in recovery from communication deficits. He is also active in philanthropic organizations and is author of *Relentless: How a Massive Stroke Changed My Life for the Better.*

Ted Baxter had what many people would consider a charmed life. He had an MBA from a prestigious school and traveled the world for his job at a top hedge-fund company.

Then, in 2005, at age 41, Ted's life collapsed when he had a massive ischemic stroke (due to a blood clot)—a life-threatening and often disabling condition that strikes nearly 700,000 people in the US each year.

Extensive damage on the left side of Ted's brain resulted in limited muscle control over the right side of his body. Worse, Ted was left with global aphasia—he couldn't speak, write or read.

Remarkably, Ted is now thriving. We spoke with him about his relentless drive to recover—and why he believes that the stroke changed his life for the better.

What did you think when you were told that your stroke had caused global aphasia?

I was terribly frightened. Global aphasia means that all communication is broken. It was difficult for me to understand what people were saying unless they spoke slowly and clearly. Because of the aphasia, I couldn't speak—the words weren't there—nor could I read or write.

What steps have you taken to recover?

Like most stroke survivors, my recovery involved physical therapy, occupational therapy and speech therapy. Working to regain my words has been much harder than regaining the use of my body. I've had to focus and practice constantly.

In the beginning, I had to start with kindergarten-level worksheets that paired simple nouns like "house" or "banana" with pictures. I moved on to exercises that had me work through various parts of a sentence—subject, verb, etc. I practiced for at least an hour every morning and an hour every night.

What role did acceptance play in your recovery?

It took months for me to finally understand and accept my new reality, but that's when my recovery took off. What I learned is that accepting reality doesn't have to mean losing hope.

How did you get through your down days?

The thing that saved me from disappearing into darkness and depression was getting a dog, a pug named Sullivan. I was never a dog person, but Sullivan saved me. A dog doesn't care if you can't remember his/her name or read a book. When Sullivan passed away, I got my dog Zorro.

It's also important to talk about your feelings and experiences. If you can't talk, find other ways to keep from growing apart from family and friends. Let them know that you'd like someone to come read to you or just watch TV with you.

You say your life is better now. In what ways?

I approach everything with a fresh appreciation, and I'm doing things that I never had the chance to do before.

I volunteer at hospitals and universities where they focus on strokes, traumatic brain injuries and aphasia. I run and attend group sessions with people who are experiencing the stages of trauma and tell them what helped me.

In my old life, I didn't make time for things like art, but now I'm visiting galleries and museums regularly. I have discovered that I love modern art!

Do you have any advice for caregivers?

The most important thing a caregiver can bring is patience. As stressful as it was for me to hunt for words, it was a crucial part of my recovery to let my brain do the work instead of loved ones filling in the blanks for me.

Also, do research so you can understand what is happening to your loved one, and locate your own support groups. Knowledge makes you more confident, and your loved one needs to feel that strength within you.

Where are you at today in your recovery?

I continue to work on my recovery every day—even 14 years later. My speech is not always smooth, but that doesn't stop me from giving public talks.

I still do physical therapy four times a week. I will never get back everything I lost, but I discovered that I have different facets of me that make my life fuller.

Any words of advice for people after stroke?

Hope and positive attitude come first. Determination is second. Doctors told me I had a two-year window for improvement in speech. After that, I would be stuck with whatever disability lingered. But I wanted to defy expectations. I continued to practice and continued to improve. For anyone who has had a stroke, just keep challenging yourself. When you get stronger, set new goals and keep doing more!

New Approaches for Aphasia

Susan Wortman-Jutt, MS, CCC-SLP, a certified speech-language pathologist in the outpatient speech department at the Burke Rehabilitation Hospital in White Plains, New York. She is involved in both patient care and research, with a special interest in rehabilitative speech and language therapies for adults.

About one million people in the US have aphasia. Some people with this condition have just a little trouble finding the right words. But others lose virtually all of their ability to speak, read, write and understand language. Most cases fall somewhere in between.

The cause of aphasia is most often a stroke or head injury. But brain tumors and other neurological disorders such as frontotemporal dementia also can lead to aphasia.

Latest news: Exciting new treatment approaches are being developed. *Best options now...*

Intensive Programs

In traditional speech-language therapy for aphasia, patients typically have 30-to-60-minute appointments two or three days a week for a limited period of time. In contrast, with a new type of treatment program called an Intensive Comprehensive Aphasia Program (ICAP), many types of therapy for aphasia, including individual, group, computer-based and sometimes cutting-edge or experimental therapies, are provided for at least three hours a day, four to five days a week for two to six weeks.

Scientific results increasingly support the role of intensive therapy programs for boosting aphasia recovery.

There are currently only a handful of ICAPs in the US, mostly at universities or hospitals, but the number is growing. Ask your speech-language pathologist for locations and if an ICAP would be appropriate for you.

Other Treatment Advances

Even if you can't participate in an ICAP, some of the latest treatments are available in traditional therapy programs. *Breakthrough and experimental approaches...*

•**Constraint-induced aphasia therapy (CIAT).** With this treatment, the patient is urged to use only spoken words—with no compensatory strategies such as gestures or writing—during therapy sessions that might last for two or more hours per day. Scientific results on its effectiveness are encouraging.

•**Computer software programs and apps can allow patients to work on speech skills independently**—whether at a speech clinic or at home.

Examples: In one software program called AphasiaScripts from Shirley Ryan AbilityLab in Chicago, a virtual therapist gives patients scripts for handling a variety of common situations, such as ordering a cup of coffee. Practice can give patients the confidence to use these words outside of therapy. And Constant Therapy is an app that provides speech, language and cognitive exercises that change as you make progress. The company can send progress reports directly to a patient's therapist. Aphasia.org lists other recommended apps for aphasia.

Important: Check with your therapist to find out which apps and programs might work for you and how best to use them.

• **Noninvasive brain stimulation.** This involves using a painless electrical current to stimulate or inhibit certain areas of the brain, with the hope of enhancing speech recovery. This is currently available only through clinical trials.

On the horizon: Hybrid therapies. Combining aphasia treatment and movement therapy for stroke survivors and others who struggle with both kinds of impairments is in the early stages of investigation but holds promise for poststroke speech and movement recovery.

Handling the Costs of Therapy

Insurance typically covers only a specific number of sessions and may not cover newer or experimental treatments. However, you may be able to get free or reduced-cost therapy at a university clinic staffed by students supervised by licensed therapists...or be eligible for a clinical trial that explores innovative treatments—costs are often covered. Check ClinicalTrials.gov.

Vital for Improvement

Patients see more improvement if they practice their skills at home and in their communities and have the support of family and friends who encourage them to communicate.

To find aphasia therapy programs and speech-language pathologists near you, go to Aphasia.org or ASHA.org.

Beware This Blood Thinner

One-third of people taking an anticoagulant, such as *apixaban* (Eliquis), to prevent stroke also take one or more over-the-counter drugs or supplements that when taken with an anticoagulant can cause dangerous internal bleeding, according to a survey of nearly 800 men and women.

Examples: Painkillers such as aspirin, *ibuprofen* (Advil) and *acetaminophen* (Tylenol)...and dietary supplements, including fish oil, as well as turmeric, ginger and other herbs and herbal teas.

If you take an anticoagulant: Ask your doctor which drugs and supplements to avoid.

Derjung M. Tarn, MD, PhD, associate professor of family medicine, David Geffen School of Medicine, University of California, Los Angeles.

Stroke Danger from PTSD for Young Adults

Study titled "Posttraumatic Stress Disorder and Risk for Stroke in Young and Middle-Aged Adults," by researchers at University of North Carolina School of Medicine, Chapel Hill, published in *Stroke*.

Over the past decade, ischemic strokes have been decreasing among older people. During that period, however, such strokes have been *increasing* among young and middle-aged adults. Here's what may be driving this alarming trend...and steps that help reduce stroke risk.

Increasing age is a prime factor in risk for ischemic stroke, the kind caused by blockage of an artery that supplies blood to the brain. However, up to 14% of such strokes occur in people ages 18 to 45. While a stroke at any age is a major life-changer, having a stroke in the prime of life can be much worse than having one in your 70s or 80s. A debilitating stroke during what should be the most productive years can have a devastating impact physically, emotionally and financially not just on the stroke patient but to young families.

In older adults, research has found that stress can be a triggering factor for both ischemic stroke and transient ischemic attack (TIA)—a "ministroke" that lasts only minutes or seconds and is often a warning for full stroke. But it has not been known whether stress also makes young people vulnerable to stroke.

To learn more about the effect of stress on stroke risk in young adults, researchers at University of North Carolina School of Medicine looked at a prevalent form of severe stress in that age group, post-traumatic stress disorder (PTSD). PTSD can result from many kinds of emotional trauma, including sexual assault, exposure to gun violence and being involved in warfare. Because PTSD is especially common among veterans, the researchers looked at incidence of stroke and TIA in 13 years of Veterans Administration medical records for about one million veterans (90% of them were men) who had been deployed to Iraq or Afghanistan after 9/11.

Study: There were 766 TIAs and 1,877 ischemic strokes over the course of the study, and about 30% of the vets were diagnosed with PTSD. Average age was about 43 at the time of their stroke or TIA.

Results: After adjusting for other stroke and TIA risk factors—such as diabetes, high blood pressure, smoking, obesity, alcohol/drug abuse, depression and generalized anxiety disorder—vets with PTSD had a 61% higher risk for TIA and a 36% higher risk for stroke than vets without PTSD. Gender did not influence risk for TIA, but risk for stroke was significantly higher in men than women.

How Might Stress Cause TIA and Stroke?

Although exactly how stress may trigger stroke is not fully understood, the researchers believe that one reason may be that stress is a well-known trigger for inflammation throughout the body. Inflammation causes physical changes that increase the likelihood of blood to clot and arteries, including those that carry blood to the brain, to narrow, contributing to chances of a blockage.

PTSD is an extreme form of stress. But this study, the first to find a link to stroke in young adults, suggests that other types of stress may also boost stroke risk in this age group. The researchers also point out that this research supports another large study, the INTERHEART study, which found that general stress, stressful life events and even financial stress may affect younger adults more than older adults—and increase their risk for stroke.

While more research is needed, the study authors hope that better screening for PTSD and other kinds of intense emotional stress and targeted counseling and appropriate therapies will help reduce stroke among young adults.

Chapter 17

VERY PERSONAL

Dangers of an Ill-Fitting Bra

Even though an ill-fitting bra may sound like a trivial problem, it has been linked to a range of health complaints. Yet research has found that up to 85% of women wear the wrong size bra. The harms related to a misfitted bra tend to occur in large-breasted women most often, but women of all breast sizes can be affected. *For example…*

PROBLEM #1: **Neck and back pain.** Even though the lion's share of a bra's support comes from the bra band, which wraps around the torso just below the bust, many women find it more comfortable to opt for a larger band measurement than what they need. Without adequate support, however, large breasts fall forward, pulling the neck, shoulders and upper back with them, triggering or exacerbating neck and back pain.

To avoid it: Go down a size in the band but up a cup size—for example, from 36C to 34D—to increase support in the band while ensuring adequate space for your breasts.

Helpful: Always use the outermost hooks when trying on bras. A bra is guaranteed to stretch out with wear, so you want it to fit well—snug, but not uncomfortably so—in the loosest position. This will add several months of life to your bra. As it stretches, move to the next hook, until you get to the first.

Note: A too-loose bra band also can lead to painful shoulder grooves. That's because a band that's not snug forces the straps to do all of the work. If the band rides up in the back, the straps dig in, creating painful grooves in the shoulders of full-breasted women and uncomfortable indentations in smaller-breasted women. Shoulder grooves also can be avoided by going down a band size and up a cup size.

PROBLEM #2: **Heartburn.** An overly tight band can aggravate heartburn—especially in fuller-figured women who already suffer from this condition. The problem happens mainly when sitting, which pushes the stomach upward, constricting the band and pressing on the diaphragm, the muscle that separates the chest and abdomen.

Because the diaphragm is positioned where the esophagus and stomach meet, pressure there can make it easier for stom-

Elisa Lawson, a certified prosthesis specialist and certified mastectomy fitter (CMF) who operates the Women's Health Boutique at Mercy Medical Center's Weinberg Center for Women's Health & Medicine in Baltimore. Lawson has fit bras for more than 40 years.

ach acid to move into the esophagus, causing discomfort and exacerbating heartburn.

To avoid it: Try a bra extender. These are small strips of fabric—roughly two inches in length—with hooks on one side and loops on the other. They lengthen the circumference of your bra to give some extra breathing room and cost far less than a new bra (you can find three-packs on Amazon.com for $6).

A bra extender isn't meant to be worn for months on end—think of it as a stopgap solution. If you use one and your indigestion improves, that's a sign you need to purchase a new bra with a looser band.

Also helpful: Try bumping up the band size and downsize the cup size—for example, go from a 36D to 38C.

Problem #3: **Rashes and skin irritation.** A poorly fitting underwire is often the culprit here. The problem typically stems from the wire resting on breast tissue and the chest wall. Additionally, breasts that rest on the torso can trap perspiration, possibly causing rashes or even fungal infections.

To avoid it: Consider a bra without an underwire. Many women think a wire lifts, but a good-fitting bra—with or without a wire—is what lifts and shapes. If you prefer an underwire bra, go up a cup size so that all breast tissue fits within the frame of the wire. Underwire bras shouldn't rub against your skin, and your breasts shouldn't be touching your torso.

If you notice redness, irritation or itchiness underneath your breasts, see your healthcare provider. He/she may prescribe an antibacterial or antifungal cream. And switch to a bra that holds your breasts up!

How to Get the Right Size Bra

To get the correct bra size, the first step is to measure before shopping.

What to do…

STEP #1: **To calculate your band size, snugly wrap a tape measure around your rib cage just beneath your bust,** where the bra band would normally rest.* If the number is odd, add five inches to the band size—for example, if you measure 33 inches add five inches, and your band is 38 inches. If the number is even, add four inches—for example, if you measure 32 inches add four inches, and your band size is 36 inches.

STEP #2: **Then loosely measure your chest at the level of your nipples.**

STEP #3: **To determine your cup size, subtract the band measurement from the bust measurement.** For example, if your bust is 38 inches and the band 35, then the difference is 3. Refer to the chart below. That corresponds to a "C" cup size, or a 38C.

FINDING YOUR CUP SIZE				
The difference in inches	0	1	2	3
Your cup size is:	AA	A	B	C
The difference in inches	4	5	6	7
Your cup size is:	D	DD	DDD, F	G

Important: Measurements are a good starting point. But bras are as irregular as jeans in sizing, so they should always be tried on. Sometimes a particular style is just not right for you. Also, it's important to remember that the size you arrive at through measuring may not apply to all bras.

Note: Good-fitting bras can be found in all price points. The longevity of the bra, however, depends on quality and care. To extend the life of a bra, wash it in a lingerie bag with a mild detergent that contains no bleach and hang it to dry. Professional bra fitters typically can be found in lingerie shops or women's clothing stores.

*For both measurements here, round up to the next whole number in inches.

Apps to Recharge Your Sex Life

Free Android and iOS phone apps to help boost your sex life…

•**With Kindu,** you and your partner separately swipe through romantic and erotic suggestions. You then separately see the suggestions that each of you have rated as "yes" or "maybe," which helps reduce any awkwardness.

•**Desire is a sex game for sending your partner a dare**—there are thousands in the app's database or couples can write their own.

•**With Honi,** you take quizzes to learn more about each other's likes and dislikes, send dares to your partner, share fantasies and learn Kama Sutra positions.

Mashable.com

The Other Reasons Why Women Lose Interest in Sex After Menopause

The study "I Want to Feel Like I Used to Feel": A Qualitative Study of Causes of Low Libido in Postmenopausal Women," led by researchers at the University of Pittsburgh and published in *Menopause: The Journal of The North American Menopause Society.*

Menopause—and the hormonal changes that accompany it—can definitely put a damper on a woman's libido. In fact, up to 40% of women over age 60 report having low libido.

To find out why so many women lose interest in sex after menopause—and determine if there are other factors beyond menopausal changes that make sex less appealing to postmenopausal women—researchers at University of Pittsburgh recently conducted a qualitative study. (This type of research involves a small sample of participants to gain a thorough understanding of a topic.) A total of 36 women ages 60 to 71 with low libido were interviewed privately or in group sessions.

Not surprisingly, vaginal symptoms, a well-known by-product of menopause, were a common complaint among the study participants. The symptoms, including vaginal dryness and a feeling of tightness, often made intercourse painful, which dampened the women's sexual desire. While some of the study participants were helped by vaginal estrogen or natural lubricants, such as coconut oil, the results were not consistently positive. However, women who tried pelvic floor exercises—also known as Kegels—on their own or with a trained physical therapist reported generally good results.

Other factors that contributed to the study participants' low libido…

•**Erectile dysfunction (ED) in male partners.** When a woman's partner has sexual difficulties, it often causes her to lose interest in intimacy. For some women in the study, their partners couldn't maintain an erection long enough for satisfying sexual intercourse. For other study participants, the partner was unwilling to discuss his problem, which led the woman to put aside her own sexual needs. When women encouraged their partners to take an ED drug, such as *sildenafil* (Viagra), the planning involved in using medication often eroded the romance. Successful alternatives to ED drugs involved other forms of intimacy, such as manual pleasuring, oral sex or using a vibrator.

•**Fatigue and pain.** Painful physical conditions, such as spinal cord issues or diabetic neuropathy, joint pain or having less stamina, in general, curbed sexual desire for many of the study participants. To address these issues, some women said they got an adjustable bed and/or tried different sexual positions.

•**Life stressors.** External demands, such as caregiving for older parents, made sex less of a priority for some of the study participants. Being retired didn't necessarily free up time for sex, and the stress levels sometimes got worse—not better—over time. Scheduling time for sex was helpful for some, but this strategy took away some of the romance for others. Taking vacations and using mental focus to ignore stressors during sex also helped.

•**Poor body image.** While some study participants noted that age made them less concerned about added weight and other body changes, others were troubled by their physical appearance and said they felt less attractive, which thwarted their interest in sex.

New Libido-Enhancer for Women

The FDA approved a libido-enhancer for premenopausal women with hypoactive sexual desire disorder (HSDD)—low desire that causes distress and that is not due to medications or health conditions. The drug *bremelanotide* (Vyleesi) excites sexual interest in about 50% of HSDD sufferers. It's self-administered by injection 45 minutes before intimacy. Do not use if you have high blood pressure or cardiovascular disease because it can raise blood pressure for up to 12 hours.

Anita H. Clayton, MD, chair of the department of psychiatry and neurobehavioral sciences, University of Virginia School of Medicine, Charlottesville.

Hysterectomies Increase Risk for Anxiety

Hysterectomies increase risk for anxiety and depression even when ovaries are not removed. Risks are greatest when hys-

terectomies were performed prior to age 35. It was previously believed that anxiety and depression risks rose only when the ovaries were removed, triggering hormone changes. If your doctor recommends a hysterectomy, ask whether there are other options.

Lisa Larkin, MD, a practicing internist and founder of Ms.Medicine, an organization for women's health clinicians, and a member of the advisory council of HealthyWomen. HealthyWomen.org

Good News: A Pill to Treat Uterine Fibroids

Jennifer Griffin, MD, MPH, associate professor, residency program director, department of obstetrics and gynecology, University of Nebraska Medical Center, Omaha.
US Food and Drug Administration press release.

While uterine fibroids are unlikely to be as serious as cancer, having them can still be a pain—literally. Up until now, treatment options leave a lot to be desired for some women. Now, though, there may be a way to stop the excessive blood flow—without surgery or injections.

Elagolix (Orilissa) is an oral drug that has already been approved by the FDA for severe-to-moderate pain associated with endometriosis.

Good news: The FDA recently approved the oral capsule Oriahnn, which is a combination of *elagolix, estradiol* and *norethindrone acetate,* for treating excessive blood flow with uterine fibroids.

About 80% of women develop uterine fibroids, usually in their 40s or 50s. Most of these lumps that grow on the uterus never cause symptoms. In fact, women usually learn they have them only when the fibroids are found during an exam. For some women, though, the symptoms can be terribly disruptive, such as excessive menstrual bleeding.

Fibroid Relief Up to Now

The first line of treatment for troublesome fibroids has been birth control pills or IUDs containing the progesterone-like hormone progestin. If these don't improve symptoms, more aggressive treatments are tried—destroying a thin layer of the lining of the uterus (endometrial ablation)...or surgery to remove the fibroids (myomectomy). Some women may choose surgery to remove the uterus completely (hysterectomy). Injectable drugs called gonadotropin-releasing hormone agonists (GnRH agonists) may also be tried. These injections into the abdomen or arm need to be repeated every three months.

The efficacy of Oriahnn was established in two clinical trials in which a total of 591 premenopausal women with heavy menstrual bleeding received the drug or placebo for six months. Heavy menstrual bleeding at baseline was defined as having at least two menstrual cycles with greater than 80 mL (about a third of a cup) of menstrual blood loss (MBL). The primary endpoint was achieving MBL volume less than 80 mL at the final month and 50% or greater reduction in MBL volume from the start of the study (baseline) to the final month. In the first study, 68.5% of patients who received Oriahnn achieved this endpoint (compared to 8.7% of patients who received placebo). In the second study, 76.5% of patients who received Oriahnn achieved this endpoint (compared to 10.5% of patients who received placebo).

Oriahnn may cause bone loss over time, and the loss in some women may not be completely recovered after stopping treatment. Because bone loss may increase the risk for fractures, women should not take Oriahnn for more than 24 months. Health care professionals may recommend a bone density scan (called DXA scan) when starting women on Oriahnn and periodically while on treatment. Oriahnn does not prevent pregnancy.

More Hope on the Horizon?

Several other drugs are still in trials and may expand fibroid treatment even further, but other drugs have fallen by the wayside because of safety issues. Most recently, *ulipristal acetate* (Ella, Esyma), which is available in the US, Europe and Canada for emergency birth control. This drug was denied initial approval for treatment of fibroids in the US because of concerns about liver damage in the dosing regimen required for fibroids.

Note: Oriahnn can cost more thn $800/month. Insurance will likely cover the cost. It is expected to be available to the public by the end of 2020.

What If You Have a Pelvic Mesh Implant?

Cheryl B. Iglesia, MD, director, Female Pelvic Medicine and Reconstructive Surgery (FPMRS), MedStar Washington Hospital Center, and professor, departments of obstetrics/gynecology and urology, Georgetown University School of Medicine, both in Washington, DC.

Now that the FDA has halted use of transvaginal pelvic mesh for repair of pelvic organ prolapse—stating that the risks of serious health problems outweigh the benefits—women who already have these pelvic mesh implants are understandably concerned. If you have a pelvic mesh implant, you need to talk to your surgeon. What you should do about it depends on how the mesh was surgically put into place.

Pelvic organ prolapse (POP) is caused by muscles, ligaments and connective tissue supporting the pelvic organs becoming damaged, such as through childbirth or injury...or weakening as a result of age and menopause...allowing the uterus, rectum or bladder to drop (prolapse) into the vagina. The usual repair for POP has been to restore anatomy by shoring up the torn ligaments. This is done using sutures...or by surgically implanting permanent (pelvic) mesh, a netlike medical device typically made from polypropylene, to permanently support the torn ligaments and muscles and help hold these organs in place.

The Problem with Mesh Implants

The surgical procedure to repair prolapse can be done using mesh placed either through the vagina or through an abdominal incision. Mesh placed through the vagina carries more risk than mesh placed abdominally for prolapse.

Reason: The vaginal approach requires a larger piece of mesh and is placed through incisions made inside the vagina. Mesh placed this way is more likely to lead to infection or contraction, and can move out of place and/or damage tissues that attach to it—for instance, it can perforate the vaginal tissues or erode into nearby organs.

In 2018, the FDA decided that surgery using polypropylene mesh was unsafe for repair of rectum prolapse (rectocele). In 2019, the FDA said that synthetic mesh repair of bladder prolapse (cystocele), the most common type of pelvic organ prolapse, was also unsafe—saying that they have not "received sufficient evidence to assure that the probable benefits of these devices outweigh their probable risks" and concluding that "these products do not have reasonable assurance of safety and effectiveness." The companies that sell the mesh were told to stop.

Note: The FDA action does not apply to surgical mesh slings to support the urethra for stress urinary incontinence or synthetic polypropylene mesh implanted abdominally or with laparoscopic/robotic surgery. No direct incisions are made on the vagina for these procedures, and the mesh used is much smaller and lighter weight compared with transvaginal mesh products.

If You Have Pelvic Mesh

If your repair is working and you don't have any problems, the mesh can stay. But do continue regular checkups annually with your gynecologist or surgeon. *Also be alert to signs of trouble, such as...*

• **Vaginal bleeding or discharge**
• **Pelvic or groin pain, discomfort or pressure**
• **Pain during sexual intercourse**
• **Pain for a partner during intercourse** (could indicate exposed mesh protruding into the vagina)

• **Frequent urinary tract infections**
• **Leaking of urine** (incontinence)
• **Bulge inside or protruding from your vagina.**

If you are having health problems caused by your pelvic mesh, you may need to have it removed and a new POP repair done. This is a challenging procedure and should only be done by a specialist in female pelvic medicine and reconstructive surgery called a urogynecologist. Check the American Urogynecologic Society website (AUGS.org) to find one near you.

Safer POP Options

If you have been diagnosed with POP but have not had surgery, you should work with a pelvic medicine specialist to determine the most appropriate treatment for you. Surgery is usually not the first option. *A specialist may advise...*

• **Kegel exercises to strengthen your pelvic muscles**
• **A pessary,** a soft, flexible device that can be inserted (and removed) into the vagina to support prolapsed organs
• **Losing weight if you are overweight.**

If you do need surgery, there are options other than using the synthetic mesh. These include transvaginal surgery using your own (native) tissue and sutures...laparoscopic and

Painting Class Can Be Sexy

In a recent study, 20 couples spent an hour playing board games or sitting side-by-side in a painting class. While men and women released the bonding hormone oxytocin during both activities, men released twice as much as women when they were painting. The novelty of the class and the opportunity to touch their partner appeared to be key.

Karen Melton, PhD, assistant professor of child and family studies at Robbins College of Health and Human Sciences, Baylor University, Waco, Texas, and leader of a study published in *Journal of Marriage and Family.*

robotic procedures…abdominal surgery with light-weight mesh mostly attaching to your tailbone…or a new technique that uses incisionless suture devices. Clinical trials are currently under way with new innovations for making grafts using your own tissues or other biologic tissues.

Do You Drool When You Sleep?

Michael Breus, PhD, a sleep specialist based in Manhattan Beach, California, and author of *The Power of When: Discover Your Chronotype.* TheSleepDoctor.com

It's nothing to be embarrassed about. Many people drool during their slumber. That's because our muscles relax during sleep, and a slackened jaw can allow the mouth to open—especially during the deep stages of sleep. Breathing through an open mouth then dries out the tongue, so the salivary glands produce even more saliva to keep the mouth moist. The extra saliva often drips out of the mouth and onto the pillow. This is even more likely to occur if you sleep on your stomach or side. If the drooling bothers you, all you may need to do is switch sleep positions so that you're on your back.

That said, drooling also can be a sign of a medical condition. Obvious causes include allergies or a cold that leads to nasal congestion, or the inflammation of chronic sinusitis could make it hard to breathe through the nose. Another possibility is a deviated (off-center) nasal septum (the bone and cartilage in the nose that separates the nostrils). This condition can block air flow through the nasal passages and cause mouth breathing. An ear, nose and throat specialist (otolaryngologist) can advise you on treatment for a deviated septum, which may include a relatively simple surgical procedure. You may also want to check any medications that you're taking. Some drugs can cause excessive saliva production, such as *clonazepam* (Klonopin), a seizure medication that is also used to treat anxiety, or certain antipsychotics.

Drooling also can be a sign of sleep apnea, a disorder in which breathing briefly stops during sleep. Symptoms include snoring, gasping for breath during the night and excessive daytime sleepiness. If you have any of these symptoms, you should be evaluated by a sleep specialist. Treatment may include a continuous positive airway pressure (CPAP) device that delivers air via a mask covering the nose during sleep.

Note: Even though sleep apnea is more common in men, it can also occur in women.

If you have a condition that makes it difficult to swallow, such as Parkinson's disease, you may notice drooling—not only at night but during the day. The FDA recently approved a drug, *incobotulinumtoxinA* (Xeomin), for such patients who often experience excessive drooling.

For most people, however, drooling isn't that serious—and can be addressed by treating any underlying condition (such as those described above) or switching your sleep position.

The Secret Ingredient That Causes Digestive Distress

Laurie Steelsmith, ND, LAc, licensed naturopathic physician and acupuncturist in private practice in Honolulu. She writes Bottom Line's "Natural Healing Secrets for Women" blog and is coauthor of three books—*Natural Choices for Women's Health*, t*Great Sex, Naturally* and *Growing Younger Every Day*. DrSteelsmith.com

The patient: "Patrice," a 55-year-old massage therapist.

Why she came to see me: Patrice appeared to be the epitome of health when she stepped into my office for the first time. Radiant and fit, it was clear she treated herself with tremendous care. Right off the bat, however, she told me that she'd spent the last month battling digestive distress that had ranged from mild to severe. Gas, constipation, bloating, and diarrhea had come to rule her days—so much so her symptoms determined her wardrobe while her ability to maintain her list of massage clients was starting to wane. She wanted to get to the bottom of her intestinal issues, and to address them without the use of pharmaceuticals.

How I evaluated her: I began my assessment as I always do: With a long and in-depth discussion about Patrice's medical and personal history.

A former civil rights attorney in Chicago, Patrice had recently moved to Hawaii after giving up her high-stress job and a marriage that had stopped working over a decade earlier. Shortly after landing in the islands, she decided to revamp her life from the inside out—and from the outside in. "A month ago," she said, "I'd never felt healthier or happier."

In the last four weeks, however, her new-found vitality had been compromised by a slew of digestive issues.

This made "zero sense" to her, as she put it: Six months earlier, she'd become a vegetarian, and five weeks earlier she'd given up gluten and dairy after reading about the potential benefits of a gluten- and dairy-free diet. And yet, almost immediately after eating a meal or snack, she felt besieged with bloating, which was then followed by gas, constipation or diarrhea. She'd also experienced soft tissue and joint pain.

To get to the root of her problem, I conducted a full physical exam, as well as a food and chemical sensitivity blood test.

What my evaluation revealed: While Patrice's physical exam underscored the fantastic health I believed her to be in, her food and chemical sensitivity test revealed an allergy that many may have never heard of: Guar gum. (She also tested positive for gluten and dairy allergies, confirming that Patrice had done the right thing

in removing those foods from her diet prior to meeting with me).

Patrice's immediate response? "I don't even chew gum!" But like several other gums—xanthan gum, acacia gum (also called gum Arabic) and locust bean gum (or carob bean gum)—guar gum is often a hidden ingredient, not only in processed foods but also in an increasing number of "natural" foods and personal care products. In particular, baked gluten-free foods often rely on guar gum to stabilize, emulsify and thicken their products. Yogurt (including dairy-free yogurt), almond milk, soup, vegan protein powders—even the non-dairy Coconut Bliss ice cream Patrice loved—also frequently contain this additive (or another gum). Guar gum is derived from the Indian cluster bean, which sounds wholesome enough; it's also sometimes used to treat irritable bowel syndrome. This may benefit some; for others, however, it can lead to digestive complications.

Why? Because guar gum is a type of soluble fiber, it can result in the benefits—and side effects—of fiber itself. Meaning, on one hand, it may organically support ideal cholesterol levels, help one feel sated longer and naturally encourage stable blood sugar levels. (Indeed, given its capacity to promote a sense of fullness, as well as the laxative effect it can have, guar gum was used in weight-loss medications until the FDA banned its inclusion in weight-loss pills in 1992.) On the other hand—particularly if one is unaccustomed to consuming fiber, or has an allergy to guar gum—the additive can cause a range of gastrointestinal problems, including gas, nausea, abdominal pain, constipation and diarrhea—the very symptoms Patrice was experiencing. In extreme cases, high doses of guar gum may also result in small bowel obstruction, pulmonary embolism, esophageal tear and even death. Lastly, guar gum, in rare cases, can engender the soft tissue and joint pain from which Patrice was suffering.

How I addressed her problem: The excellent thing about Patrice's diagnosis was that it was simple to treat—and, to her delight, we were able to do so naturally.

First, I asked Patrice to toss any foods in her kitchen that contained dietary gums. (While she did not test to having an allergy to other gums, data reveals that xanthan gum can exacerbate digestive issues, while carrageenan—a gum derived from seaweed and used in the likes of soy milk and salad dressing—can cause inflammation and lead to IBS and ulcerations. Meanwhile, locust bean gum, which is from carob, may cause increased flatulence, and gellan gum has been linked to intestinal abnormalities.) Out went the brand of coconut milk she typically used in her coffee, as well as the gluten-free bread she typically used to make toast. In their place, I suggested she reach for foods that did not come in a package—fruits, vegetables, seeds and nuts.

I then suggested she start rebuilding the healthy bacteria in her gut through a mix of probiotic and prebiotic foods. For the former, I suggested sauerkraut and kimchi, both of which could be added to salads or sandwiches; for the latter, I urged her to fill her plate with foods that would act as "fertilizer" for the probiotics in her gut (such as bananas, asparagus and sweet potatoes).

To be on the safe side, I also encouraged Patrice to take a look at the ingredients in her personal care products—lotions, cosmetics—and even paper products. (Guar gum is more ubiquitous than one might think!)

Finally, I asked Patrice to consider adding cardio and yoga to her daily wellness practice. While tai chi has a wealth of benefits, the gut—literally—needs a work out. Even a gentle walk after a meal would help alleviate her symptoms.

The patient's progress: Four weeks later, Patrice returned to my office with terrific news: Her digestive issues have gone from agonizing to significantly reduced. She's stopped grazing on gluten-free muffins and crackers and has become smitten with Brazil and macadamia nuts.

The Lowdown on Laxatives

Joshua Levitt, ND, naturopathic physician and medical director at Whole Health Natural Family Medicine, Hamden, Connecticut. He is a clinical preceptor for Yale School of Medicine and author of *The 21-Day Revival, The Science-Based Truth About CBD* and *The Honey Phenomenon.*

If you're 60 or older, chances are one in three that you have occasional or chronic constipation. For people under age 60, the odds are one in six, and women of all ages are 50% more likely to have constipation than men.

But not all constipation is created equal. It occurs for several reasons, and different causes call for different treatments. Use the wrong treatment, and your problem may only get worse. *Naturopathic physician Joshua Levitt, ND, explains what you need to know…*

Chronic Constipation

An aging colon is a major culprit when it comes to chronic constipation. Reduced muscle function in the large intestine makes defecation more difficult. The smooth muscles in the wall of the colon become weaker, impairing peristalsis, the automatic muscular contractions that propel stool through the bowel.

Other causes: You may not be getting as much exercise as you used to. Less physical activity results in less intestinal motility—the movement of the stool. Or your diet may be low in fiber. You need roughage from fruits, vegetables, beans, grains, nuts and seeds to add bulk to your stool.

Growing problem: Chronic constipation is a side effect of certain medications.

Worst offenders: Pain relievers such as opioids and nonsteroidal anti-inflammatory drugs (NSAIDs)…antidepressants…and proton pump inhibitors for heartburn.

Note: There also are a number of diseases that cause constipation, including Parkinson's and hypothyroidism. If you have disease-caused chronic constipation, see your doctor.

The Right Laxative for Chronic Constipation

It's important to understand your unique type so that you can choose the laxative that will work best for you. *At the most basic level, there are two types of chronic constipation…*

• **Spastic.** This is characterized by pellets or thin ribbons of stool that require you to strain to pass them. This happens because of a tense bowel—the smooth muscles of the colon are overly tight.

• **Atonic.** This is characterized by large, hardened stools that accumulate in the bowel. It happens in people who have been constipated for a while—they have trouble squeezing out the stool due to an atonic, or flaccid, bowel.

What to do…

For spastic constipation: There are osmotic or softening laxatives, some with magnesium, such as Phillips' Milk of Magnesia, and some using other compounds, such as polyethylene glycol (MiraLAX).* So-called "stool softeners" usually are osmotic laxatives, such as docusate (Colace, Surfak). They work by drawing water into the bowel, softening stool.

But my favorite osmotic laxative—because it's the most effective due to higher absorbability and better muscle relaxation—is magnesium citrate, a nutritional supplement taken as a powder, pill, capsule or liquid. To find your tolerance level, start with a dose of 300 milligrams (mg) of magnesium citrate, taken with dinner, to hopefully produce a morning bowel movement. Because magnesium requires digestive acid and digestive enzymes for absorption, it's best taken with a meal. Take the 300-mg dose for three days. If it doesn't produce results, increase the dose to 450 mg. Continue to increase the dose by 150 mg every third day until you produce

---

*Check with your doctor before taking any supplement—especially if you have a chronic medical condition or take medication.

Keep Everything Moving

The following good habits help to prevent constipation…

• **Go when you need to go.** Delaying defecation stretches the bowel, creating and worsening atonic constipation. When your body is telling you it's time to go—go.

• **Use a toilet footstool.** The optimal position for effortless defecation is squatting, not sitting. A way to mimic this pose is to use a footstool in front of your toilet, which raises your knees, creating a squatlike position that helps open the rectum. (Squatty Potty is a popular brand.)

• **Don't sit around.** To prevent constipation and for general health, the pelvic floor should be toned and tight. Unfortunately, sitting too long on the toilet relaxes the pelvic floor—stretching layers of muscle and tissue like a hammock. If defecation isn't happening, come back later. If you're finished, don't hang around. —Joshua Levitt

---

a laxative effect. If you get to the point of watery diarrhea, cut back to the previous dose. Magnesium citrate can be taken on an ongoing basis as long as it's 150 mg below your tolerance level. I suggest Magnesium Citrate by Vital Nutrients or Natural Calm by Natural Vitality.

Another option for spastic constipation is enteric-coated peppermint oil. Peppermint is an antispasmodic, making it ideal for spastic constipation.

My advice: I favor Mentharil from Integrative Therapeutics. Take one capsule (0.2 milliliters of enteric-coated peppermint oil) at bedtime. If that doesn't work, take two the next night. If that doesn't work, take three the next night. If it still isn't working, it's not the right laxative for you.

Note: For mild constipation, a cup of peppermint tea is a great option.

For atonic constipation: While there are many fiber-rich (bulking) laxatives—wheat dextrin (Benefiber), methylcellulose (Citrucel), calcium polycarbophil (FiberCon) and psyllium (Metamucil)—the most effective "laxative" is simply high-fiber food.

Try a daily breakfast of one-half cup of oatmeal, a tablespoon of ground flaxseed, a handful of slivered almonds or walnuts and a sprinkling of berries. Throughout the rest of the day, eat five servings of fruits and vegetables and plenty of beans, legumes, whole grains and/or nuts and seeds.

Alternative: Add ground flaxseed to a smoothie. The optimal dose is two tablespoons—but don't start at that level because it can produce increased gas. Instead, start with one-half tablespoon for three days, increasing it to one tablespoon on day four...to one-and-a-half tablespoons on day seven... and to two tablespoons on day 10.

• **Stimulant laxatives.** Popular stimulant laxatives include *bisacodyl* (Dulcolax) and sennosides, the active ingredient in the herb senna (Senokot, Ex-Lax). These over-the-counter products work by stimulating the bowel to contract and expel stool—but I suggest trying a gentler, natural alternative with fewer side effects first. Drink one-half cup of senna tea daily. Try Traditional Medicinals Smooth Move senna tea.

For Occasional Constipation

If you want quick relief from a bout of constipation that is not chronic, try this protocol, which helps prevent rectal tears caused by passing stool that has accumulated in the colon over several days.

DAY 1:

1. Drink one cup of prune juice and eat three to four prunes (dried plums). Prunes contain naturally occurring sorbitol, which works like an osmotic laxative.

2. Take magnesium citrate—from 300 mg to 500 mg.

DAY 2: If bowels have not moved...

Continue the steps above and...

3. Drink one cup of senna tea. Steep two bags for five minutes.

4. Take an aloe vera extract, which "greases" the bowels, helping stool move.

Try one 450-mg capsule of Super Aloe from Ortho Molecular Products.

Caution: If there is an abrupt change in bowel movements...you're constipated for more than a week...constipation is accompanied by severe abdominal pain...or you see blood in your stool—see your doctor.

Digestive Supplements— Here Are the Ones That Really Work...

Tamara Duker Freuman, RD, CDN, an expert in digestive health in private practice and a clinical preceptor for the Dietetic Internship Program at Teachers College, Columbia University, both in New York City. She is author of *The Bloated Belly Whisperer: See Results Within a Week and Tame Digestive Distress Once and for All.* TheBloatedBellyWhisperer.com

Many products for bloating, constipation and gas don't work as claimed— and might contribute to other health problems. In spite of rave reviews, scientific evidence does not back the claims of many digestive supplements. Dietary supplements do not need Food and Drug Administration (FDA) approval that they are safe, nor do supplement makers need to test their products to prove marketing claims.

To help ensure that you get the digestive support you need, here's a quick primer on products that really can help...

• **Magnesium—for constipation.** This essential mineral plays a critical role in maintaining nerve and muscle function...regulating blood pressure and blood sugar levels...and may help prevent migraines and stroke. Doses of 350 mg or more stimulate bowel movements by drawing water into the gastrointestinal tract.

Use any form of magnesium (citrate, sulfate, oxide, hydroxide). Typically, 400 mg taken at night with a full glass of water (with or without food) produces an easy, cramp-free bowel movement the next morning. If it doesn't, increase the dose by 200 mg/night up to 1,000 mg. If 1,000 mg isn't helpful, talk to your doctor about other options.

Good product to try: Phillips' Milk of Magnesia (500 mg magnesium per liquid or caplet dose).

• **Lactose-digesting enzyme (lactase)— for lactose intolerance.** Digestion of the milk sugar lactose requires lactase, an enzyme that is deficient in about 65% of adults worldwide. Lactase supplements allow people who are deficient in lactase to still enjoy dairy foods.

Key: Consume enough lactase with the first bite of dairy-containing food to handle the full amount of lactose in the dairy meal/snack. Lactase products on the market typically recommend 9,000 acid lactase units (ALU) per dose, which should be sufficient for most dairy-containing meals.

Good product to try: One that does not contain the gas-producing sugar alcohols sorbitol or mannitol, such as Puritan's Pride Lactase.

• **Alpha-galactosidase—for gas, bloating and abdominal discomfort from eating certain foods.** In order to digest the highly fermentable fibers in certain healthy foods, including legumes (chickpeas, beans), cabbage, broccoli and brussels sprouts, you need to have enough of the enzyme alpha-galactosidase. If these foods cause you excess gas, bloating and abdominal distress, you may be able to comfortably eat them if you also consume alpha-galactosidase, the active ingredient in Bean-zyme and Beano.

Note: This enzyme may reduce the effectiveness of the diabetes medication *acarbose* (Precose).

Research finding: In a small study from University of Pavia in Italy, participants who consumed alpha-galactosidase while eating a meal that contained about two cups of beans produced significantly less gas afterward, compared with those who received a placebo with their beans.

A serving size of Beano (two capsules) or Bean-zyme (one capsule) contains 300 alpha-galactosidase units (GalU). Participants in the study who got the most intestinal relief consumed 1,200 GalU—but they also ate a lot more beans than you're likely to eat in one meal. How much to take varies by individual. Try 300 GalU with your first bite of a problem food. I often recommend two Bean-zyme pills per half cup of beans, adjusting as needed.

Note: Look for alpha-galactosidase supplements that do not contain sugar alcohols, such as mannitol (or other ingredients that end in ol). As noted earlier, these can cause gas.

Vitiligo: Treatments for a Mysterious Skin Disorder

John E. Harris, MD, PhD, director of the Vitiligo Clinic and Research Center at University of Massachusetts Medical School in Worcester. UMassMed. edu/vitiligo

Michael Jackson may be the most famous person ever to have vitiligo, but he's definitely not alone. The autoimmune disorder, in which the body attacks cells that give skin its pigment, affects roughly one out of every 100 people in the world—regardless of race or gender.

In the US, it's estimated that up to five million people have this condition. Even though vitiligo ("vittle-eye-go") occurs most commonly before age 30, it can develop at any age. People with certain other autoimmune disorders, such as the thyroid condition known as Hashimoto's disease and type 1 diabetes, are at greater risk.

Good news: While vitiligo is still incurable, recent scientific advances are uncovering important facts about the condition that are leading to more—and better—treatment options than ever before. *What you need to know...*

The Mystery of Vitiligo

A malfunctioning immune system has been implicated as the cause of vitiligo. Scientists theorize that the immune system attacks melanocytes, the cells that make pigment (aka melanin) in our skin, hair and eyes, mistaking them for a disease. When this occurs, pigment is lost and white patches develop.

In a person with vitiligo, pigmentation can be lost anywhere on the body, but common areas include the face, neck, scalp, hands and arms. Sometimes vitiligo affects the armpits, mouth and genitals.

Vitiligo is highly individualized. One person might lose all pigment in his/her body over the course of a lifetime, while another develops a single white patch later in life. For some, the condition remains stable for decades, until something triggers the immune system and it spreads again. Triggers can include a bout of severe stress...a cut or burn...or environmental exposure to certain chemicals, including phenols found in permanent hair dyes and some detergents.

Are You at Risk?

Vitiligo is an equal-opportunity disorder, but the most common risk factor seems to be genetic. Up to 25% of people with vitiligo also have a relative with the disorder. The fact that identical twins—who share the same genes—don't have the same risk for vitiligo suggests that the cause isn't completely genetic.

Having another autoimmune disorder also increases risk. When researchers looked at nearly 1,100 people with vitiligo, close to 20% had another autoimmune disease, such as alopecia, inflammatory bowel disease, lupus or Sjögren's syndrome, according to research published in *Journal of the American Academy of Dermatology*.

Treatment Options

At this time, there are no FDA-approved medical treatments to reverse vitiligo—but that could be changing as promising new treatments are now in clinical trials. In the meantime, people with vitiligo are prescribed treatments "off label," meaning that the medication was originally intended for another condition. Most insurers cover these treatments for people with vitiligo, but check first. *Current treatment options…*

• **Prescription topical steroids can help restore the pigmentation in smaller areas of the body.** The cream provides moderate improvement, and side effects may include stretch marks and thinning of the skin.

Note: When a person's vitiligo is rapidly expanding, a low-dose oral steroid is sometimes used until the disease has stabilized.

Topical tacrolimus is a newer treatment that can be applied to parts of the body that are more sensitive to the side effects of long-term use of steroid cream, such as the face, genitals, breasts and underarms.

• **Narrow-band UVB phototherapy is recommended when depigmented areas are too extensive (typically more than 5% of the body) for topical treatment alone.** In most cases, it requires two to three visits per week with each treatment lasting only about one to four minutes. However, the treatment may take up to a year to be effective and must be continued indefinitely to maintain results.

Note: This type of phototherapy uses UV radiation that does not increase risk for skin cancer.

What happens: This treatment is administered in a booth in which the patient stands with the affected areas of the body exposed to UVB light. UV goggles are worn to protect the eyes. The treatment usually is covered by insurance and is offered at dermatologists' offices throughout the US.

Note: A laser therapy, similar to narrow-band UVB phototherapy, is highly effective on small areas of the skin. Brand names include XTRAC and Pharos.

• **"Bleaching" therapy, *monobenzone* (Benoquin), is a topical "depigmenting" cream that can be used if a person has extensive vitiligo (covering more than 80% of the body).** With this treatment, skin is permanently lightened in unaffected areas of the body so that the spots caused by vitiligo are no longer noticeable. The treatment may take one to two years to complete. Side effects may include burning, itching and redness of the treated skin.

•**JAK inhibitors are drugs that are already on the market to treat conditions such as rheumatoid arthritis and bone marrow disease.** The drugs, tofacitinib and ruxolitinib, can be used both orally and topically. These medications block the cellular pathway that fuels vitiligo.

Impressive study result: In the first-ever, large-scale clinical trial for vitiligo treatment, study participants used either a medicated cream containing a JAK inhibitor or a placebo. After six months, about half of the people who used a higher dosage of the medicated cream saw pigment return to 50% of the vitiligo on their faces, compared with just 3% of those who used the placebo. Researchers expect even greater improvement with further treatment, and larger trials are expected. Until it is approved by the FDA, this treatment can be prescribed off-label and produced by a compounding pharmacy.

Living with Vitiligo

Because vitiligo is so visible, it impacts a person's self-esteem and quality of life. Strangers may stare or make rude comments. Up to one-third of people with vitiligo experience symptoms of depression. Because melanocytes are found not just in skin but also in the eyes and ears, vitiligo can, in rare cases, affect those areas, too. Hearing loss can occur if the immune system attacks the melanocytes in the inner ear.

For people with vitiligo, lifestyle changes (such as diet, exercise, vitamins or supplements) have not been shown to help much. However, there is one step that should be followed at all times—wearing sunscreen. Patches of skin without pigment burn easily.

Skin damage also can trigger an autoimmune response that may lead to more vitiligo, so take particular care with cuts and burns. For the same reason, people with vitiligo may not want to get tattoos, especially if the disease is actively spreading or existing spots are getting larger. Makeup can help.

Good brands: Dermablend and Cover FX.

Support groups for individuals with vitiligo are a good resource for coping with the psychological effects of the disorder. To find such a group, consult the website of Vitiligo Friends, VITFriends.org, a nonprofit dedicated to enhancing the quality of life for people with vitiligo. Global Vitiligo Foundation, GlobalVitiligoFoundation.org, is another good resource to learn about research and local support groups.

INDEX